AF615397

Radiology of Occupational Chest Disease

A. Solomon L. Kreel
Editors

Radiology of Occupational Chest Disease

With 225 Illustrations

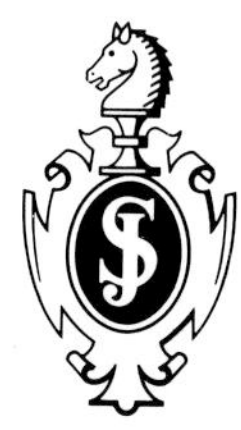

Springer-Verlag
New York Berlin Heidelberg
London Paris Tokyo

Albert Solomon, M.D.
Professor and Head of Department of Radiology, Tel-Aviv Medical Center, Ichilov Hospital, 64-239 Tel-Aviv, Israel

Louis Kreel, M.D.
Professor, Newham Hospital, Plaistow, London NW11 7JB, U.K.

Library of Congress Cataloging-in-Publication Data
Radiology of occupational chest disease / A. Solomon, L. Kreel, editors.
p. cm.
Includes index.
1. Lungs—Dust diseases—Diagnosis. 2. Lungs—Radiography.
3. Occupational diseases—Diagnosis. I. Solomon, A. (Albert)
II. Kreel, Louis.
[DNLM: 1. Lung Diseases—radiography. 2. Occupational Diseases.
WF 600 R129]
RC773.R23 1989
616.2'40757—dc19
DNLM/DLC 88-38205

Typeset by Publishers Service, Bozeman, Montana.
Printed and bound by Arcata Graphics/Halliday, West Hanover, Massachusetts.
Printed in the United States of America.

9 8 7 6 5 4 3 2 1

ISBN 0-387-96877-6 Springer-Verlag New York Berlin Heidelberg
ISBN 3-540-96877-6 Springer-Verlag Berlin Heidelberg New York

Introduction

This text is in no danger of incomplete identification of where it should fit in the bibliographical spectrum of radiological monographs. It can be placed in many areas—radiology of the chest, occupational diseases, pneumoconioses, clinical medicine. In each, it would be informative and helpful.

In part, this is inherent in the subject but, equally, it reflects the good judgment of the editors in selecting both subjects to be covered and contributors who could succeed in their delineation in terms of current usage and current issues.

Radiology of lung diseases has deep roots. Roentgen announced his discovery of x-rays in 1895. By the next year, the new technique was used to study lung disease. On October 1, 1896, Francis H. Williams was able to report in the Boston Medical and Surgical Journal, "I have examined about 40 cases of pulmonary tuberculosis . . ." In his classic text, *The Roentgen Rays in Medicine and Surgery*, published in 1901, thoracic diseases took pride of place in the 658-page volume. It is of further interest that just as Glyn Thomas here emphasizes the importance of technique, so did Williams in his writings.

Solomon and Kreel are perceptive descendants in another way, to our immense advantage, with their clear judgment that the radiological descriptions be focused on and judged by their clinical applicability. This takes us back even further. The first monograph on illness in an occupational group was Paracelsus' monograph *Diseases of Miners*, written during the 1530s (but not published until 1567). The first group of occupational diseases reported, then, were the pneumoconioses and their status more than 400 years later is detailed here.

Laced through the pages that follow are three governing themes that not only make their study profitable in terms of data and knowledge but also encourage their practical utilization for clinical management, public health, and prevention of disease.

A central perspective is the epidemiological background against which observations are presented and evaluated. With occupational lung disease, as with pulmonary medicine in general, we have learned not only to judge radiological findings in relation to the individual patient but also to see where they fit in broader population terms. The radiologist, as do the pathologist and the clinician, frequently now contributes to epidemiological research. Witness the extensive discussion in this volume of the International Labour Office (ILO) Classification, where the radiologist voluntarily accepts the constraint of describing what is seen in statistical terms and is concerned not only about what is seen on the film but also about selective bias in the population studied.

This has long been a concern of the ILO in its efforts to provide suitable classifications for radiographs of the pneumoconioses. This was true for the 1930 Johannesburg classification's emphasis on silicosis, the later 1950 Sydney and 1958 Geneva classifications' focus on coal workers' pneumoconiosis, as well as the 1971 and 1980 classifications extending radiological categorizations to encompass asbestos-associated disease. Indeed, the ILO has clearly stated the purpose of its Classifications – "for epidemiological use."

The capable authors have seen to it that clinical relevance is no mere correlation of associations between clinical abnormalities and x-ray shadows. Rather, significant current issues are presented, with the potential contributions of radiological findings. [Williams had, in a way, promised this (in 1901), with his remark that "X-rays are a most effective method of showing how great a role the imagination may play when using auscultation and percussion."]

Thus, we have discussion of the critically important concepts of latency; dose/disease response relationships (quite different in coal workers' respiratory disease and asbestotic pleural pulmonary disease); the recent recognition of the importance of small airways disease even in the absence of cigarette smoking; differentiation between diseases included in "chronic obstructive pulmonary disease" and the pneumoconioses; discrepancies between radiological, clinical, and pathological changes; the importance of neoplasms, especially bronchogenic carcinoma and pleural mesothelioma; and similar problems. Radiological/clinical discussions include the relationship between the microscopic fibrosis seen in cigarette smokers' lungs and the pneumoconiotic fibrosis observed in dust diseases, debated for a decade and clarified only recently by the radiological studies of Castallan and his colleagues and the analytical discussions in 1988 of Blanc and Gamsu. Issues such as the possible importance of different fiber types; "Caplan's syndrome" and rheumatoid pleural-pulmonary disease among dust-exposed individuals; the growing recognition of the clinical and functional importance of pleural fibrosis, particularly when diffuse; the functional importance of visceral pleural fibrosis (as well as parietal); pseudotumors or "folded lung;" and the occurrence of pneumoconioses with less widespread exposure to such dusts as bentonite, talc, kaolin, and beryllium. Brief exposure potentially producing mesothelioma is noted with the concomitant knowledge that fibrotic changes in the lung parenchyma or pleura may be minimal or absent. There is also discussion of such less commonly acknowledged differences between silicosis and asbestosis as acute pneumoconiosis in the former, but very rare in the latter, as well as the same generalization for pulmonary tuberculosis complicating silicosis but not increased with asbestos exposure.

I well remember the first meeting, at Mount Sinai, of the Working Group established by the International Union Against Cancer (IUCC). Clinicians and radiologists such as Eugene Pendergrass, G.K. Sluis-Cremer, and Benjamin Felson were gently guided along epidemiological lines by the skill and good humor of John Gilson, toward the development of an extended Classification of Radiographs of Pneumoconiosis. After additional meetings in Cincinnati at the U.S. Public Health Service's laboratories, this became the U/C Classification (UICC/Cincinnati), and later evolved into the ILO's 1971 and 1980 Classifications.

This volume brings us many steps further, to the integration of clinical and radiological understandings. In this, it is a culmination of almost 100 years of medical advances and, by its example of continuity, provides the foundation for the additional progress that will be made.

Irving J. Selikoff, M.D.
Mount Sinai School of Medicine
of the City University of New York

Preface

The chest radiograph is crucial in monitoring the effect of occupational exposure. Not all radiographic changes are accompanied by pulmonary impairment, nor in fact are the changes necessarily a result of inhalation of offending particles; for example, advancing age and smoking, in the absence of dust exposure, may lead to the development of irregular opacities in the lung and cause confusion in monitoring the worker at risk. Although the body can adapt to most minor respiratory insults encountered daily, there are still many occupations where workers are exposed to high concentrations of inhaled agents, causing a pathological lung response and associated radiographic changes. The chest radiograph in the pneumoconioses is valuable because there is a relationship between the extent and the profusion of opacities present in the radiograph and the retention of lung dust. This relationship is particularly reliable in coal worker's pneumoconiosis. Immunological responses may occur as a result of inhaled organic and nonorganic particles; in this regard the host reaction is unpredictable. Accurate assessment of the chest radiograph requires an awareness of these variations.

An international coding system for recording lung changes following occupational exposure has been provided by the International Labour Organization classification. Familiarity with the classification and its application permits a standard reporting of chest radiographs and a universal means of communication.

The contributors to this book are well versed in the interpretation of chest roentgenograms associated with occupational diseases. Their collective expertise is offered to encourage both clinicians and radiologists to expand their interest in the complexities of occupational chest diseases.

Acknowledgments: The editors wish to acknowledge the Medical Bureau for Occupational Diseases, Johannesburg, South Africa, Vincent Wright Radiologic Museum of the Bureau for Occupational Diseases, and Mr. Cecil M. Weintraub, Surgeon and Photographer, for their assistance in the preparation of this book.

Albert Solomon

Contents

Contributors

Gerald L. Baum

Professor of Medicine, Sackler School of Medicine, Tel-Aviv University; Director, Pulmonary Division of the Chaim Sheba Medical Center, Tel-Hashomer, Israel

D. Caillaud

Assistant Professor in Pneumology, Consultant in Respiratory Disease, University de Clermont-Ferrand I, Clermont-Ferrand, France

David S. Feigin

Clinical Professor of Radiology, University of California, San Diego; Assistant Chief, Radiology Service, Veterans Administration Medical Center, San Diego, California, USA

Stephanie Flicker

Chairman, Department of Radiology, Deborah Heart and Lung Center, Brown Mills, New Jersey, USA

R. Glyn Thomas

Honorary Lecturer in Radiology, Faculty of Medicine, University of Witwatersrand, Johannesburg, South Africa; Chief Radiologist, Rand Mutual Hospital and Chamber of Mines of South Africa, Johannesburg, South Africa

Jeffrey A. Golden

Clinical Consultant in Pulmonary Diseases, and Adjunct Associate Professor of Medicine, University of California, San Francisco, California, USA

Jan Lieber

Professor of Occupational Medicine, College of Medicine and Dentistry of New Jersey Rutgers Medical School, Piscataway, New Jersey, USA; Formerly Professor of Occupational Medicine, Jefferson Medical College, Thomas Jefferson University, Philadelphia, Pennsylvania, USA

W.K.C. Morgan
Professor of Medicine, University of Western Ontario, Ontario, Canada; Director, Chest Disease Service, University Hospital, London, Ontario, Canada; President, Canadian Thoracic Society

C. Molina
Professor of Pneumology and Clinical Immunology; Head, Department of Respiratory Diseases, University de Clermont-Ferrand I, Clermont-Ferrand, France; Chief of Research Center for Respiratory Allergy; Member of the Ministry Committee for Occupational Diseases in Agriculture, France

Howard Naidech
Department of Radiology, Deborah Heart and Lung Center, Brown Mills, New Jersey, USA

Gerhard K. Sluis-Cremer
Director of Epidemiology Research Unit, Medical Bureau for Occupational Diseases, Johannesburg, South Africa

Albert Solomon
Director, Radiology Department, Tel-Aviv Medical Center, and Associate Professor of Radiology, Sackler School of Medicine, Tel-Aviv University; Member of Pneumoconiosis Panel of the Ministries of Health and Labor, Tel-Aviv, Israel; Previously Chief Radiologist, Baragwanath Hospital, and Professor of Radiology, University of Witwatersrand, and part-time Consultant of the Medical Bureau for Occupational Diseases, Johannesburg, South Africa

Robert M. Steiner
Professor of Radiology, Associate Professor of Medicine, and Chief of Section of Thoracic Radiology, and Co-Director of the Division of Diagnostic Radiology at Thomas Jefferson University, Philadelphia, Pennsylvania, USA

A.B. Zwi
Epidemiology Unit, National Center for Occupational Health, and Department of Community Health, University of Witwatersrand, Johannesburg, South Africa

S. Zwi
Professor of Pulmonology, Department of Medicine, Johannesburg Hospital, and University of Witwatersrand Medical School, Johannesburg, South Africa

1

Radiography of Occupational Chest Diseases

R. Glyn Thomas

The quality of a chest film depends on a number of factors, not least is the radiography. In turn, radiography depends on equipment, kilovoltage, film, screens, processing, positioning of the subject, and whether a grid or air gap is used. Over decades, experience and detailed research have shown how the best results can be obtained. Nevertheless, there is no absolute, universally applicable method that allows for the fat and the lean, the muscular and the puny, calcifications and soft tissue. However, an effective compromise is possible.

The technologist is therefore crucial in obtaining the best results. A professional, dedicated, and knowledgeable approach allows not only for subject variations of size and possible deformities such as scoliosis, but also for pathological variations such as overdistended lungs, the prediction of a high diaphragm, or dyspnea. Initial viewing is of extreme importance for it will determine if a repeat film or extra view is indicated.

It is possible that many of the technical problems may be overcome in the not too distant future with computed techniques. Digital radiography can theoretically remove overlying rib shadows or show only bone and calcifications. Windowing of the data can prevent repeat examinations and maximize the information by a single exposure. Storage of radiographic information is greatly facilitated.

The chest radiograph, often thought of as the simplest of techniques, is in fact yet another example where the best results can only be obtained by matching enthusiasm with reliable, effective equipment.

Technical Factors

Choice of Peak Kilovoltage (kVp)

Only about 25% of each lung is visible unobscured by overlying bone shadows.[1] Any technique that makes more of the lung visible through the overlying bone must be regarded as highly desirable.[2]

Figure 1.1 shows clearly the advantage of using higher kilovoltages in chest radiography. The mass absorption coefficient of bone is appreciably smaller relative to that of soft tissues in the higher kilovoltage ranges. The result is the thoracic cage components become less obscuring. Although increasingly high kilovoltage does diminish the contrast between soft-tissue structures/fluid/blood vessels and the surrounding air-filled acini of the lung, it does allow increased visibility by lowering the bone density on the radiographs.

Visibility of the lesion depends not only on the contrast between the lesion and the surrounding structures but also on the complexity of the surrounding structures, which in the chest are the ribs and blood vessels. The term "structured noise" has been given to this complex shadowing, which can conceal what might be considered obvious abnormalities.[3,4]

Another effect of high kilovoltage is the flattening of contrast, ie, the range of densities of the thorax from bone to lung is reduced. By reducing the complexity of the shadows of the surrounding structure, a lesion is more easily seen, even though the contrast of the lesion itself may be reduced. Increasing peak kilovoltage affects both variables—the contrast of the abnormality

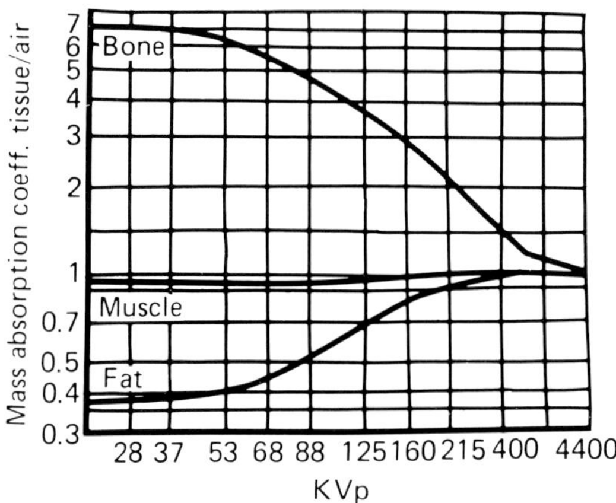

Figure 1.1. With the use of higher kilovoltage the mass absorption coefficient of bone is appreciably smaller relative to that of soft tissue. The result is that thoracic cage components do not obscure lung detail. From Glyn Thomas, R: Chest Radiography at 200 kV. S.A. Medical Journal 1973;47:2466.

is reduced but so is the surrounding contrast and its complexity.

Depth resolution is a measure of the thinnest layer of tissue that casts a detectable shadow. On chest radiographs it increases with increasing peak kilovoltage.[5] The improvement is due mainly to more images being recorded at middle densities where film contrast is high and the film blackening is optimum for comfortable viewing on a standard viewer.

Much experimental work has been done on the optimum kilovoltage for chest radiography. Christensen et al[6] showed that nodule detectability in a chest phantom improved with increasing peak kilovoltage up to 200 kVp; however, from 100 kVp and up the improvement was fairly small, and there was an increase in false-positive readings with the higher peak kilovoltages. For example, 300 kVp conferred no advantages, nodule detection decreased, and patient x-ray dose increased compared with 200-kVp films.

Using isolated human lung specimens[7] radiographed at 90, 140, and 350 kVp, it was shown that nodules of less than 3-mm diameter and lines of less than 3 mm in width were poorly seen at 350 kVp, probably owing to the large focal spot of the 350-kVp apparatus. It was no surprise that the 90-kVP images were better than 140 kVp in nodule demonstration, but this was due to the absence of the overlying bone of the thoracic cage. There is some trade-off between the optimum peak kilovoltage for nodule detection and the optimum peak kilovoltage required to lower the density of the bony structures to enable lung to be seen through them.

Another study[8] showed that 140 kVp was superior to 120 and 75 kVp in the detection of lung abnormalities (mainly cancers) in patients. The reduced structural complexity of the surrounding lung more than outweighed the reduced object complexity. This can be expressed as[4]

$$\text{conspicuity} = \frac{\text{lesion contrast}}{\text{surround complexity}}$$

This explains how a prominent background of the vascular pattern, for example, may obscure fairly obvious pathological lesions on the chest film.

At the Medical Bureau for Occupational Diseases in Johannesburg we have used 125-, 150-, 200-, and 350-kVp chest radiographs in a large series of men. Our own experience parallels that of Haus et al[9] who, when comparing conventional and 350-kVp chest radiographs, found that the large focal spot used with 350 kVp significantly limited resolution.

Our experience with 200-kVp chest radiographs[2] using an anode focal spot of 0.6 mm was most rewarding in that lung detail, as well as the peripheral pleural and retrocardiac areas, was superbly displayed.

Although 150 kVp showed a slight advantage over films exposed at 125 kVp, the 125 kVp is almost universally available; therefore, we now use 125-kVp films routinely at the Medical Bureau for Occupational Diseases, and as far as possible for all chest films routinely done on the gold mines in South Africa.

A major advantage of high kilovoltage technique is the great exposure latitude. Tuddenham[10] summarizes the peak kilovoltage situation succinctly. The characteristics of the various structures of the chest are so dissimilar that ideal imaging of all structures on a single radiograph is simply not possible. The radiologist must adopt a technique that selectively optimizes the recording of the type of structure of greatest diagnostic interest in a particular situation. The high peak kilovoltage techniques do this satisfactorily for the lung pertinent to diagnosis of pneumoconiosis.

Radiation Scatter Cleanup

With higher peak kilovoltage, scatter increases, and these scattered photons striking the fluorescent screens of the x-ray cassette in a random manner give an overall "fog" level that severely degrades the image.

At 125 kVp a 12:1 fine-line grid or Bucky diaphragm is necessary. High ratio Bucky diaphragm and high ratio grids, which are always of focused type, are extremely sensitive to malalignment. If they are not accurately aligned to the focal spot of the x-ray tube, one gets falloff in density across one side of the film, giving hazy slight opacification of one or the other lung.

Artifacts mimicking "p" or "q" shadows may be produced by the very short high kilovolt (peak) exposure time, only allowing minimal movement of the reciprocating Bucky. This results in ill-defined faint vertical white lines crossing horizontally disposed lung shadows, eg, fine peripheral vessels, thus creating spurious nodules. The source of these artifacts can be verified by finding the telltale vertical stripes above the soft tissues of the lung. Adjustment of the grid and exposure time synchronization will eliminate the problem.

An air-gap technique, where the front of the chest stand is separated from the film plane by a moderate distance, can be used to reduce the random scattered radiation from the patient, which is then dissipated in the air gap. Trout et al[11] compared an air gap and a grid in radiology on the chest, using a pneumoconiosis test phantom. Their conclusion was that an air-gap technique could provide contrast equivalent to that obtainable with a grid, but with lower patient x-ray exposure than that of grid techniques, and with less precise centering of the x-ray tube to the film. The optimum air gap was shown to be 15 cm (6 in.) with focus-film distance of 305 cm (10 ft). A considerably larger x-ray room is needed because of the long focus film distance.

In our experience, an air-gap technique is suitable for small-to-average-sized men using 125 kVp, but a grid (Bucky) technique is essential with large men, where the air-gap technique produces grey "fog-o-grams." Slit-beam techniques have successfully been used to decrease the amount of scattered radiation.[12,13] The principle is simple. A collimating device produces a narrow slit beam of x-rays that is moved across the object or patient being radiographed (with usually a synchronously moving matching slit orifice between the patient and the x-ray cassette) with the result that only direct radiation is recorded on the film. Slit-beam methods produce excellent air/soft-tissue contrast in the 120- to 125-kVp range. The major disadvantage is the impossibility of obtaining slit movements sufficiently fast to "freeze" heart movement, pulmonary artery and cardiac pulsation transmitted to the adjacent lung areas. An experimental rotating disk slit device has been used with good results.[14]

Filtration

A 2-mm total aluminum equivalent filtration between the x-ray source and the patient is regarded as being most suitable for chest radiography. Consisting of intrinsic filtration of the x-ray tube envelope plus added external aluminum filtration, it gives a good range of densities to the lung fields, but is deficient in showing mediastinal structures at 125 kVp.

Additional filtration "hardens" the x-ray beam by filtering out the softer long wavelengths of the x-ray beam and is advantageous in demonstrating lung detail through the bones of the thoracic cage; the more the rib detail is washed out, the more lung detail becomes visible through the bone shadows.

Filters have been devised that not only give better visualization of those parts of the lung usually hidden behind the heart, but also give better demonstration of the mediastinal structure. A "trough" filter of thick aluminum has a vertical concavity or trough running down the center, ensuring a higher x-ray exposure to the central chest structures than to the peripheral lung fields without significant degradation of the lung portion of the image.[15] Such filters, however, have the disadvantage of a fixed shape central trough while cardiac and mediastinal shapes and sizes are very variable; these filters are therefore not entirely satisfactory.

Proper beam filtration with high kilovolt chest radiography can shape the energy distribution of the beam so that the radiograph is unaltered but patient exposure is reduced by two to three times that given by conventionally filtered x-ray beams.[16]

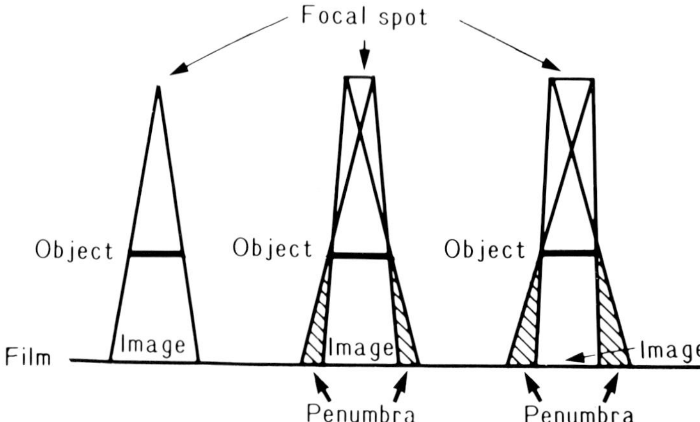

Figure 1.2. A demonstration of how the smallest focus improves the sharpness of lung and bone structures by reducing the blur due to the penumbra.

Focus Size

Modern rotating anode tubes usually have dual foci (some have three foci), with the smallest focal spot varying from 0.3 mm (a "microfocus" tube) to 1.2 mm and the large focus from 0.6 to 2 mm. The x-ray tube focal size is seldom a limiting factor in the resolution of chest images at ±125 kVp. Small foci cannot be loaded as heavily by the x-ray generator and longer and longer exposure times are necessary. The potential improvement in resolution could be completely negated by movement blurring.

The major advantage of a small focus is the increase in sharpness of the edges of lung and bone structures. The increase in sharpness is particularly valuable when tiny structures, such as pneumoconiotic nodules, are being demonstrated; the circumferential "blur" due to the surrounding penumbra is reduced (Fig. 1.2).

The accuracy in detecting abnormalities is unaffected in the range of focal spot size from 0.3 to 2.0 mm, but the false-positive rate within this range decreases with increasing focal spot size.[17] A good compromise of x-ray tube focus size is 1.2 mm for high peak kilovoltage work, where exposures are much shorter than with low kilovolts (peak). Haus et al[9] state that the total resolution of a chest radiography system can be improved by using a 1.0-mm nominal focal spot size, but limited tube output and long exposure times can make such combinations impractical.

Heel Effect

An almost forgotten and certainly much neglected factor in chest radiography is the heel effect. The intensity of x-radiation is not uniform, but diminishes toward the anode end of the x-ray tube—the "heel." With focus film distance of 180 cm, this effect is minimal. However, there may be occasions where the x-ray tube position may have to be reversed to eliminate the anode heel effect and to allow a lesser exposed area of the chest to be better exposed (Fig. 1.3).

Film-Screen Combinations

The x-ray film/intensifying screen combination is important but some compromise is necessary. High-resolution fluorescent screens necessitate longer exposures for adequate radiographs, and with medium to low-powered x-ray generators the improvement in resolution (clarity of small structures) is offset by movement blurring due to pulsation of the heart and pulmonary vessels, transmitted heart movement to the lungs, and to the inability of the patient to remain motionless in full inspiration for the requisite time.

With "fast" screens the exposures are much shorter, but quantum mottle can degrade any advantage given by the ultrashort exposures used. Quantum-mottle is due to random variations in the particles of x-ray energy reaching the fluorescent screens in the cassette. Longer exposures minimize the quantum effect.

Another source of error is the inadvertent mismatching of x-ray film with a spectral sensitivity different to that emitted by the fluorescent screen. Green-emitting screens, for example, work best in conjunction with special films having photographic emulsion and dye coatings designed for sensitivity to the green part of the light spectrum.

Some improvement in chest-image quality can be obtained with the use of films and screens developed for "wide contrast," but increased cost is often a prohibiting factor.

Screen-Film Contact

Poor film-screen contact is a frequent cause of substandard chest images. Minor degrees of poor contact are seldom recognized, although the loss of detail information can be substantial. Testing for good screen-film contact is done by radiographing a fine-mesh wire grid in contact with the cassette. Areas of poor screen-film contact show degradation of resolution—the tiny wires of the mesh become blurred.

Optimum Density of Films

Appendix A of the "Guidelines for the Use of the Classification of Radiographs of Pneumoconioses"[18] gives recommendations for the optimal range of densities for chest radiographs. The range of optical densities of the region of interest should fall between 0.3 and 1.7 units, and the difference in optical density between the darkest and lightest regions of interest should not exceed 1.0. Below 0.3, inherent contrast is poor. Above 1.7, special lighting methods such as bright lights are necessary to perceive detail and relative contrast of structures. The physical criteria for density state that[18]

1. Hilar regions should exhibit a minimum of 0.2 unit of optical density above fog.
2. Parenchymal regions should exhibit a maximum of 1.8 units of optical density above fog.

For *gross image contrast*, the difference in optical density between the darkest segment of the lung parenchyma and the lightest portions of the hilar regions should fall within the range of 1.0 to 1.4 units of optical density. Well-exposed chest radiographs taken at 125 to 150 kVp easily fulfill these criteria.

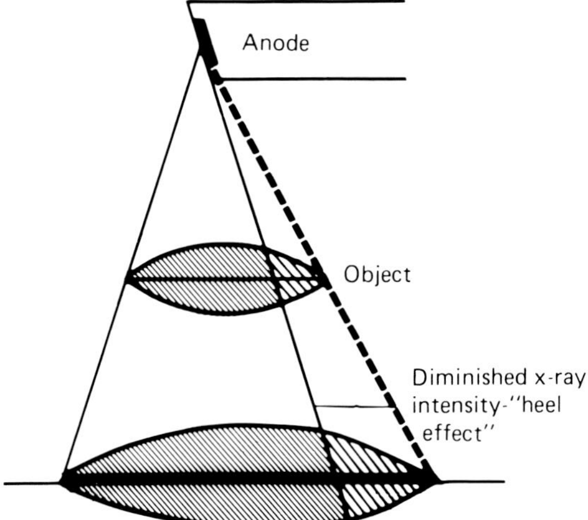

Figure 1.3. The diagram demonstrates the influence of focus size on penumbra and the loss of sharp resolution with increasing focal size.

Other Imaging Methods

Xeroradiography

We have used xeroradiography at 200 kV in the investigation of asbestos- and silica-exposed men as a research procedure.[19] This was very successful in demonstrating the earliest basal lung changes of asbestosis because of the effect of edge enhancement at density boundaries, which is a most useful property of xeroradiography systems. Pleural changes were also well shown; however, the demonstration of silicotic nodules was poor. Both the small size of the xerographic record paper (22 × 34.5 cm) and the relatively high radiation dose make xerographic techniques unsuitable for routine use. There is justification in exposing a xeroradiograph of the lung base where standard radiographs show equivocal changes of asbestosis and a diagnosis is essential.

Computed Tomography

Computed tomography (CT) produces axial images of the body, with a slice thickness that can be varied from about a millimeter up to a centimeter. Computed tomography is both too costly and too time consuming for suveillance of the chest in dust-exposed individuals, but it is a valuable adjunct in clarifying particular clinical problems.

Characteristic features are found in pulmonary asbestosis,[20,21] and CT is particularly valuable in showing pleural thickening and distinguishing it from other causes of pleural or chest wall shadowing.[22] Some features of asbestos-related disease are better shown on CT scans than on conventional roentgenograms, and occasionally features not shown at all on conventional films may be demonstrated on CT scans.[23]

Digital Radiography

In digital radiography of the chest, the stored image is displayed on a cathode-ray-tube monitor. The image can be manipulated by the viewer to provide optimum density for bones, mediastinum, lungs, or soft tissues. Electronic edge enhancement can be used, and the image can be changed from the conventional negative mode to the positive mode by the flick of a switch. It is interesting that many readers prefer the positive image where lung vessels appear black and the lung air, white ("clear").[24] The resolution of a prototype system is excellent,[25,26] but inferior to conventional silver halide emulsion x-ray film and fluorescent screen combinations.

A recent development in digital-image storage has been the use of the laser disk, which enables vast amounts of digitized data to be stored in a very limited space and which permits rapid access. This might bring the eventual replacement of film by electronic images closer.

References

1. Evans RJ, Lewis CJ, Moorson D: The radiographic visibility of the lung fields. Br J Radiol 1968;41: 801–803.
2. Glyn Thomas R, Sluis-Cremer GK: Chest radiography at 200 KV. S Afr Med J 1973;47:2465–2468.
3. Revesz G, Kundel HL, Graber MA: The influence of structured noise on the detection of radiologic abnormalities. Invest Radiol 1974;9:479–486.
4. Kundel HL, Revesz G: Lesion conspicuity, structured noise and film reader error. Am J Roentgenol 1976;126:1233–1238.
5. Dyke WP, Barbour JP, Charbonnier FM: Depth resolution: A mechanism by which high kilovoltage improves visibility in chest films. Radiology 1975; 117:159–164.
6. Christensen EE, Dietz GW, Murray RC, et al: Effect of kilovoltage on detectability of pulmonary nodules in a chest phantom. Am J Roentgenol 1977;128: 789–793.
7. Herman PG, Goldstein J, Balikian J, et al: Visibility and sharpness of lung structure at 90, 140 and 350 KV. Radiology 1980;134:591–597.
8. Revesz G, Shea FJ, Kundell HL: The effects of kilovoltage on diagnostic accuracy in chest radiography. Radiology 1982;142:615–618.
9. Haus AG, Meyer J, North LB: Effects of geometric and screen-film unsharpness in conventional and 350 KVp chest radiography. Radiology 1980;137: 197–202.
10. Tuddenham WJ: Rationale for high KVp chest radiography. The optimization of chest radiography. Am J Roentgenol 1980;134:199–205.
11. Trout ED, Kelley JP, Larson VL: A comparison of an air gap and a grid in roentgenography of the chest. Am J Roentgenol 1975;124:404–411.
12. Sorenson JA, Nelson JA: Investigations of moving-slit radiography. Radiology 1976;120:705–711.
13. Barnes GT, Cleare HM, Brezovich IA: Reduction in scatter in diagnostic radiology by means of a scanning multiple slit assembly. Radiology 1976;120: 691–694.
14. Sorenson JA, Nelson JA, Niklason LJ, et al: Rotating disk device for slit radiography of the chest. Radiology 1980;134:227–231.
15. Wieder S, Adams PL: Improved routine chest radiography with a trough filter. Am J Roentgenol 1981; 137:695–698.
16. Sieband MP: Equipment limitations and filtration. The optimization of chest radiography. Am J Roentgenol 1980;134:199–205.
17. Gray ME, Taylor KW, Hobbs BB: Detection accuracy in chest radiography. Am J. Roentgenol 1978; 131:247–253.
18. Guidelines for the Use of ILO International Classification of Radiographs of Pneumoconioses. Revised Edition, 1980. Occupational Safety and Health Series No 22 (Rev), International Labour Office, Geneva.
19. Glyn Thomas R, Sluis-Cremer GK: 200 KV xeroradiography in occupational exposure to silica and asbestos. Br J Ind Med 1977;34:281–290.
20. Kreel L: Computer tomography in the evaluation of pulmonary asbestosis. Acta Radiol [Diagn] 1976; 17:405–411.
21. Katz D, Kreel L: Computed tomography in pulmonary asbestosis. Clin Radio 1979;30:207–213.

22. Sargent EN, Boswell WD Jr, Ralls P, et al: Subpleural fat pads in patients exposed to asbestos: distinction from non-calcified pleural plaques. Radiology 1984;152:273–277.
23. Sluis-Cremer GK, Glyn Thomas R, Schmaman IB: The value of computerised axial tomography in the assessment of workers exposed to asbestos. Am J Ind Med 1984;6:27–35.
24. Fraser RG, Breatnach E, Barnes GT: Digital radiography of the chest: Clinical experience with a prototype unit. Radiology 1983;148:1–5.
25. Sashin D, Sternglass EJ, Slasky BS, et al: Diode array digital radiography: Initial clinical experience. Am J Roentgenol 1982;139:1045–1050.
26. Sherrier RH, Chiles C, Wilkinson WE, et al: Effects of image processing on nodule detection rates in digitized chest radiographs: R.O.C. study of observer performance. Radiology 1988;166:447–450.

2

Classifying Radiographs of the Pneumoconioses

R. Glyn Thomas

The chest radiograph remains a crucial tool in the assessment of pneumoconioses. Sophisticated lung function tests, however important, do not provide sufficient indication of altered gross morphology, nor of possible complications, especially of the pleura, or infections.

Although neither lung function tests nor chest radiographs are pathognomonic within the context of dust inhalation, they are effective in monitoring the harmful effects of exposure both immediate and long term. The accurate assessment of the chest radiograph is, however, by no means simple. A detailed knowledge of normal variations and of the many nonindustrial diseases of the chest are crucial in reading chest films. Even more important is intimate familiarity with the International Labour Office Geneva (ILO) classification, conceptually and in practice. Although variations in reading cannot be completely eliminated, close agreement between readers and of an individual reader is attainable.

As the radiographic changes can be accurately recorded, correlation with changed morphology has improved, providing a better understanding of the pathogenesis of dust-inhalation disease. Although the added hazard of cigarette smoking is well recognized, it is as yet not possible to separate its effects from that of inhaled dusts on either lung function tests or on the chest radiograph with any degree of certainty.

Classifying Radiographs of the Pneumoconioses

The international classification is primarily a means of communication between doctors working within a center as well as with film readers in other centers or other countries. The classification, however, should be rigidly adhered to, its use requiring frequent referral to the standard films radiographs.

The ILO classification may be used in "short" or "complete" forms (Table 2.1), or in combinations of both to suit the circumstances.[1] For standardization and accuracy of communication, particularly in epidemiologic surveys where multiple reader groups are involved and often in different countries, it is essential as a preliminary to indicate which parts of the classification used are the "complete" and which are the "short." An example cited by the Guidelines[1] is the reading of coal worker's pneumoconiosis, where the full classification is used for the changes frequently shown in the lungs and the short classification for the occurrence of rare pleural changes.

Such a scheme would be inappropriate for reading films of asbestosis where pleural changes are frequent and tend to be related to duration of exposure.[2] For routine use, the short classification is suitable, but for epidemiological and statistical survey, the complete classification should be used. Before the classification is used, a decision as to exactly what information may be required in the long term must be made. A great deal of valuable

Table 2.1. The ILO classification.

The complete classification records:

1. Technical quality of the radiograph
2. Parenchymal abnormalities
   - Small opacities – profusion
     - shape and size
     - extent
   - Large opacities – categories
3. Pleural abnormalities
   - Pleural thickening – chest wall – types, site, width, extent
     - diaphragm – left or right
     - costophrenic angle obliteration – left or right
   - Pleural calcification – site
     - extent
4. Symbols of radiographic features of importance
5. Comments

The short classification is a simplification of the complete classification and records:

1. Technical quality of the chest radiograph
2. Parenchymal abnormalities
   - Small opacities – profusion
   - Shape and size – rounded
     - irregular
   - Large opacities
3. Pleural changes – pleural thickening
   - pleural calcification
4. Symbols
5. Comments

information can be lost forever if an inappropriate classification is employed; studies of progression of radiologic silicosis, for example, may not be suitable for analysis if the brief "short classification" is used.

Exposure to dusts may cause opacities in the lungs. The classification defines the profusion of these opacities and their types and sizes. The opacities may be nodular, easily measured and circular, or linear, or ill-defined. The sizes of opacity are categorized for both well-defined lesions and poorly defined lesions, and there is provision for indicating shadows of different sizes or of different types in the same chest radiograph.

Profusion is considered to be more important than size or type of opacity and is therefore expressed first, followed by the symbol for the type(s) of opacity. The predominant type and size are expressed first, followed by the symbol for the less dominant lesions if present, or duplication of the first symbol if only one type of opacity is present.

Silicotic nodulation could, for example, be expressed as 2/2 q/q when the nodules are all in the size range of 1.5 to 3 mm and the profusion with that shown on the standard radiographs for 2/2. In the 1980 classification profusion is defined solely by comparison with the standard films rather than by features, such as obscuring of the lung vessels as used in the earlier classification.

The classification is not intended to define the amount of compensation for lung disease, nor is the classification in any way related to lung function or loss of working capacity. It is an accurate, reproducible system to define specific appearances on the chest radiograph. Information contained in the classification may be used by various bodies in association with clinical and pulmonary function tests to formulate acceptable standards for compensation and legal purposes.

The classification is designed for use with posterior anterior (PA) chest films, although additional films, oblique or lateral for example, can be classified, provided that the views are specified. The radiographic appearances vary considerably between low kilovolt (peak) direct chest films and high kilovolt (peak) Bucky films. Prior to any correlative survey using the ILO classification, we believe it essential that the radiographic technique be standardized. Chest films of 125 kVp are now routine, having generally replaced low kilovolt (peak) direct (nongrid) techniques for pneumoconiosis surveillance.

No features of a chest radiograph are pathognomonic of pneumoconiosis, there is always a differential diagnosis; but if any features in the parenchyma or pleura are consistent with pneumoconiosis, the films should be classified. If it is possible that the chest film might represent pneumoconiosis, but there is some doubt, the features should be categorized according to the classification and a note made of the other causes considered. If the appearances are thought to result from some other pathology, the radiograph should not be classified, but comment should be made using the appropriate symbols and any other *remarks* necessary. This course of action would clarify apparent major discrepancies between readers, particularly if there are differences of

Table 2.2. Details of the classification.

Findings	Short classification	Complete classification
Film quality		
Grade	1, 2, 3, 4	1, 2, 3, 4
Comment made	Y/N	Y/N
Normal parenchyma	0	0/– 0/0 0/1
Abnormal parenchyma		
Small opacities		
Profusion	1, 2, 3	1/0 1/1 1/2 2/1 2/2 2/3 3/2 3/3 3/+
Type		
Rounded	p/p q/q r/r or combinations of p, q, r	p/p q/q r/r or combinations of p, q, r
Irregular	s/s t/t u/u or combinations of s, t, u	s/s t/t u/u or combinations of s, t, u
	Combinations of well-defined rounded opacities (p, q, or r) with irregular opacities (s, t, or u) would also be recorded when appropriate	
Extent	–	Lung zones involved RU LU RM LM RL LL
Large opacities	A, B, C	A, B, C
Pleural abnormality		
Pleural thickening	pt	Chest wall Circumscribed plaques Y/N Site R L Face on Y/N Width a, b, c Extent 1, 2, 3 Diffuse Y/N Site R L Face on Y/N Width a, b, c Extent 1, 2, 3 Diaphragm Y/N Site L, R Costophrenic angle obliteration Y/N Site L, R
Pleural calcification	pc	Presence Y/N Chest wall R, L Diaphragm R, L Other R, L and specify (eg, mediastinal site or pericardial)
Symbols	Y/N Up to 6 of: ax bu ca cn co cp cv di ef em es fr hi ho id ih kl od pi px rp tb (+pt, pc with short classification) Record further symbols (if > 6) in "Comments" section.	
Comments	Y/N Written comments	

opinion as to whether the appearances could or could not be pneumoconiosis. A 0/0 reading with suitable comment by one reader, for example, is then comparable with a 3/3 reading on the same radiograph by another observer who believes the condition to be pneumoconiosis.

Explanation – Complete Classification

The technical quality is graded as follows:

1. Good.
2. Acceptable – no technical flaw that would impair classification.
3. Poor – film with defects but still classifiable.
4. Unacceptable.

If quality is not grade 1, comment should be made about the deficiencies of the film. The "Explanatory Notes" of the 1980 classification point out that a better radiograph might not be available in circumstances such as an epidemiological survey and more detail about the technical deficiencies should be recorded. If, for example, the parenchyma is visible but the pleura not, or vice versa, only part of the complete classification may be usefuly available for statistical purposes.

Parenchymal Abnormalities

Small Opacities

Profusion. The profusion of small opacities is categorized by comparison with the standard radiographs available from the International Labor Office in Geneva. Category 0 represents normal. Categories 1, 2, and 3 represent increasing profusion as defined by the standard radiographs. The symbols are used in this unchanged form for the short classification. The complete classification uses those symbols expanded to a 12-point scale as follows:

The radiographs are classified into one of the above four grades of profusion. If a grade of profusion above or below that which was decided on was seriously considered as an alternative, it is recorded. For example, if a film is categorized as 2, but 1 was seriously considered, this is encoded as 2/1; but if 3 was considered, it is recorded as 2/3, the additional symbol coming immediately *after* that decided upon as the correct category. The midcategory where there is no doubt whatever is categorized as, say, 1/1, 2/2, 3/3. Within category 3, a radiograph that shows a greater profusion than expected for the midcategory is recorded as 3/+.

In the 0 category, 0/1 indicates that the possibility of nodules was seriously entertained but discarded; 0/– is used when the absence of any possible abnormality is particularly striking – a sort of "super-normal." The complete scale of profusion evolved in this way is as follows:

0/–	0/0	0/1
1/0	1/1	1/2
2/1	2/2	2/3
3/2	3/3	3/+

Shape and Size. The shape of small opacities may be clear-cut and rounded, or irregular or linear.

In the category of clear-cut, well-defined opacities and irregular opacities that can be linear or irregular in outline, there are three designated sizes. These are illustrated on the standard radiographs, which take precedence over the written definitions.

Well-defined, rounded opacities are indicated by p, q, and r: p = a diameter of up to 1.5 mm (Figs. 2.1 and 2.2), q = 1.5 to 3 mm in diameter (Figs. 2.3 to 2.6), and r = a diameter of more than 3 mm and up to 1 cm (Figs. 2.7 to 2.9).

The letters s, t, and u represent irregular opacities that include irregular nodules as well as linear shadows: s = width up to 1.5 mm (Figs. 2.10 to 2.12), t = width 1.5–3 mm (Figs. 2.13 to 2.15), and u = width more than 3 mm up to 1 cm.

Opacities on a chest radiograph may be all of one size and shape or the radiograph may have opacities of mixed sizes and shapes (Figs. 2.16 and 2.17).

The predominant opacity pattern is represented by a letter, and – following an oblique stroke after the letter – a second letter, which may be either the same letter if the lesions are all of the same size and shape or a different letter representing the less dominant opacity pattern.

Thus, p/p, q/q, r/q, p/s, etc represent the types and sizes of opacities that are all of one sort, or mixed. The first letter represents the dominant opacities in a mixed pattern and the second letter the less profuse types of lesions.

Experience and judgment are required to categorize pattern types, with frequent reference made to

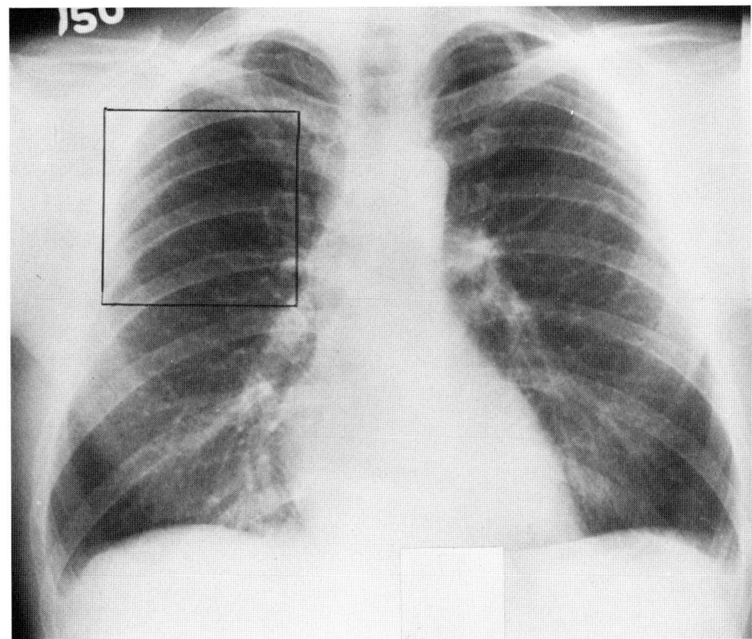

A

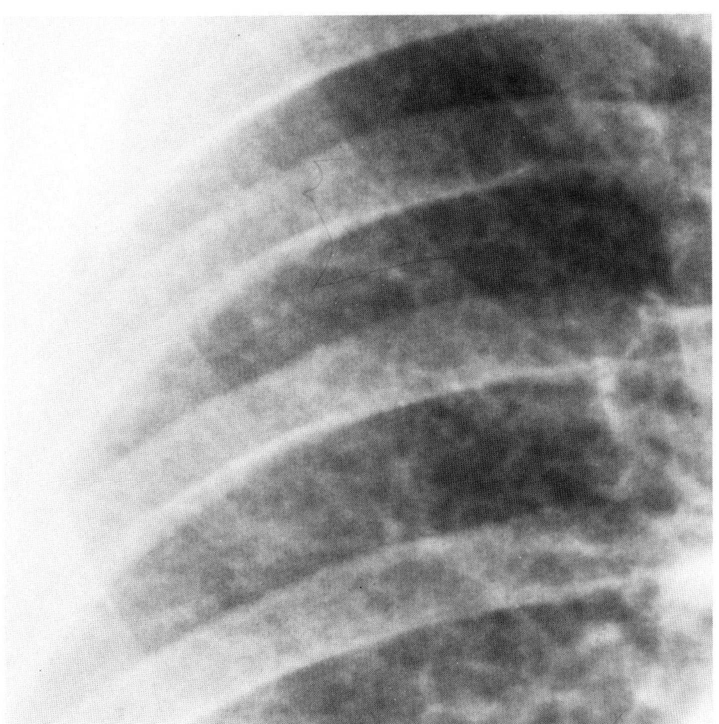

B

Figure 2.1. Well-defined rounded opacities (up to 1.5 mm diameter) are shown, ie, corresponding 1/0 p/p. Insets are full size.

the standard films. It is inappropriate, for example, to classify a radiograph as r/q if only a couple of q-sized nodules are found on the film. It should be clearly apparent that there is a mixture of the sizes in the various zones—the wording in the Guidelines[1] is "significant" numbers of the second type of opacity.

Extent. Each lung is divided into upper, middle, and lower thirds by horizontal lines drawn at one third and two thirds of the distance along a vertical from the dome of the diaphragm to the lung apex. The zones affected are recorded. The maximally affected zones are categorized by comparison with the standard films and this constitutes profusion.

A

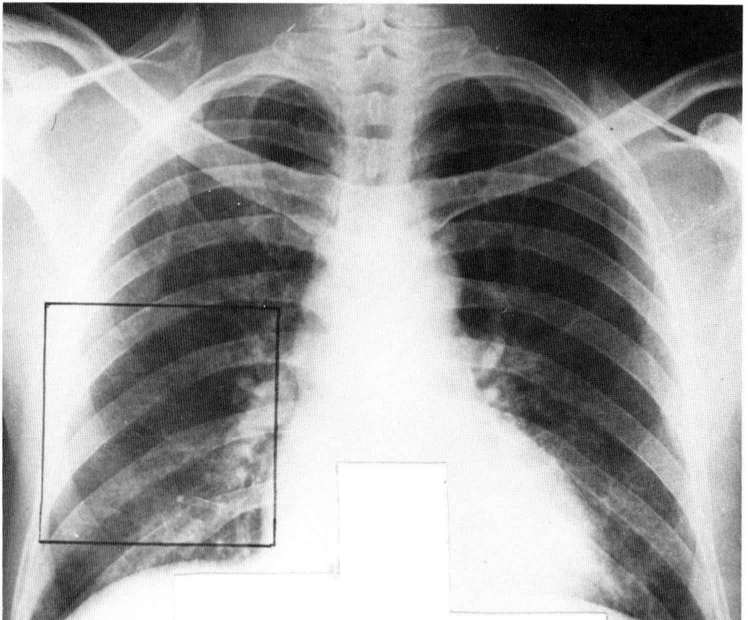

B

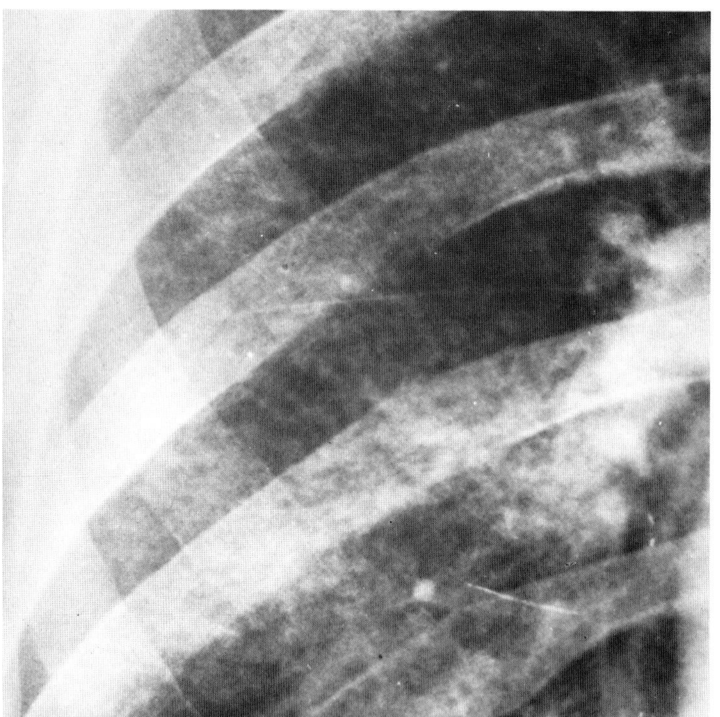

Figure 2.2. Pronounced, well-defined rounded opacities up to 1.5 mm, ie, 1/1, p/p.

If profusion in any other zone is three or more subcategories lower than this, these zones of lesser involvement are *not* recorded as positive. As an example, if the profusion is 3/3 in the right and left upper zones and only 2/1 in the midzones, *only* the upper zones are recorded as positive.

It is obvious that the complete classification can be modified to record separately the types and profusions of densities in each of the six zones, but this is not part of the standard ILO classification, and any such nonstandard modifications must be carefully annotated. The readings cannot then be

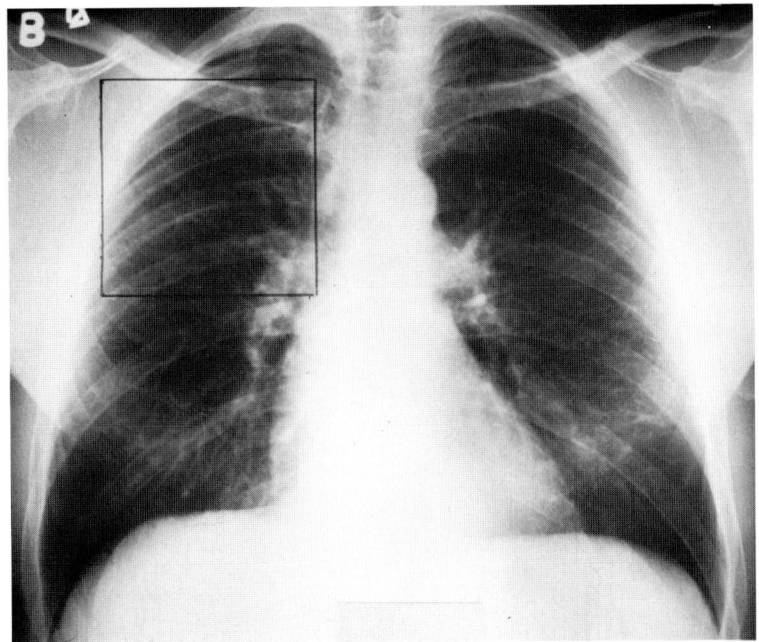

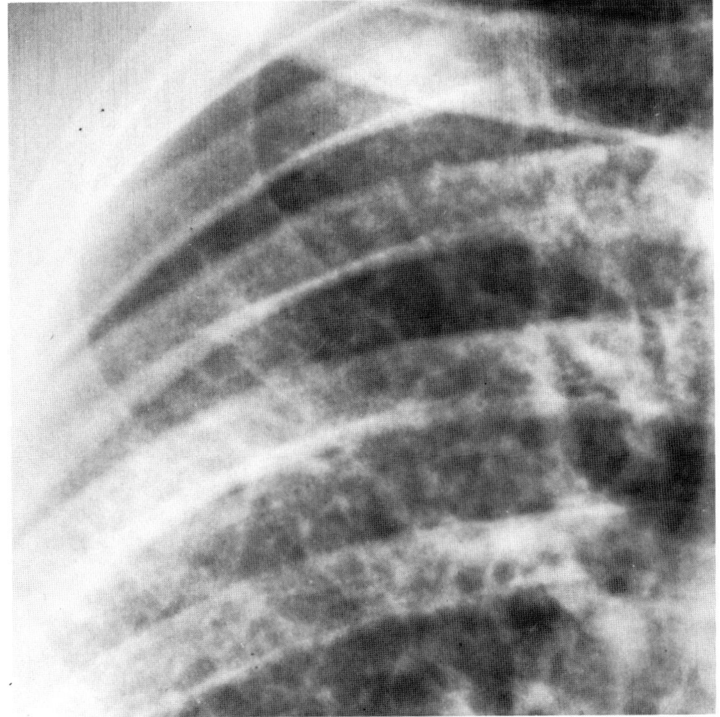

Figure 2.3. Well-defined rounded opacities from 1.5 to 3.0 mm are present, ie, 1/0 q/q.

directly compared, for example, with readings from another center using the classification precisely as defined in the Guidelines.

Classification for profusion of small opacities requires a mental process of integrating profusion over the affected zones and comes only with considerable experience; nevertheless, there will still be occasions when the same reading on two different radiographs of a patient, or chest radiographs of two different patients, will not represent the same thing. Taking the case of 3/3 in two upper zones, the one film may have only this,

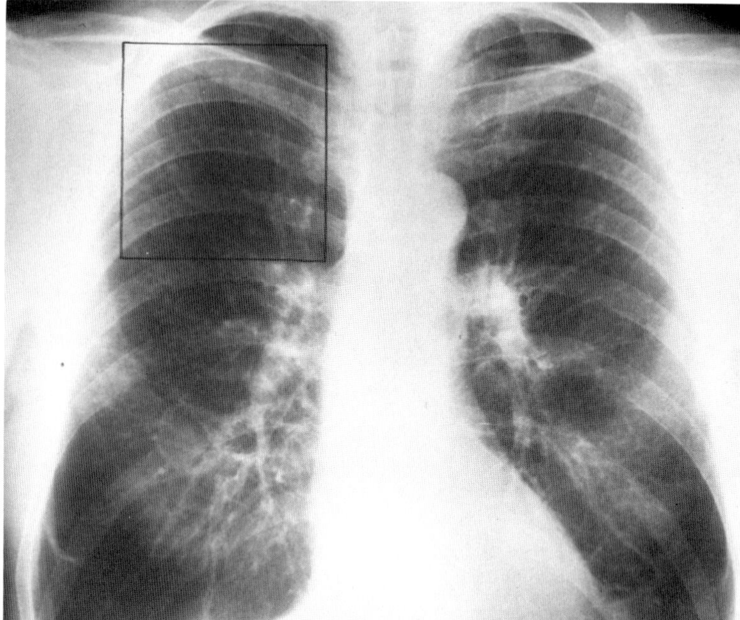

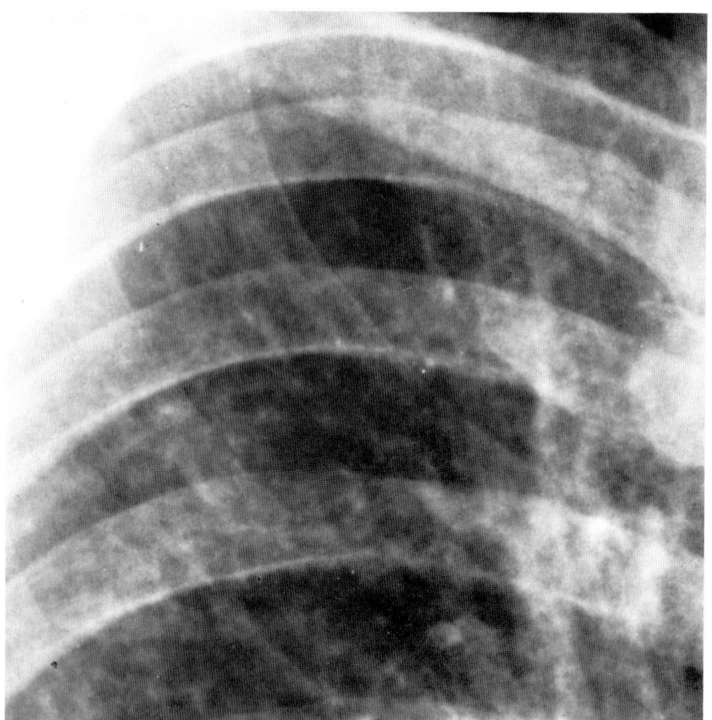

Figure 2.4. In the right upper zone well-defined rounded opacities are of 1.5 to 3.0 mm in size, ie, 1/1 q/q.

whereas the other film will have extensive opacities over the other four zones, but of category 2/1 or lower.

Large Opacities

These are opacities of greater than 10 mm in diameter. They are classified as follows:

Category A: An opacity having a greatest diameter of more than 10 mm but less than 50 mm, or the sum of the greatest diameters of several opacities that does not exceed 50 mm.

Category B: One or more opacities larger or more

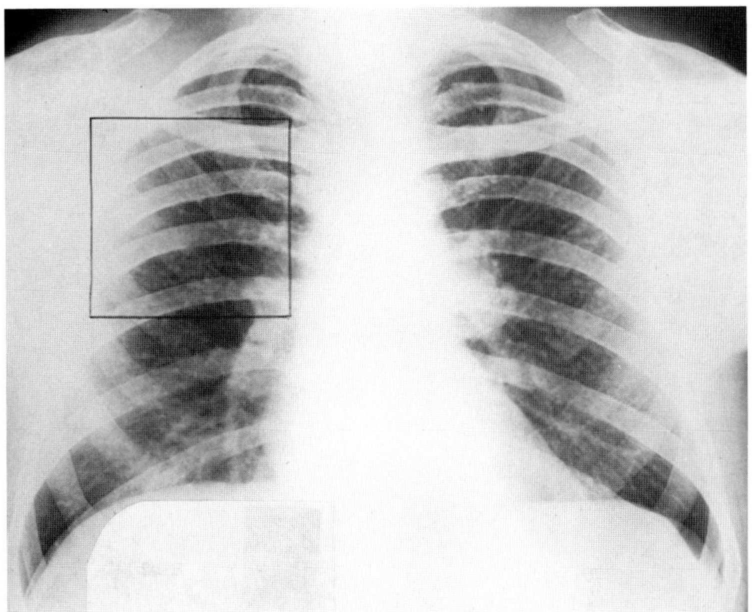

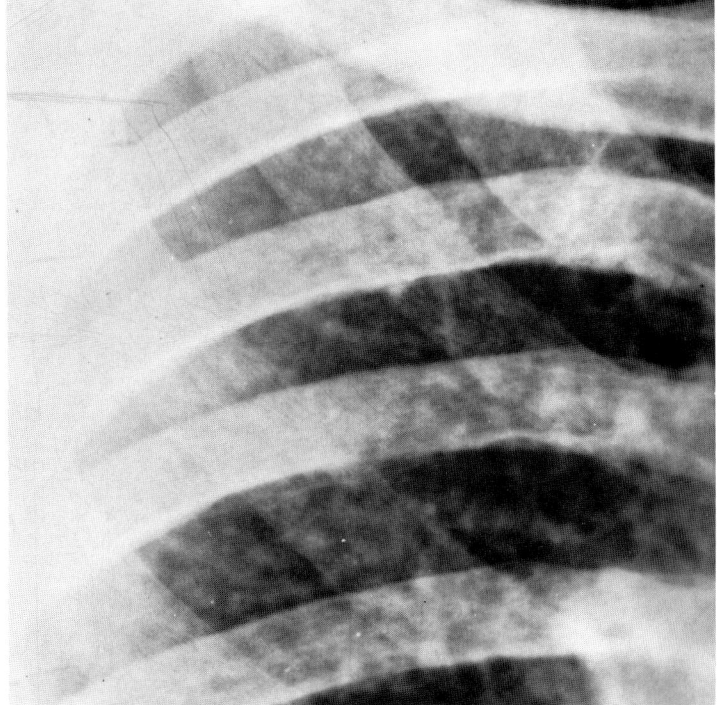

Figure 2.5. The rounded well-defined opacities are between 1.5 to 3.0 mm in size, ie, 2/2 q/q.

numerous than category A whose combined area does not exceed that of the right upper zone.

Category C: One or more opacities whose combined area exceeds the equivalent of the right upper zone.

Note that the large opacity categories refer to lesions of more than 1 cm each in diameter. Below this the densities would correspond to r or u.

It is readily apparent that lengths are defined by category A, but as the total length or sum of lengths exceeds 50 mm, there is then a translation into the concept of area. The "right upper zone" for

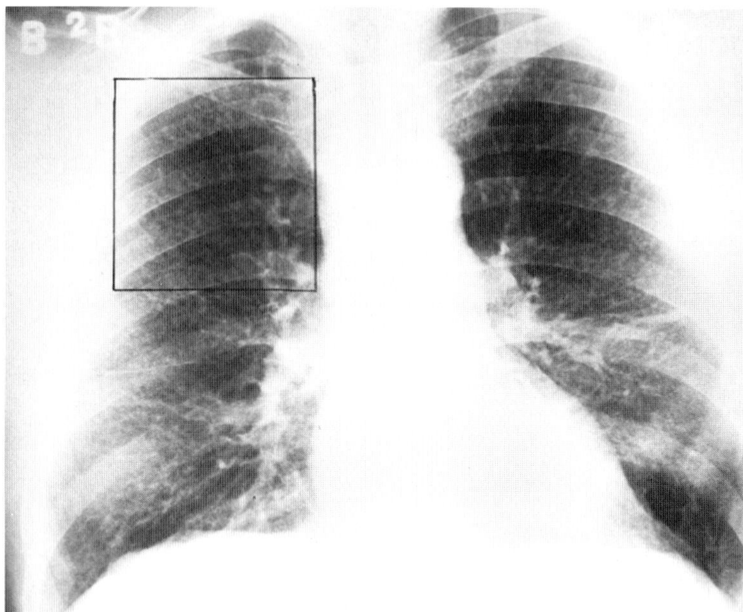

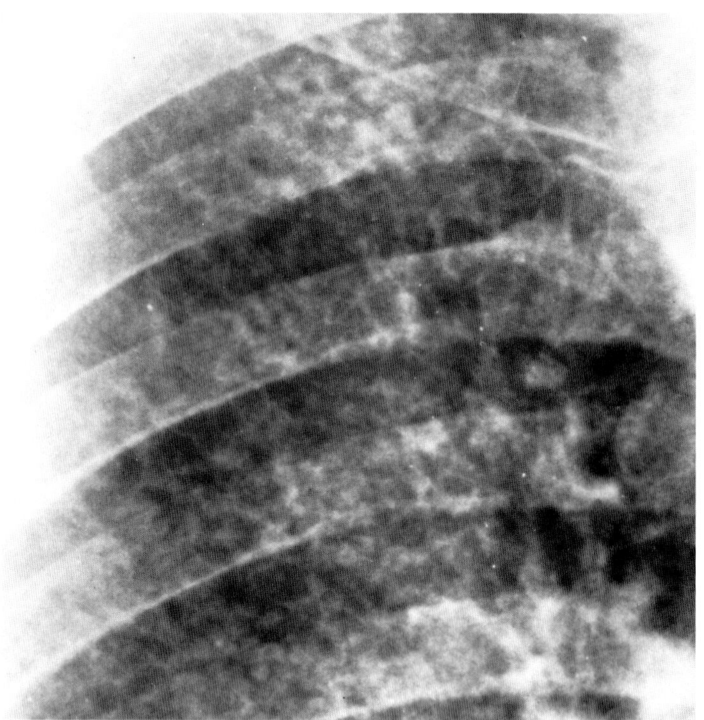

Figure 2.6. Pronounced, well-defined rounded opacities between 1.5 to 3.0 mm in size, ie, 3/3 q/q.

purposes of classification is defined as the upper one third of the lung measured by dividing the vertical distance from the dome of the diaphragm to the apex into three and drawing a horizontal line to divide off the upper third from the lower two thirds. "Rib counts" and other arbitrary methods are not used in the 1980 classification.

Large opacities can represent either areas of coalescence of smaller pneumoconiotic nodules, or, more frequently, progressive massive fibrosis (PMF) where the areas of density may have few or no visible nodules within them.

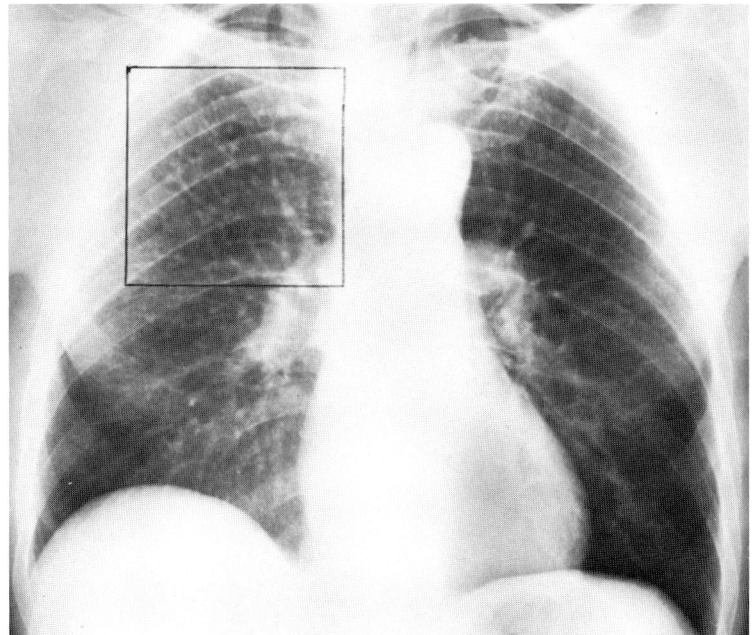

A

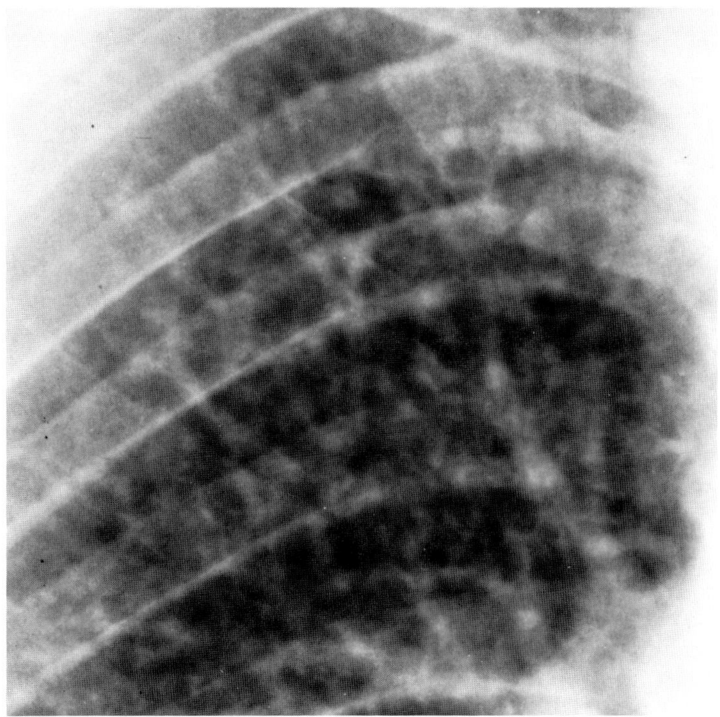

B

Figure 2.7. The rounded opacities are greater in size than 3 mm and below 1.0 cm, ie, 1/1 r/r.

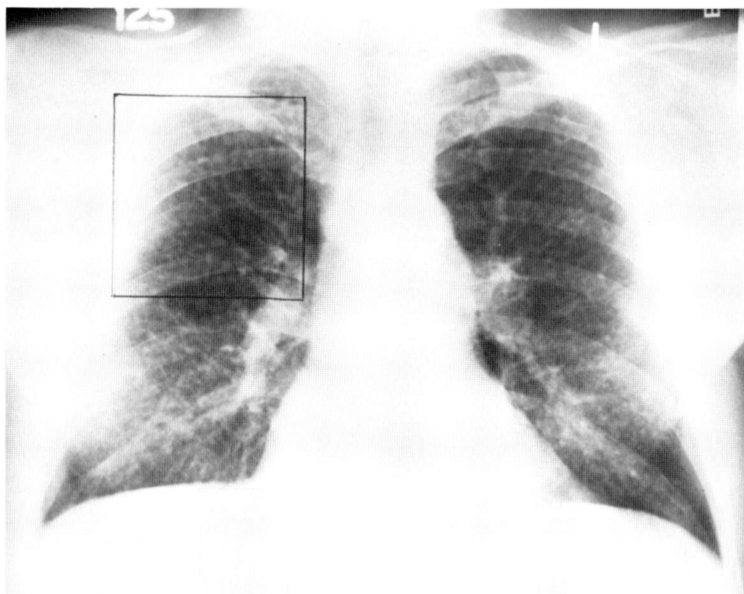

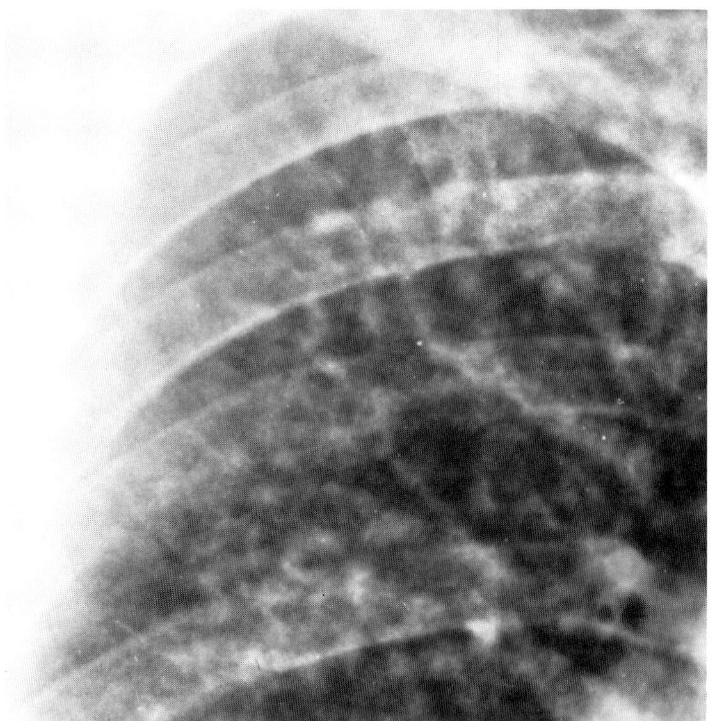

Figure 2.8. Pronounced, well-defined rounded opacities exceeding 3.0 mm but not greater than 1.0 cm. They correspond to 3/2 r/r ILO classification.

Figure 2.9. Profuse, well-rounded opacities varying in size from 3.0 mm to 1.0 cm, ie, 3/3 r/r.

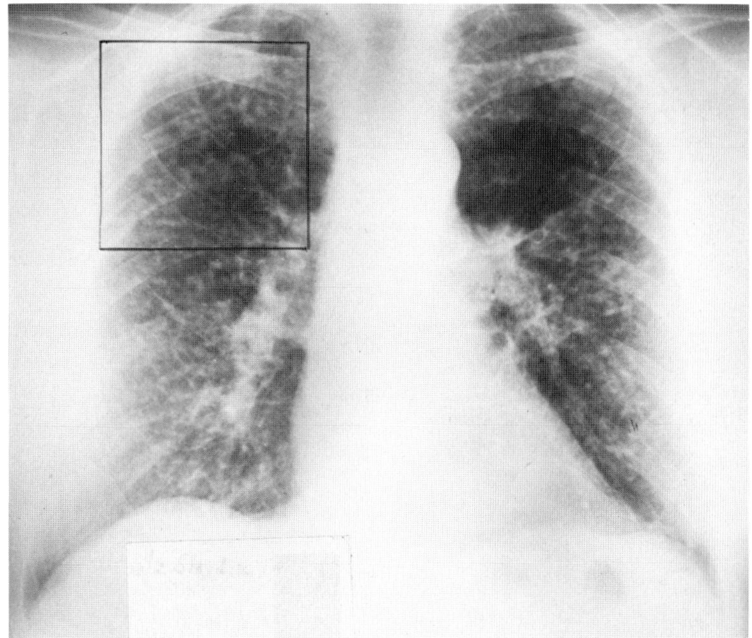

A

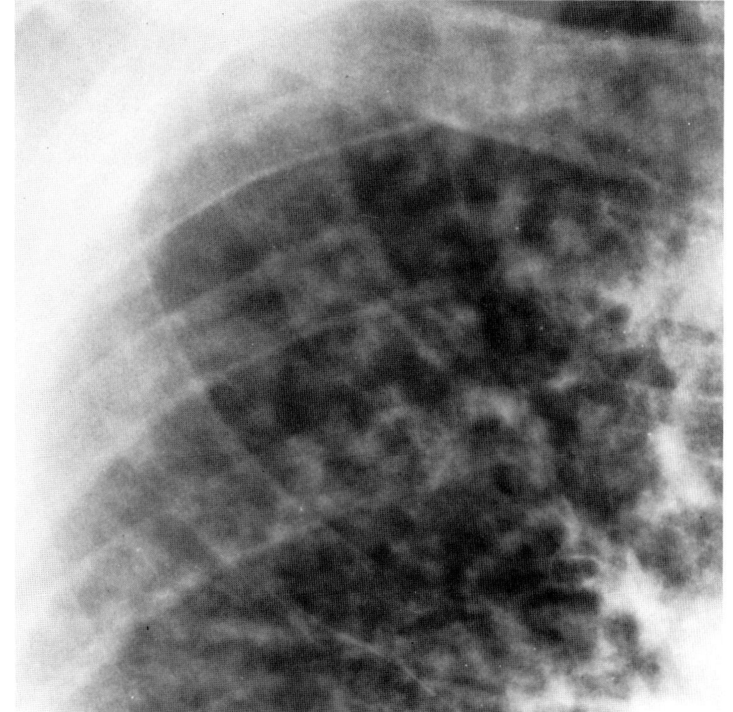

B

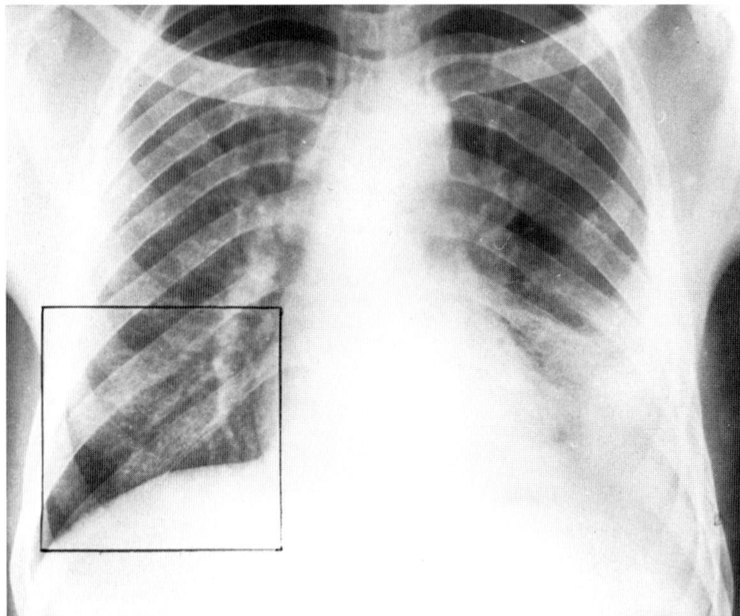

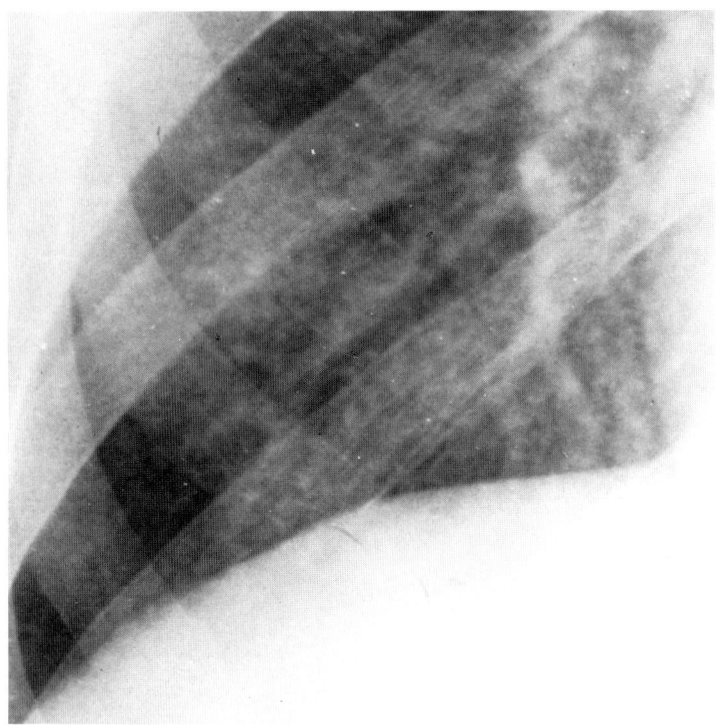

Figure 2.10. Basally disposed irregular opacities and irregular nodules with a width up to 1.5 mm, ie, 1/1 s/s.

Figure 2.11. Pronounced, irregular linear shadows and irregular nodules whose width does not exceed 1.5 mm, ie, 2/2 s/s.

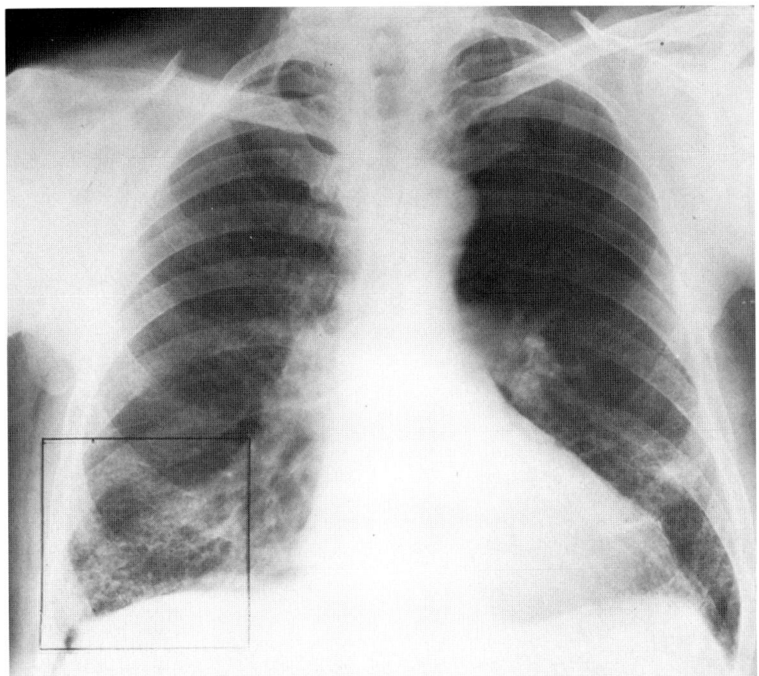

A

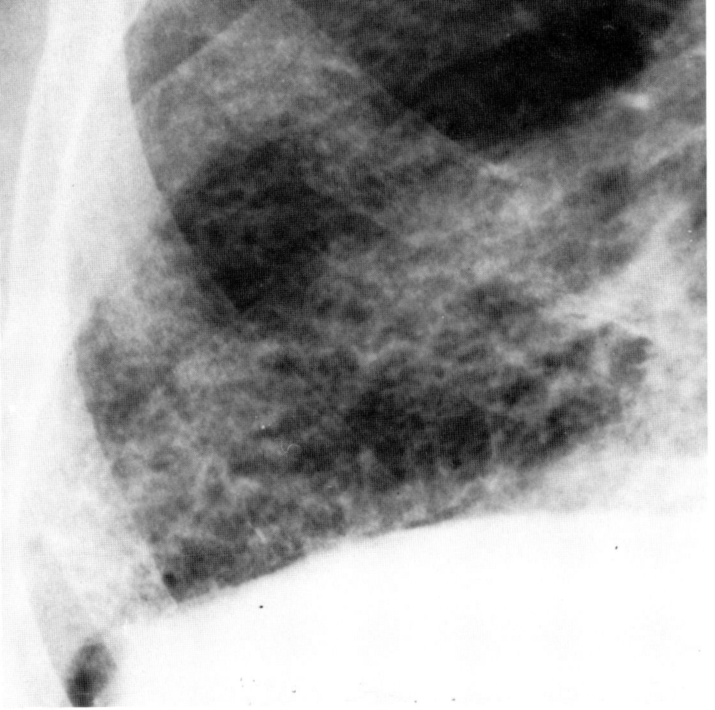

B

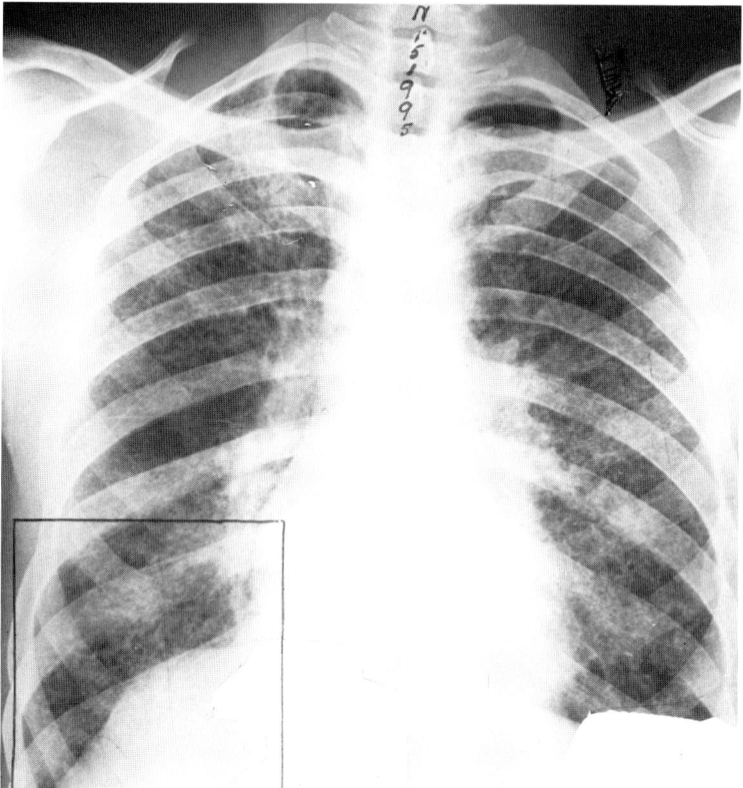

A

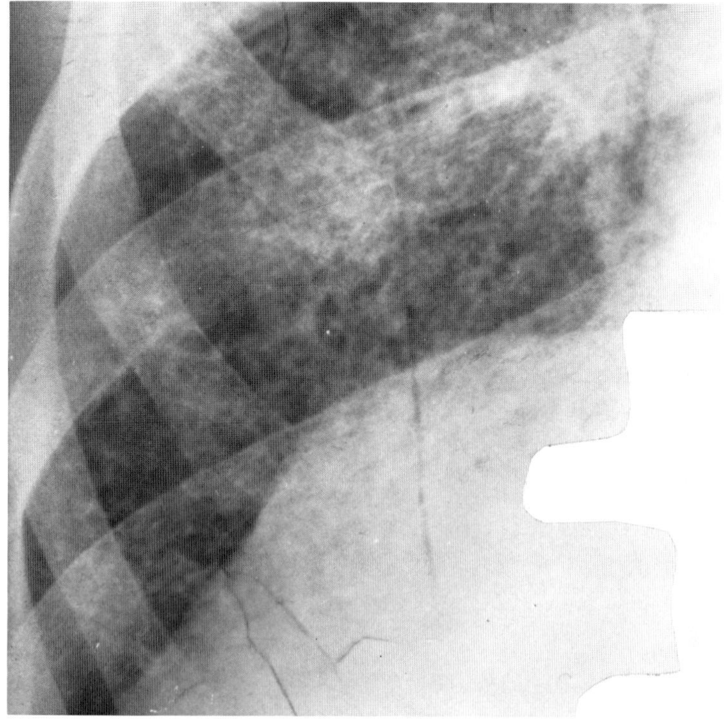

B

Figure 2.12. Extensive irregular linear nodules and lines not exceeding 1.5 mm in width, ie, 3/3 s/s.

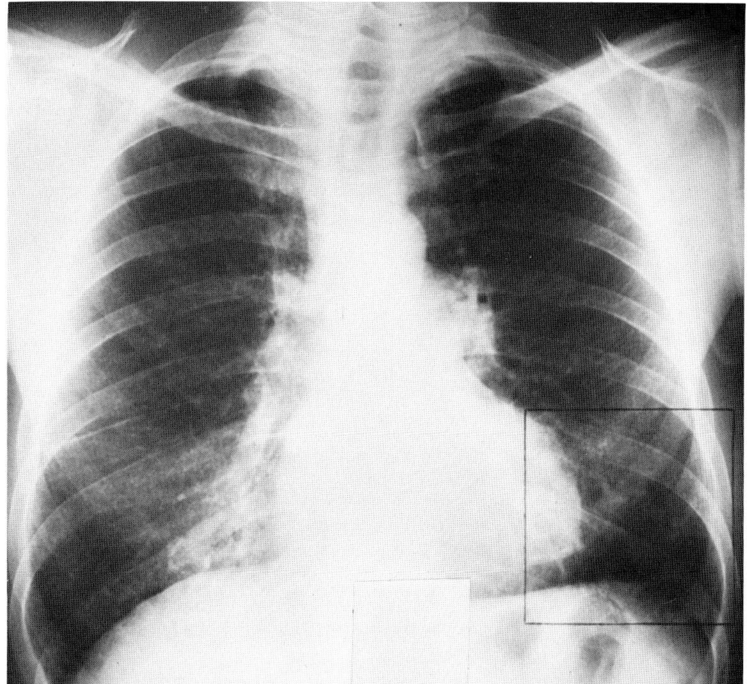

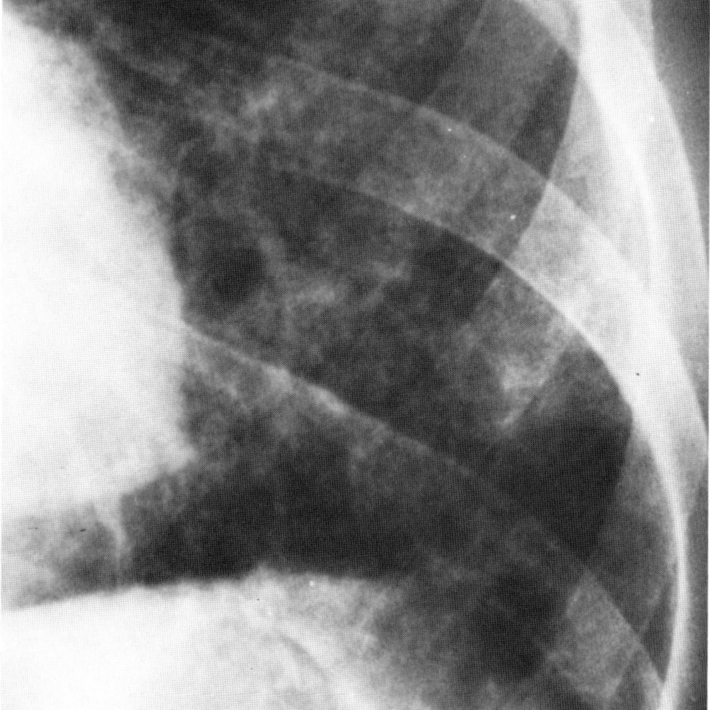

Figure 2.13. The basal irregular linear opacities and irregular nodules vary between 1.5 to 3.0 mm in size, ie, 1/0 t/t.

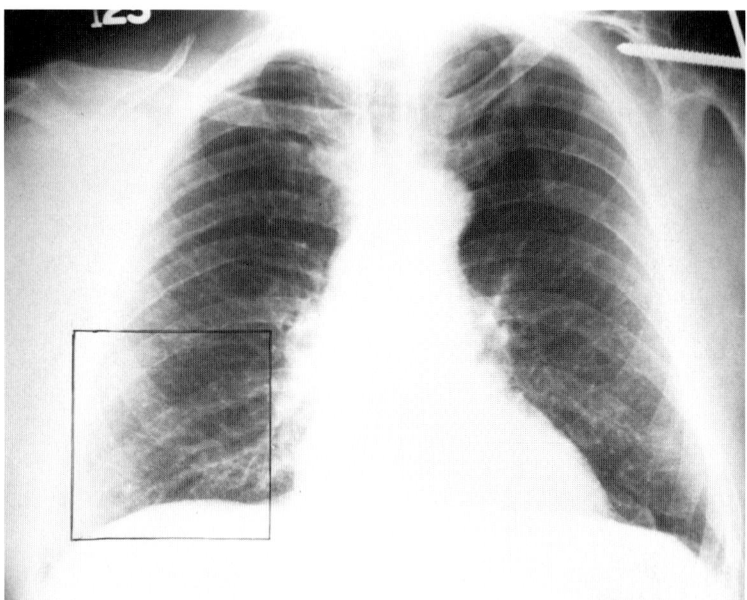

A

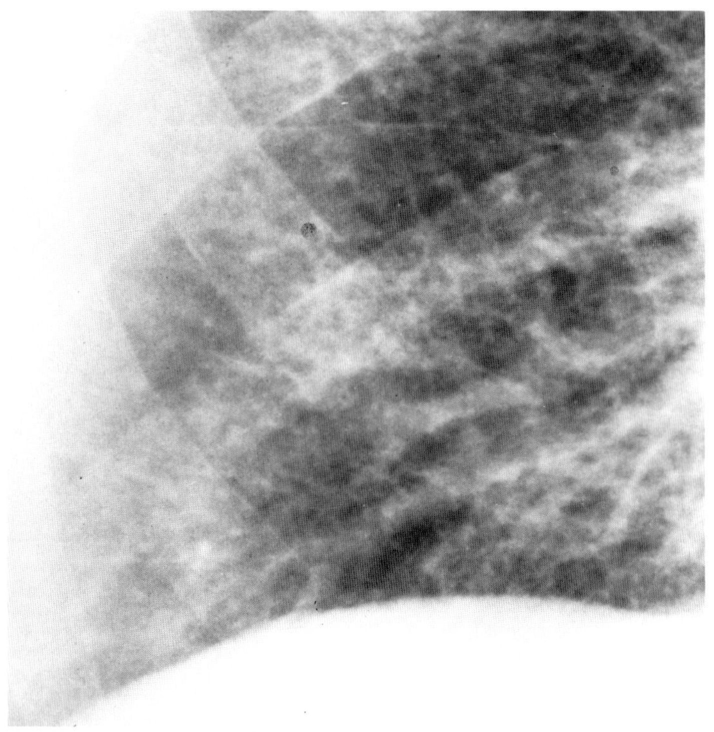

B

Figure 2.14. The irregular lines and nodules are between 1.5 to 3.0 mm in size and correspond to 1/1 t/t category.

Figure 2.15. Profuse basal and irregular linear shadows and irregular nodules with size varying between 1.5 to 3.0 mm, ie, 3/2 t/t.

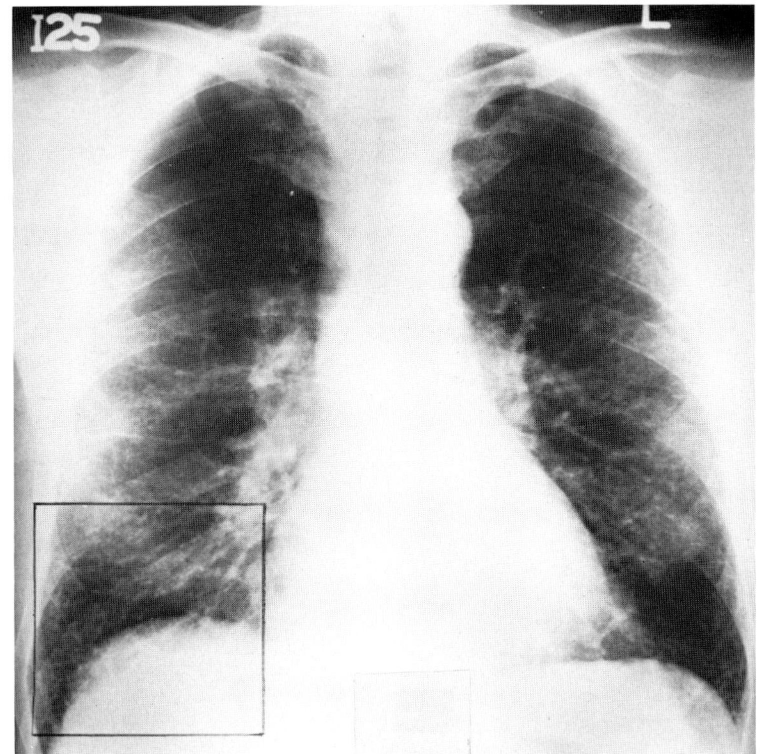

A

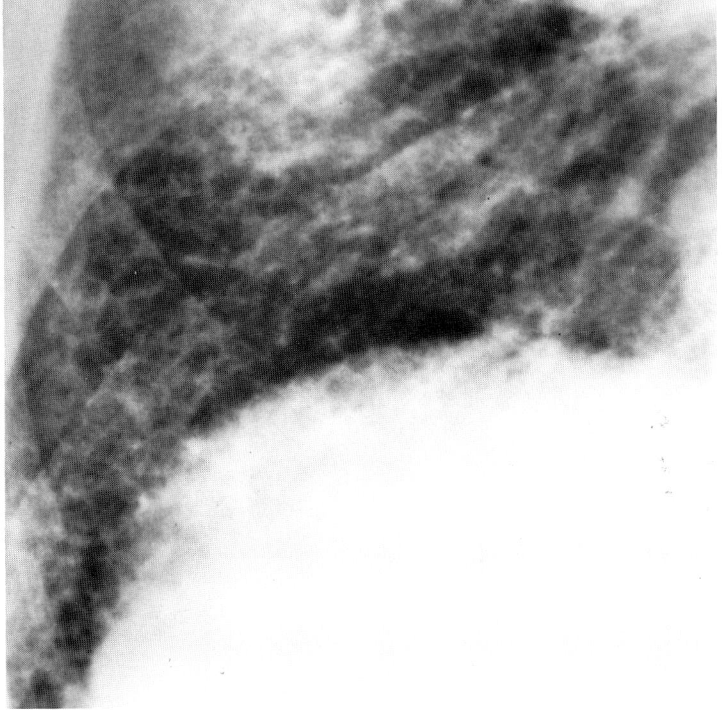

B

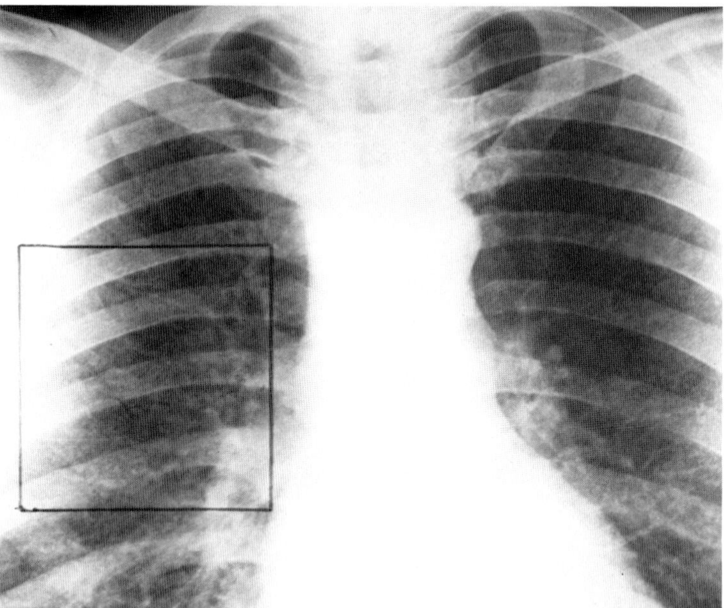

A

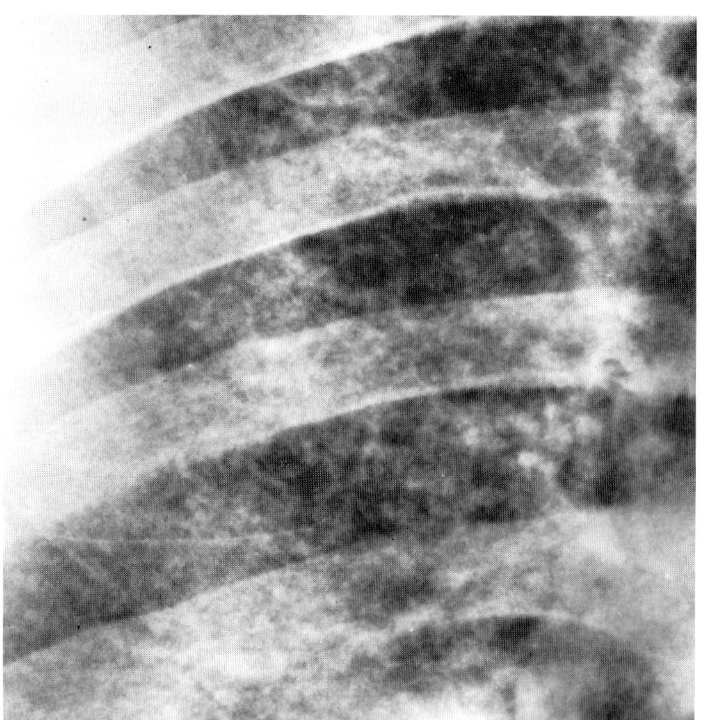

B

Figure 2.16. Pronounced, well-defined nodules of mixed sizes (below 1.5 mm and up to 3.0 mm), ie, 2/3 p/q.

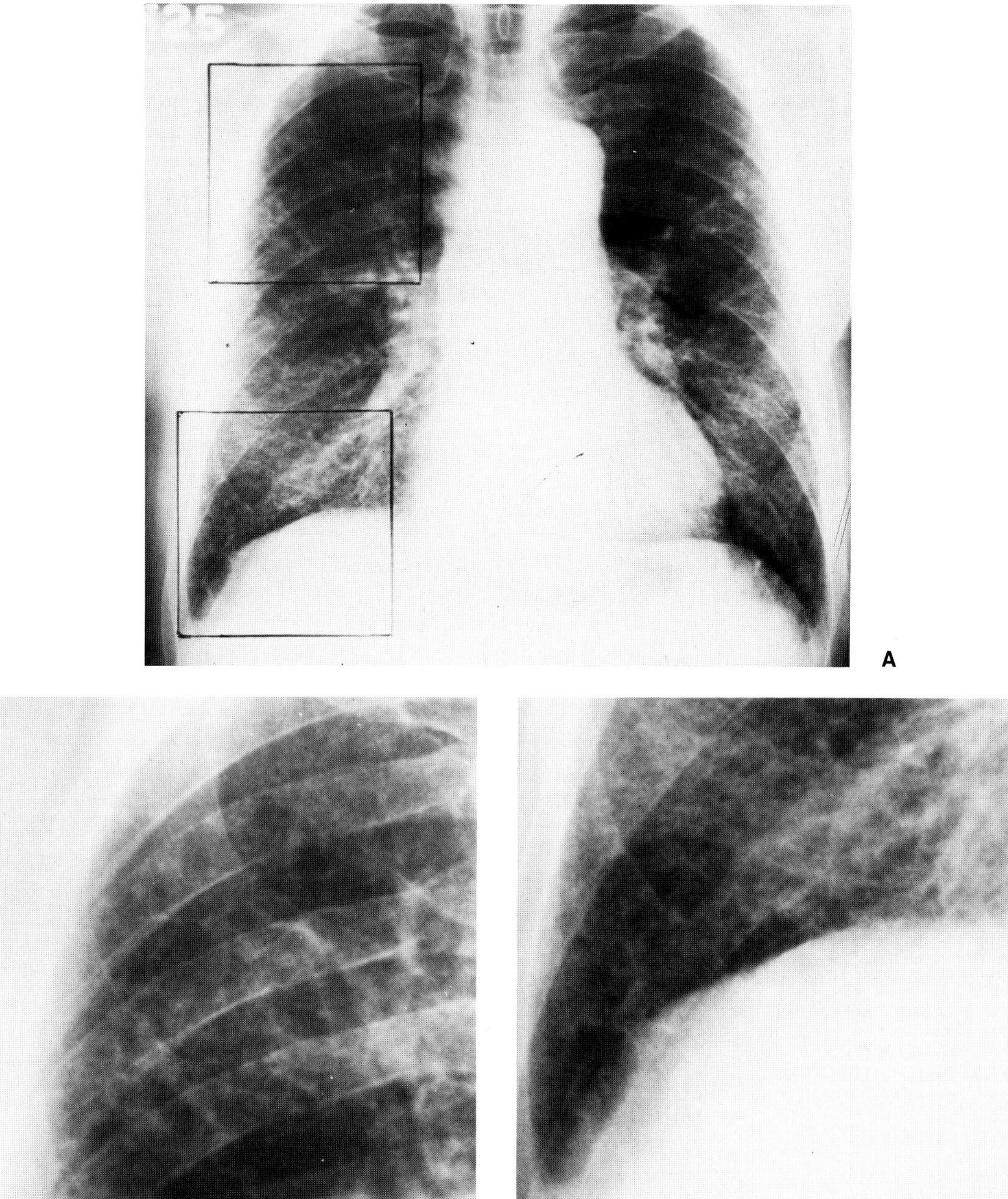

Figure 2.17. The lesions in the upper zone are between 1.5- and 3.0-mm well-defined opacities, whereas in the lower zone the more pronounced irregular opacities are 1.5 to 3.0 mm, ie, 2/2 t/q. Insets B and C are reduced in size.

Pleural Abnormalities

Site, width, and extent of pleural thickening are recorded separately.

Pleural Thickening

Chest Wall. Types, circumscribed or diffuse; site, left or right chest wall or both; width, this can only be measured along the lateral chest wall and is the maximum width from the inner line of the chest wall to the inner margin of the clear-cut parenchymal-pleural boundary. Pleural thickening seen face-on is recorded as present even if it is *also* seen in profile. Width *cannot* be measured when only face-on plaque or diffuse area of pleural thickening is seen. a = maximum width up to 5 mm; b = maximum width between 5 and 10 mm; and c = maximum width over 10 mm.

Extent is defined by maximum length of pleural involvement, or as the sum of maximum lengths, whether seen in profile or face-on, or both:

1 = Total length equivalent to up to one quarter of one lateral chest wall.
2 = Total length exceeding one quarter but not one half of the projection of the lateral chest wall (Fig. 2.18).
3 = Total length exceeding one half of the projection of the lateral chest wall.

As the lateral chest wall length varies considerably not only with patient size, but with thoracic cage configuration, body habitus, and inspiratory diaphragm position, these recordings of extent are specific to the particular x-ray of the chest and are not absolute measurements.

Diaphragm. A hyaline plaque or pleural thickening involving the diaphragm is recorded separately as present or absent, left or right.

Costophrenic Angle Obliteration. The lower limit of pleural thickening across the costophrenic angle that should be recorded is defined by the 1980 Standard Radiograph (radiograph "1/1 t/t"). Costophrenic angle thickening is recorded separately from any other form of pleural thickening and is noted to be either present or absent, and right or left sided, or both. If the thickening extends above the angle onto the lateral chest wall, this is separately recorded under "chest wall."

Costophrenic angle loss is an extremely common nondust-related finding, hence the separate reading. The diaphragmatic muscle digitations are a common cause of blunting or obliteration of the angle in a man who breathes particularly deeply and should not be confused with abnormality.

Pleural Calcification

Site and extent are recorded separately for the two lungs.

Site. Chest wall, right or left; diaphragm, right or left (Fig. 2.19); other includes pericardial and mediastinal pleura.

Extent. This is defined as follows:

1 = An area of calcified pleura with greatest diameter up to 20 mm or a number of areas the sum of whose greatest diameter does not exceed 20 mm.
2 = An area of calcified pleura with greatest diameter exceeds 20 mm and up to 100 mm, or a number of such areas, the sum of whose greatest diameters exceeds 20 mm but not above 100 mm.
3 = An area of calcified pleura with greatest diameter exceeding 100 mm or a number of such areas whose sum of greatest diameters exceeds 100 mm.

The measured length in pleural calcification takes precedence over the examples in the Standard Radiographs.

Asbestos calcification is usually bilateral and is linear when seen end-on or "geographic" and map-like when seen face-on. Extensive unilateral calcification is more likely to follow old hemothorax, empyema, or tuberculosis than asbestos exposure.

Figure 2.18. The basal irregular nodules and lines are up to 1.5 mm in width, ie, 2/2 s/s. The bilateral pleural thickening is of a "b" width (ie, between 5 and 10 mm). The extent of the pleural change exceeds one quarter but is not more than half of the lateral chest-wall projection (ie, extent 2).

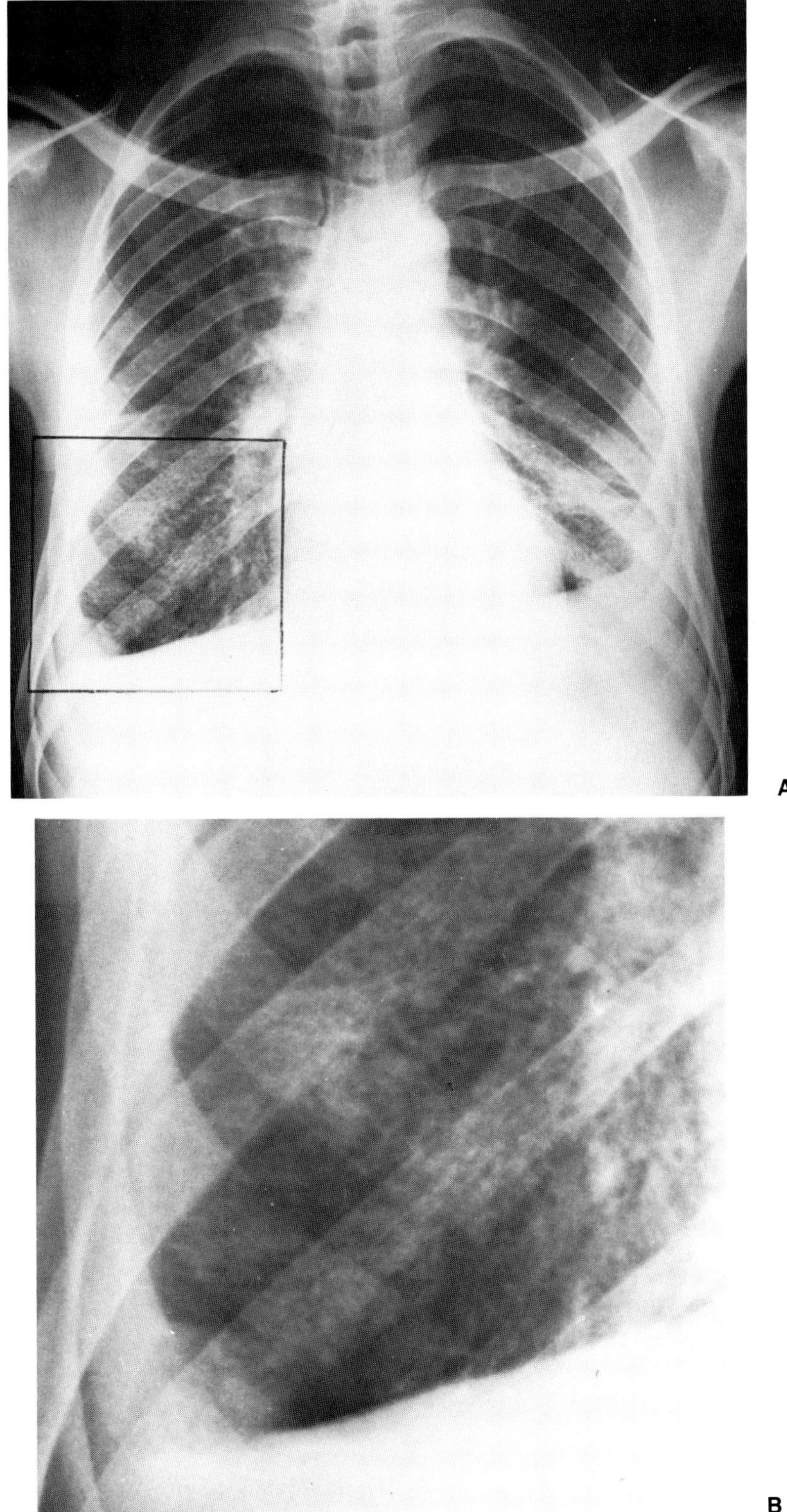

Figure 2.18

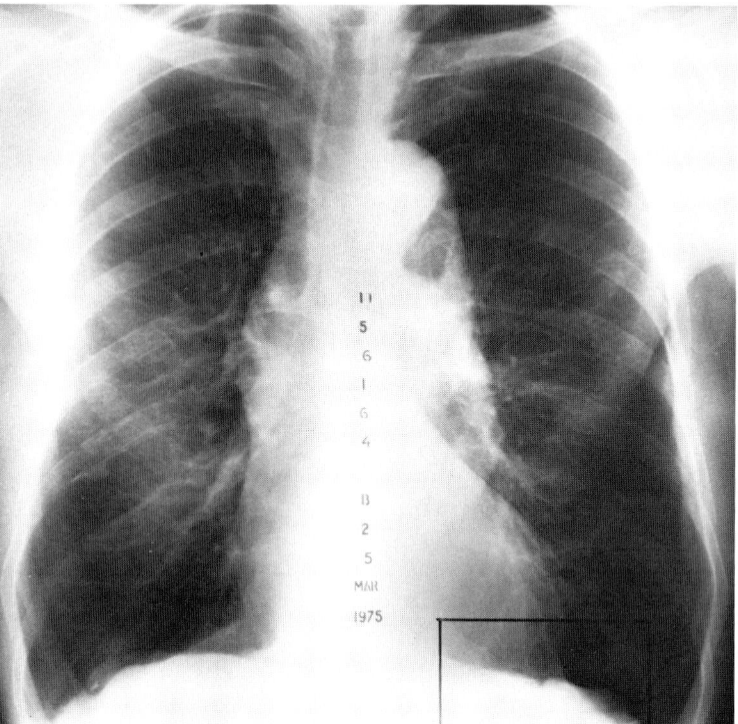

A

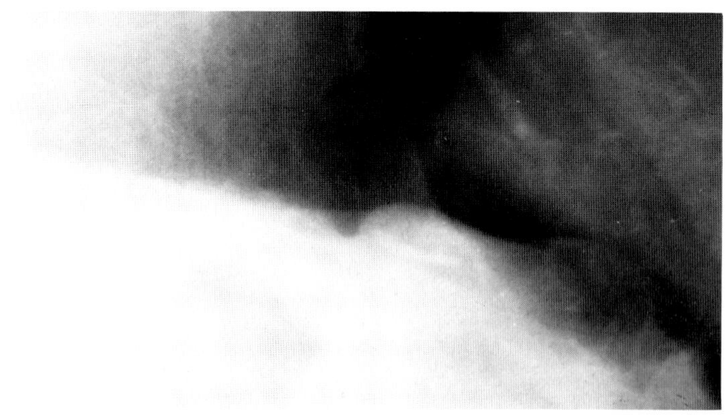

B

Figure 2.19. The left-sided diaphragm has a well-circumscribed calcified pleural plaque present.

Symbols

The use of symbols is obligatory. Noting the symbol as present makes the assumption that the words "suspect," "changes suggestive of," and the like precede the condition indicated by the symbol. The use of the symbol accordingly does *not* indicate an unequivocal positive diagnosis of the condition.

ax = coalition of small pneumoconiotic opacities
bu = bulla(c)
ca = cancer of lung or pleura
cn = calcification in small pneumoconiotic opacities
co = abnormality of cardiac size or shape
cp = cor pulmonale
cv = cavity
di = marked distortion of intrathoracic organs
ef = effusion
em = emphysema
es = eggshell calcification of hilar or mediastinal lymph nodes
fr = fractured rib(s)

hi = enlargement of hilar or mediastinal lymph nodes
ho = honeycomb lung
id = ill-defined diaphragm if more then one third of one hemidiaphragm
ih = ill-defined heart outline if a length of more than one third of left heart border
kl = septal (Kerley) lines
od = other significant abnormality
pi = pleural thickening in the interlobar fissure or mediastinum
px = pneumothorax
rp = rheumatoid pneumoconiosis (Caplan's syndrome)
tb = tuberculosis
Y/N = yes/no

The calcified primary complex of tuberculosis or other granulomatous processes such as coccidiodomycosis or histoplasmosis should not be coded under "tb." Such appearances should be noted under "Comments."

Comments

Comments pertaining to the classification of the radiograph should be recorded, particularly if some other cause is thought to be responsible for a shadow that could be thought by others to be due to pneumoconiosis, and for identifying radiographs where the technical quality may have affected the reading materially.

The details of the short classification are the same as the complete classification, but with simplification.

Technical Quality. Recorded 1, 2, 3, and 4, as for the complete classification.

Normal Parenchyma. Recorded as 0 profusion.

Abnormal Parenchyma. Small opacities: Profusion is recorded as 1, 2, and 3, by comparison with the standard radiographs. Shape and size are recorded by comparison with the Standard Radiographs: Rounded, p, q, r; irregular, s, t, and u, as for the complete classification, including combinations when appropriate. *Large opacities*: Categories A, B, and C, as for complete classification.

Pleural Abnormality. Pleural thickening, symbol pt; pleural calcification, pc.

Symbols. As for the complete classification, together with pt, pc as above. The use of symbols is obligatory.

Comments. They should be recorded as for the complete classification.

Experience With Use of the Classification

We use a modified short classification. In addition to the use of 0, 1, 2, and 3, we have added 0/1 and 1/0 with a clear line of division between the two. A reader has therefore to make up his/her mind: "I have considered category 1/0 profusion—minimally but definitely positive x-ray signs but have rejected it—record 0/1" or "this is minimally positive—record as 1/0 profusion." The "symbols" have also been modified for local use, eg, od—"other significant abnormality"—must *always be defined.*

Profusion grades are defined by comparison with the standard films, and a good rule of thumb for day-to-day use is to think of 0 = absent, 1 = mild, 2 = moderate, and 3 = severe degrees of profusion.

The classification instructs one to record as p, q, r, s, t, and u any instance that could be pneumoconiosis and to record in the comment any cases where other conditions are causing the appearances. The most important correlative feature in the use of the classification is the history of dust exposure.

Unexposed populations may have positive ILO classification features, some due to other disease, but a good proportion being idiopathic in otherwise clinically fit individuals in whom one would be reluctant to recommend lung biopsy.[3] In a study of chest radiographs of hospital admissions, Epstein et al found that 18% of 200 patients had category 1/0 or higher profusion of opacities, and included in this number were 22 cases (11%) with neither a history of dust exposure nor a medical condition that could cause opacities.[3]

In the dust exposed person many conditions can masquerade as pneumoconiosis[4] and the recording of an appropriate positive ILO reading should not lead one to ignore the possibility that the individual may be suffering from another disease requiring elucidation and treatment. Vigilance should be especially directed to those cases with symptomatology inappropriate to the radiograph, or atypical presentation such as very rapid development of nodules or opacities in unusual situation, such as, for example, predominantly basal category r nodules.

Some misconceptions regarding the classification have been published. In a paper discussing the use of the ILO classification to describe diffuse interstitial lung disease,[5] the authors state, "However the 1980 classification intends that p/s should mean p and s in different locations with p predominating. . . ." This is, of course, incorrect. The classification makes no distinction as to whether opacities are in the same or different areas of the lung. In practical use, for example, r/q usually indicates nodules of both sizes in the same area, usually the upper halves of the chest, while t/q, for example, would most frequently represent basal "t" shadowing due to asbestosis, with the "q" nodules in typical situation, ie, predominating in the upper lungs.

We have found the 1980 classification to be a significant improvement on the 1970 version and, used intelligently, an excellent system of recording and communication.

The Standard Radiographs have improved, but there are still deficiencies, and we substitute local examples when we believe they are better or more clearly representative of the intended profusion and type of opacities.

A recent test of using the ILO classification to compare the reading results of digitized chest radiographs with the original radiographs revealed that even though performance and observer variation were considered adequate, the readers themselves still preferred the simplicity of the viewing box.[6]

References

1. Guidelines for the use of ILO International Classification of Radiographs of Pneumoconioses. Revised edition 1980. Occupational Safety and Health Series No 22 (Rev) International Labour Office, Geneva.
2. Irwin LM, du Toit RSJ, Sluis-Cremer GK, et al: Risk of asbestosis in crocidolite and amosite mines in South Africa, in Selikoff IJ, Hammond EC (eds): Health Hazard of Asbestos Exposure. Ann NY Acad Sci 1979;330:35–79.
3. Epstein PM, Miller WT, Bresnitz EA, et al: Application of ILO classification to a population without industrial exposure: Findings to be differentiated from pneumonconiosis. Am J Roentgenol 1984;142: 53–58.
4. Pendergrass EP, Kainhart WS, Bristol LJ, et al: Roentgenological patterns in lung changes that simulate those found in coal worker's pneumoconiosis. Ann NY Acad Sci 1972;200:494–501.
5. McLoud TC, Carrington CB, Gaensler EA: Diffuse infiltrative lung disease: A new scheme for description. Radiology 1983;149:353–363.
6. Kundel HL, Mezrich JL, Brickman I, et al: Digital chest imaging: comparison of two film image digitizers with a classification task. Radiology 1987; 165:747–752.

3

Clinical and Functional Aspects of Occupational Chest Diseases

Jeffrey A. Golden and Gerald L. Baum

Introduction

Identifying, characterizing, and quantifying occupational lung disease based largely on radiographic evidence has logically been a priority, but clearly the toxic or allergic factor must be defined as well as the resulting impairment of lung function following dust inhalation. It is the intent of this chapter to define the clinical characteristics of these diseases and to describe the physiological consequences of inhaling the noxious materials.

There are some important points common to all forms of occupational lung disease. First, there is, in general, a linear relationship between the likelihood of developing a pulmonary reaction to contact with a toxic substance and the length of time that contact was maintained. Second, there appears to be a minimum concentration of the materials below which no disease would result despite prolonged contact; that concept, however, is currently under serious scrutiny since there is evidence, at least in the case of asbestos-related disease, that there may be no safe level of exposure. Third, personal factors, most not identified, appear to determine the likelihood of development of disease after exposure to almost all of the agents discussed in this book. Last, it is essential to sample the air of the workplace and determine with accuracy the levels of dust to which the worker is exposed and how consistently these levels are found. In addition, the physical characteristics of the workplace, including temperature, humidity, ventilation, and general cleanliness, are important factors that must be carefully documented.

The importance of a careful clinical and occupational history cannot be overemphasized. A meticulous radiographic technique is required together with the clinical history emphasizing chronological order of symptoms, associated illnesses, and factors tending to modify pulmonary symptoms. The details, in finicky completeness, of environmental exposure to all manner of dusts and noxious substances, including those encountered at the worksite and at other locales where the patient has lived, are also of critical importance.

The clinical history has traditionally been obtained directly from the patient by the physician. In the recent past, however, epidemiologists have begun to study environmental diseases and have evolved a questionnaire approach to obtaining data. Although this appears to be less desirable than the personal encounter with a physician, experience has shown that a well-constructed questionnaire administered by a person trained in its use (not necessarily a physician) obtains very nearly the same data, and perhaps even more, than the physician-patient interview. Without considering in detail the relative merits of an individual case, the questionnaire is the only practical way of obtaining the necessary information to evaluate environmental risk factors and the occurrence of industrial disease.

Physical examination and routine laboratory testing are of lesser importance because their results are relatively nonspecific, but the abnormalities should be documented even though these studies do not give us critical diagnostic information. However, pulmonary function studies have become crucial in assessing the functional impact of past exposure to noxious substances and/or abnormal findings on chest radiography. The chest radiograph and, to a lesser extent, history of symptoms were until the 1950s the main data used by industrial commissions around the world. Since then, pulmonary function studies have played a more and more important role, even though many governmental agencies have been slow to recognize their importance.

Cigarette smoking is an important cofactor in the pathogenesis of certain diseases resulting from exposure to occupational dusts. In particular, the relationship between smoking among asbestos workers and the development of lung cancer is dramatic. A direct relationship between smoking and the development of pulmonary fibrosis has not been shown, but there is a higher morbidity in cigarette smokers from acute respiratory infections than in workers exposed to a variety of industrial dusts. This finding comes as no surprise since the adverse effect of tobacco smoke in inhibiting clearance from both upper and lower respiratory tracts is well known.

The association of chronic obstructive airways disease with industrial exposure to dusts on the one hand, and with cigarette smoking on the other, is well documented. In asbestos exposure chronic bronchitis appears to be more common (certainly bouts of acute bronchitis are), but whether silicosis and coal workers' pneumoconiosis are associated with obstructive lung diseases is still an open question. Tobacco smoke must seriously augment the suspected susceptibility of dust-exposed workers to obstructive lung disease.

Before discussing significant clinical findings and physiological abnormalities in specific diseases, contamination of the home environment must be mentioned. The families of workers can be exposed to dusts adhering to shoes, clothes, and hair, especially from working clothes brought home for laundering. Furthermore, urban areas can have 10 to 1,000 times the concentration of asbestos fibers in the air compared with the countryside because of fibers being freed into the environment during manufacture, construction, or demolition.

Asbestos-Related Pulmonary Disease

The radiological manifestation are detailed in Chapter 4.

Asbestos is a family of naturally occurring silicate fibers, including amosite, chrysotile, and crocidolite, with an insulating capacity of tremendous industrial and commercial value. The inimical effects of asbestos exposure result from the inhalation of these fibers, leading to a variety of pulmonary sequelae such as asbestosis (interstitial fibrosis), benign pleural processes (plaques, effusion, and diffuse fibrosis), as well as mesothelioma and bronchogenic carcinoma. These potential sequelae of asbestos exposure are dose related where dose is calculated in terms of the number of fibers in lung tissue rather than exposure history. However, other factors are also important, such as individual host susceptibility, as well as coexposures such as cigarette consumption in the case of bronchogenic carcinoma.[1] In evaluating a patient for the presence of a possible asbestos-related sequelae, it is important to obtain a precise occupational history including details of summer employment, even in the very remote past, as well as possible neighborhood and household exposure.

Asbestosis

The only pneumoconiosis consequent to asbestos exposure is asbestosis, defined as fibrosis of the lung parenchyma due to inhalation of fibers, and in such terms lung cancer and disease of the pleura are not pneumoconioses.[2] Asbestosis or interstitial fibrosis was the earliest noted asbestos-related disease; Cook described a female textile worker with asbestosis in 1927.[3] The clinical presentation of asbestosis is nonspecific and similar to any diffuse peripheral disease of the lung parenchyma. The most common presenting symptom is shortness of breath. Initially, dyspnea occurs only with exertion, but with time patients complain of shortness of breath even at rest, which is often described as an inability to "get anough air" and not as fatigue or weakness. A nonproductive cough is often present, but wheezing is not a feature. Rapid shallow breaths are observed on physical examination, and on auscultation, dry and "velcro" rales are heard. Initially such rales are heard only in mid or late inspiration, but with time, as the process progresses, they are heard throughout inspiration. Dry respiratory rales are generated in fibrotic lungs with the opening of closed airways. In some patients such rales can only be detected after a cough at low lung volumes, which closes peripheral airways, so with reopening on a subsequent inspiration, dry rales become more apparent. Finding inspiratory rales, however, is not specific for asbestosis. In a study by Epler et al, patients with significant interstitial disease often had no rales.[4] Finger clubbing is nonspecific for asbestosis, it is not a universal finding in patients with asbestosis,[5] and its presence does not parallel the radiographic severity of asbestosis.[6]

Routine laboratory data are nonspecific, including high titers of antinuclear antibody or rheumatoid factor. Although there is a dose-exposure relationship for mild and moderate asbestosis, the progression from moderate severe disease does not relate to the number of asbestos fibers found in the lung.[1,7] Host factors or susceptibility seem important, including the development of positive high titers to antinuclear antibody (ANA), positive rheumatoid factor, abnormal number and function of peripheral blood lymphocytes, and perhaps genetic factors like the presence of human lymphocyte antigen.[8,9]

Asbestosis produces restrictive lung disease by causing small or restricted lung volumes. In addition to decreased lung volumes, like other peripheral infiltrative lesions, asbetosis results in preserved or increased flow rates, but causes a low diffusing capacity for carbon monoxide (D_{LCO}).

Whether asbestosis can cause obstructive lung disease is not settled. Many asbestos-exposed workers are cigarette smokers. Most studies purporting to show airflow obstruction were done in asbestos workers who also smoked.[10,11] When an asbestos-exposed population is compared with a nonexposed population, and the factor of cigarette smoking is controlled, there is no evidence that asbestos-exposed populations have excess airway obstruction.[12]

Animal experiments have shown asbestosis to involve small peripheral airways where the pulmonary macrophages first contact inhaled asbestos fibers.[13] Further, in recent sheep experiments the peribronchial mononuclear alveolitis resulting from inhalation of asbestos fibers caused compression of small peripheral airways.[14] Such small airway disease has been described in other interstitial lung disease.[15-17] However, flow is determined by *both* airway geometry and elastic recoil of the lungs; asbestos is associated with noncompliant or stiff lungs with increased elastic recoil, as is the case for any infiltrative lung disease.[18] In a study of asbestos workers who had never smoked cigarettes and consequently were free of peripheral airway disease due to smoking, flow rates were maintained.[19]

The D_{LCO} in asbestosis may be decreased by virtue of reduction in lung volume and consequently in the surface area of the alveolar capillary membrane, rather than to decrease in the membrane permeability itself.[1,20] In asbestosis patients the diffusing capacity correlated with lung histology better than any other measure of pulmonary function.[21] In serial studies of pulmonary function among patients with asbestosis, the fall in the D_{LCO} often preceded any significant decline in the vital capacity.[1]

It should be emphasized that studies of pulmonary function may be only slightly abnormal, if at all, despite significant asbestosis.[21] Just as patients early in their course complain of dyspnea only with exercise, pulmonary function may be abnormal only after exercise. The abnormalities on exercise testing in interstitial lung disease include an abnormal pattern of ventilation and abnormal gas exchange.[22] Ventilation for each level of exercise is increased above normal by an abnormal increase in respiratory rate due to the small lung volumes. The abnormal gas exchange results in hypoxemia or, more precisely, an increasing alveolar/arterial oxygen difference with increasing exercise load. The increased alveolar/arterial oxygen difference with exercise was the one physiologic measurement that correlated best with histology in interstitial lung disease; furthermore, significant physiologic abnormalities on exercise can occur with a normal chest roentgenogram.[23]

In clinical practice the degree of lung impairment "cannot be predicted reliably from symptoms (at rest), pulmonary physiology, or radiographic changes. It should therefore be evaluated by appropriate exercise tests."[1]

Benign Pleural Effusion

Asbestos can cause benign pleural effusions and according to Epler et al, 9% of heavily exposed asbestos workers will develop effusions[24]; 50% of asbestos effusions are asymptomatic. Acute onset of pleuritic pain with systemic manifestations such as fever, malaise, and leukocytosis may occur or there may be only chronic pleural pain. Asbestos-induced effusions can be unilateral or bilateral, first on one side and then the other, occurring soon after exposure or in less than 5 years, or as long as 6 to 15 and even 40 years after the first asbestos exposure.[25]

Physical examination reveals dullness to percussion and decreased breath sounds on the involved side(s). Effusions of 500 to 1,500 mL have been noted. The fluid is exudative and may be serosanguinous or frankly bloody. Physiologically such effusions cause decreased lung volumes.

Gaensler and Kaplan's patients with benign effusions frequently had biopsy-proved asbestosis as well.[26] Virtually all of Hillerdal's 22 patients, however, were symptom free and without pulmonary impairment on resorption of the fluid. Interstitial fibrosis was not present in his series of patients with asbestos-induced benign pleural effusion.[25]

Pleural Plaques

These are usually an incidental finding on a routine chest radiograph in an asymptomatic patient. In workers with more than 40 years since their first exposure to asbestos, 58% had calcified pleural plaques. Even household contacts of such workers developed plaques.[27] Plaques reflect prior asbestos exposure. A worker with pleural plaques does not have an increased risk of developing more significant asbestos-related problems than a similar exposed worker without pleural plaques.[1]

Thickened Pleura

One other benign pleural process that may result in pulmonary impairment is diffuse pleural thickening. In contradistinction to pleural plaques, diffuse pleural thickening is associated with adhesion between visceral and parietal pleural surfaces. Because nearly all asbestos-related benign pleural effusions are exudative and resolve with blunting of the costophrenic angle, Epler et al suggested that diffuse pleural thickening is a sequela of prior benign asbestos pleural effusion(s). Among their 35 patients with asbestos effusions, 54% had residual diffuse pleural thickening.[24]

The pleural thickening can be sufficiently diffuse to restrict the underlying lung, producing an "en cuirasse" effect with impairment and dyspnea. Wright et al described the consequent abnormality as a decrease in lung volume, but unlike parenchymal fibrosis or asbestosis, there is a preserved or even increased $D_{L_{CO}}$ when this value is corrected for lung volume.[28] The normal $D_{L_{CO}}$ as well as the normal parenchyma on computed tomographic (CT) scan indicated that normal lung was trapped, en cuirasse, causing small lung volumes.[28] There was wide variation in both severity of symptoms and time of development.[25,28] Miller et al described seven patients with severe dyspnea consequent to chest wall restriction caused by asbestos pleural fibrosis,[29] one of whom improved after decortication of the pleura. Autopsy on others showed minimal to no parenchymal fibrosis.

Asbestos-Related Lung Cancer and Other Tumors

The clinical presentation of asbestos lung cancer is no different from cancer unrelated to asbestos exposure. Asbestosis patients who present with hemoptysis should be evaluated for bronchogenic carcinoma independent of a smoking history. Although asbestos exposure plus cigarette smoking pose an extremely high risk of lung cancer, asbestos-exposed workers who do not smoke are also at increased risk of developing bronchogenic carcinoma (about 10 times) relative to nonasbestos-exposed workers.[30,31,31a] An estimated 15% of asbestos-exposed persons will develop bronchogenic carcinoma in 20 to 40 years following diagnosis of pneumoconiosis.[32]

The most frustrating asbestos-related malignancy is mesothelioma, which has an incidence of 1,000 times that expected in the general population and accounts for approximately 70% of all deaths in patients suffering from asbestos-related disease. On the basis of pulmonary asbestos fiber load, there is a dose-response relationship for the development of mesothelioma; but the culpable exposure may be extremely brief (less than 1 month) and very remote, more than 30 to 40 years following the first exposure to asbestos.[1] In addition, because these cancers arise from the pluripotential mesothelial cells of the pleura or peritoneum, the histology is often very difficult to interpret, especially when only a small amount of material is obtained by closed pleural biopsy. Open pleural biopsy that provides adequate tissue for diagnosis is associated with complication, including the development of tumor at the operative site. No therapy is effective. The course is downhill, culminating in death, usually within one year.[32]

The usual presentation of patients with mesothelioma is an insidious onset of chest pain, either dull and aching, or typically pleuritic, becoming constant and severe. Shortness of breath may develop as a consequence of the accumulation of pleural fluid. Mesthelioma has, however, been detected in asymptomatic patients on routine chest radiography.[33] In a study of 37 patients by Oels et al, a third of their patients presented without chest pain and half without dyspnea.[34] Large effusions were somewhat less frequently associated with pain than small effusions, 64% compared with 79%, but on initial presentation large effusions were more common, 56% compared with 16% in small effusions.[34] Pulmonary impairment rapidly develops as a result of the tendency of the tumor to spread along serosal surfaces encasing the lungs. Physical examination findings may be normal or, with the onset of chest pain, may demonstrate decreased breath sounds and dullness to percussion, with a smaller hemithorax on the involved side leading eventually to immobilization of the chest wall and the development of scoliosis.[35] Clubbing may develop.

The clinical presentation of mesothelioma is not unlike that for benign asbestos pleural effusions, including the development of pain, weight loss, and associated bloody pleural fluid. Two of Eisenstadt's four patients and one of Gaensler's 12 patients eventually developed mesothelioma, although none of Hillerdal's patients subsequently developed tumor.[25,26,36] It is currently not clear how many patients with recurrent benign asbestos pleural effusions subsequently developed mesothelioma or even if these two processes are related.

Peritoneal mesothelioma can also occur as a consequence of asbestos exposure producing a large mass of tissue, but is considerably less common than pleural mesothelioma.

Silicosis

Silicosis occurs only in workers exposed to silica particles of 2 to 5 μm in diameter. Physicians must, therefore, be aware of occupations associated with harmful silica exposure. Mining, sandblasting, foundry work, ceramic tile production, and the use of quartz fine dust (flour) are known high-risk occupations. Many others exist and must be identified by physicians dealing with such workers.

The clinical spectrum of silicosis includes a chronic form, an acute syndrome, and an intermediate or "accelerated" form. *The chronic or classic form* is generally asymptomatic. The development of radiographic changes takes on average 20 to 30 years and no functional abnormalities of the lung occur if there are only fine nodulations. Cough with phlegm is usually due to cigarette smoking, but if conglomerate fibrosis develops, mild restriction and moderate airway obstruction will occur together with dyspnea on exercise. In both simple nodular and conglomerate silicosis, recurrent upper respiratory tract infections are more frequent than in normal nonexposed individuals.[37,38]

Acute silicosis may develop within 6 months of the onset of massive silica exposure, and progression may be seen within 4 to 5 years.[37] The usual exposure time is 3 to 6 years. This remarkable clinical picture is associated with pathological changes of alveolar proteinosis and death is inevitable owing to a lack of effective treatment. In Buechner and Ansari's review, death occurred 77 to 455 days from the onset of symptoms.[39,40] The main symptom is dyspnea, which is sudden in onset and progresses rapidly to physical incapacity. In addition, cough, fatigue, fever, weight loss, and pleuritic chest pain are noted. Sandblasters who work indoors and laborers dealing with quartz flour are particularly at risk.

The picture of *accelerated silicosis* is characterized by the development of conglomerate masses within 6 years or less of exposure, long before this occurs in the classic case of silicosis.[37] Pulmonary symptoms in such patients are minimal until the conglomerate phase, then the clinical picture is as described above. Pulmonary function tests reveal minimal decrease in forced vital capacity (FVC) and forced expiratory volume in one second (FEV_1) as compared with a control group.[40] The more rapid development of the late stage of silicosis is probably due to exposure to small particles of silica, 2.3 to 5.2 μm, in high concentration. Exact definition of length of exposure and other physical and environmental factors leading to this pattern are not known.

Silica workers have been noted to have a high prevalence of ANA in their serum, which appears to relate directly to the severity of changes on the chest radiograph.[38] Jones et al reported that 44% of 39 silica sandblasters had positive ANA titers and that the ANA-positive subjects all had pulmonary function abnormalities.[39] There appears to be an increased prevalence of scleroderma in silicosis patients and a decreased prevalence of lung cancer.[38]

The pathology of this disease characteristically consists of nodules varying in size from 5 to 10 μm to several centimeters. Microscopically these nodules are mainly whorled collagen with occasional macrophages containing foreign particles. Necrosis is rare. In acute silicosis a picture of alveolar proteinosis may occur.[40] The polarizing microscope reveals double refractile crystals in affected tissue.

Tuberculosis has been a serious complication of silicosis, the association having been recognized in the 19th century. Previously all conglomerate silicosis was considered due to tuberculosis, but this is no longer believed, although *Mycobacterium* infections are still an important complication. Until the 1950s when effective antituberculosis chemotherapy first became available, up to 20% of persons with silicosis were said to have died of tuberculosis or to have had active tuberculosis at death. In 1974 Bailey et al reported that 22 of 83 sandblasters with silicosis had mycobacterial complications, 10 due to *M tuberculosis*, 9 to *M kansasii*, and 3 to *M intracellulare*.[41] Silicosis is clearly identified as a risk factor for developing all forms of mycobacterial lung disease.[42,43] The mechanism of the relationship is not known. The work of Gross identified an adjuvant-like effect of tuberculoprotein upon the pathologic response to silica and a prolongation and exaggeration of the response to tuberculoprotein imposed by silica,[44] suggesting an immunologic relationship.

Tuberculosis must be suspected and sputum cultures performed in any silicosis patient whose clinical status suggests the possibility of active pulmonary tuberculosis, ie, weight loss, fever, night sweats, cough and sputum, hemoptysis, or whose chest radiograph shows progression, cavitation, or sudden change. A patient with appropriate clinical and/or radiographic evidence who has a positive skin test should be treated with a currently acceptable combination of antituberculosis drugs, even if sputum culture is negative.

In 1953 Caplan described single or multiple large pulmonary nodules in 51 miners. On further investigation, 90% had rheumatoid arthritis.[45] These necrotizing nodules with rheumatoid disease occur in patients with coal workers' pneumoconiosis and in patients with silicosis, but are uncommon regardless of the type of dust exposure. Chatgidakis and Theron found at autopsy one case among 576 gold miners in whom there were 11 with rheumatoid arthritis.[46] Except for arthritic symptoms, the progression of clinical and pulmonary function abnormalities is the same as that seen in silicosis without the rheumatoid diathesis.

Treatment of silicosis is preventive only. Reduction of the concentration of silica in the workers' environment by improving ventilation at the worksite and by enforcing the use of masks are essential. There is increasing public pressure to ensure safety at the worksite, and many industries are providing good work conditions. So-called "cottage industries" are a continuing problem in this regard. Active treatment is purely symptomatic.

Coal Workers' Pneumoconiosis

In the 1940s and 1950s controversy existed over whether or not exposure to coal dust could, of itself, without quartz or other silica exposure, produce fibrotic parenchymal lesions.[37,47] Recent treatises on pneumoconiosis state clearly that it can. At least 10 to 12 years of underground mine work are necessary to cause the characteristic early radiographic changes. Exposure to anthracite coal is more dangerous than exposure to bituminous coal, and work at the exposed coal surface in a mine, is the most dangerous form of occupational exposure.[47]

Clinically, early coal workers' pneumoconiosis (CWP) is symptomless. If chronic cough and sputum occur, it is almost always due to cigarette smoking. Physical examination findings are normal or unrelated to coal exposure, and pulmonary function test findings are also normal. Morgan has presented the case for a true coal-induced bronchitis in "coal-surface" miners that could be responsible for cough and sputum production.[48]

After prolonged exposure (more than 12 years), dyspnea on exertion may develop, clearly exaggerated by cigarette smoking. When the disease is advanced and radiographs show progressive massive fibrosis (PMF; areas 3 cm or greater in diameter) dyspnea, exaggerated by exercise, is a prominent symptom with severe disability in the later stages. Physical examination reveals signs of maldistribution of ventilation and may, if infection is present, demonstrate crackles, wheezes, and ronchi. In the late stages barrel-chest deformity and cor pulmonale may develop. Cor pulmonale is seen in 20% of all CWP patients encountered, but cyanosis and clubbing are rare.

The so-called coal macule is the basic pathological finding. This may be small, with a few surrounding lymphocytes and macrophages, or there may be collagen and reticulin fiber collections as well. The black pigment is striking. Focal areas of emphysema or PMF may be seen in adjacent tissues. Such areas are similar microscopically to the smaller macules, but necrosis may occur even in the absence of infection.

At an early stage pulmonary function studies may show exaggerated frequency dependence of dynamic compliance with a normal or increased static compliance; later, the static compliance decreases. Diffusion capacity of carbon monoxide is normal early and gradually decreases with progression of the disease. Slight hypoxia is noted in the late stage with an increased alveolar-arterial oxygen pressure difference.[37] The changes due to CWP are clearly restrictive in character. If airway obstruction is found, it is due to associated chronic bronchitis and is almost always related to cigarette smoking.

Patients with PMF present a special problem when the mass becomes necrotic, liquefies, and ruptures into a bronchus. Patients cough up black sputum (melanoptysis) in varying quantities (up to a cup or more per day), and this may cause a sudden fit of choking. In contrast to the large amount of jet-black sputum found in patients with PMF, long-time coal workers produce grey-to-black phlegm in small quantities for several years after prolonged exposure in a coal mine has ended.[47]

Treatment of CWP is preventive. Attempts must be made to reduce the amount of inhaled coal dust by miners through various means such as better ventilation and the use of better filters in masks; but a major effort must be directed against the use of cigarettes by miners. No effective treatment of the lung damage is known: only supportive care of symptomatic patients, especially those with cor pulmonale, is available.

Talc, Kaolin, and Bentonite Pneumoconioses

Among the fibrogenic silicates, talc is a recognized hazardous material. The persons at risk are those employed in the mining and milling of talc, infants who may accidentally inhale large quantities of talc contained in dusting powder and drug abusers who inject intravenously a powdered suspension of a tablet containing a combination of talc (used as a filler) and the drug to which they are addicted.[49,50] Apparently among millers and miners the minimum occupational exposure is 10 years, but at least 15 to 20 years is necessary before symptomatic disease develops.[49,51]

Symptoms develop insidiously and classically consist of cough, sputum, dyspnea, and wheezing.[52–54] In one survey, comparing talc miners and millers with potash workers, cough, sputum, dyspnea, and hemoptysis were seen more frequently in the talc workers. Once again cigarette smoking was a major related factor.[55] In another study, both symptoms and radiographic changes were noted more commonly with exposure to fibrous talc than exposure to granular talc.[54]

Pulmonary function abnormalities reflect the fibrotic nature of the parenchymal disease and include decreased FVC in more than half the cases with reduction in total lung capacity (TLC) and flow rates seen less frequently. The FEV/FVC ratio is modestly reduced and the residual volume (RV)/TLC relationship is modestly increased. Airway obstruction may well be related to smoking in these subjects and not to talc inhalation. In general, it appears that pulmonary function test (PFT) abnormalities are related to cumulative talc exposure.[49]

Another silicate, kaolin, used in the paper industry, has particularly been implicated in the development of fibrotic lung disease, but Parkes questions the role of kaolinite (main silicate in kaolin) in the development of lung disease, favoring contamination by quartz as the fibrogenic substance.[51] Dyspnea is the main symptom, and in advanced cases when PMF is present, it may become severe. The relationship between radiographic changes and PFT abnormalities as well as the clinical disability is similar to that of CWP. Yet bentonite, another substance suspected of causing fibrotic lung disease, is probably not fibrogenic; disease related to its use is most likely caused by silica contaminating the product.[51]

Berylliosis

Inhalation of beryllium produces both acute and chronic pulmonary responses. Acute berylliosis is a chemical pneumonitis usually resulting from an accidental inhalation of large amounts of beryllium. Fortunately, there have been no recorded cases of acute berylliosis in the United States since 1969.[56] A recent fatal case in Finland resulted from the demolition of fluorescent light bulbs containing beryllium, which were manufactured prior to 1960.[50] Symptoms occur 72 hours after the inhalation of large amounts of beryllium and include nonproductive cough, dyspnea, bronchitis with blood-streaked sputum, retrosternal pain, and conjunctival and mucus membrane irritation. On physical examination there is tachypnea, tachycardia, and rales, but fever is uncommon. The pathology is consistent with acute chemical pneumonitis, with intra-alveolar edema, exudation of macrophages, desquamated alveolar epithelial cells, lymphocytes, and plasma cells being seen.[57]

Chronic pulmonary disease resulting from inhalation of low levels of beryllium over an extended period of time is less common since occupational standards were introduced in 1949. Cases are still being reported primarily because of persistent excessive air levels of beryllium in industries.[50,55,56] Almost half of all new cases of chronic berylliosis had their first exposure since 1949.[58] Although no longer used in fluorescent light-bulb manufacture, modern technology such as rocket thermal coatings, nuclear reactors, rocket fuel, etc has increased the demand for beryllium.[59] Most patients with chronic berylliosis give a history of occupational exposures. Neighborhood and household exposures previously linked to chronic berylliosis no longer occur. Chronic berylliosis can develop within months or as late as 20 years after cessation of beryllium exposure.[56]

The clinical presentation of chronic berylliosis is that of a systemic granulomatous disease with dyspnea, nonproductive cough, weakness, malaise, and weight loss. Other symptoms are similar to sarcoidosis: kidney stones, joint aches, parotid tenderness, central nervous system and skin lesions. Physical examination reveals conjunctivitis, tachypnea, tachycardia, inspiratory rales, restrictive cardiomyopathy, hepatosplenomegaly, and peripheral adenopathy. Routine laboratory evaluation also suggests sarcoidosis; hypergammaglobulinemia, hypercalcemia, and hypercalciuria. Bilateral hilar adenopathy on chest radiography without parenchymal involvement has also been noted. Clinical features not seen in chronic berylliosis but present in sarcoidosis include uveitis, uveoparotid fever, cystic bone lesions, cranial and peripheral neuropathies.[60]

The pathology in chronic berylliosis is diffuse interstitial fibrosis with noncaseating granulomas whose giant cells contain asteroid and Schaumann's bodies. The findings indicating a restrictive pulmonary function defect are consistent with any peripheral infiltrative pulmonary disease, namely small lung volumes, decreased diffusing capacity for carbon monoxide, and noncompliant lungs. The most consistent abnormality in chronic berylliosis is hypoxia with progressive worsening of the alveolar-arterial oxygen pressure difference on incremental exercise testing.[61] Although one study purported to show an obstructive defect in 40% of chronic berylliosis patients, the factors measured indicated only peripheral small airway dysfunction, ie, increased RV/TLC and increased helium equilibration time. Such peripheral airway obstruction is consistent with peripheral bronchial compression consequent to granuloma formation in small airways and peribronchial fibrosis but is not a cause of major airway obstruction and would not be detected by the FEV_1/FVC ratio.[61] Although debatable, the mechanism of beryllium-induced pulmonary dysfunction appears to be immunologic, and data substantiating immunologic mechanisms may be useful diagnostically. Evidence for an immune mechanism includes low attack rate, long latent period after exposure, predictable positive response to steroid therapy, and a lack of a dose-response relationship.

The immune mechanism is confirmed by studies of cellular immunity such as blast transformation of lymphocytes from patients with chronic berylliosis in the presence of beryllium sulfate.[62] In

Williams' study all patients with chronic berylliosis had lymphocyte transformation on exposure to beryllium, and all healthy beryllium workers had no such lymphocyte sensitivity. There was also good correlation between the severity of the clinical disease and the degree of blast transformation.[63,64] Bronchoalveolar lavage yielded an increased number and proportion of bronchoalveolar T cells and activated T cells from patients with chronic berylliosis compared with controls. In addition, bronchoalveolar lavage lymphocytes from patients proliferated in response to beryllium sulfate more than peripheral blood lymphocytes from the same patients.[59] Such evidence for an immune mechanism can be even more useful in establishing a diagnosis of berylliosis than open-lung biopsies, especially in ruling out sarcoid.

Finding beryllium in lung tissue is part of the definition of the disease and indicates previous beryllium exposure, but it can be misleading diagnostically. In one report, 20% of chronic berylliosis patients had beryllium tissue levels in the normal range. Beryllium is ubiquitous and is present in low concentrations in soil and water; many healthy people have beryllium measurable in their tissues. Workers who die of causes unrelated to beryllium exposure may have normal lung tissue containing as much beryllium as the lungs of workers with chronic berylliosis.[60]

Hypersensitivity Pneumonitis (HP)

Hypersensitivity pneumonitis is an interstitial peripheral infiltrative pulmonary process resulting from inhalation of various organic antigens. The two most familiar examples of HP are pigeon-breeder's lung and farmer's lung.[65] Symptoms range from acute to chronic. Typically, acute symptoms occur four to eight hours after exposure and include dyspnea, nonproductive cough, fever and myalgias and many spontaneously resolve 12 to 24 hours after termination of exposure. Physical examination after acute exposure reveals a viral-like illness with fever, tachycardia, tachypnea, nonproductive cough, and late inspiratory rales on auscultation. Wheezing is not present.[66] At the other end of the clinical continuum, patients may present with insidious chronic symptoms, especially dyspnea and weight loss. Whether the patient develops a severe or mild syndrome depends on the material inhaled, including its aerodynamic behavior, the intensity of exposure, and individual susceptibility to the inhaled material. Routine laboratory data includes leukocytosis without eosinophilia and increased serum IgG and IgA. The angiotensin-converting enzyme (ACE) is normal, in contrast to sarcoidosis, another granulomatous interstitial lung disease.[67] In addition, skin testing and serologic evaluation reveal the presence of precipitating antibody to *Micropolyspora faeni* in the case of farmer's lung, or avian protein in cases of bird breeder's HP. Unfortunately, half the bird breeders without disease also have precipitating antibody as a manifestation of exposure.[68]

Pulmonary function is as varied as the clinical presentation. When the patient is asymptomatic between exposures, pulmonary function can return to normal. Six hours after the appropriate exposure, a restrictive pattern develops, including small lung volumes, preserved FEV_1/FVC ratio, low diffusing capacity for carbon monoxide, and hypoxia as well as decreased lung compliance.[69] There is a peripheral small airway dysfunction detectable by various appropriate studies.[5] With cessation of further exposure, pulmonary function can return to normal.[65] However, with continuing exposure, restrictive disease may become irreversible.[70]

The pathology of HP varies with length of exposure. Acutely there is infiltration of the interstitium as well as of respiratory bronchial walls with lymphocytes, plasma cells, and histiocytes with foamy cytoplasm. Subsequently, a granulomatous reaction develops and, in time, fibrosis of the interstitium. Chronic HP leads to interstitial fibrosis and ultimately honeycomb lung. In addition to end-stage restrictive disease, small airways may be permanently damaged (bronchiolitis obliterans).[71,72]

The pathogenesis of HP is unknown. A farmer exposed to hay stored in moist warm silos inhales and retains 750,000 spores per minute of the thermophilic actinomycete, *Micropolyspora faeni*. These 1-μm spores may exert a direct toxic effect on the lung via the release of potent enzymes or directly activate the alternate complement pathway.[73,74] Most observations, however, implicate immune mechanisms in the pathogenesis of HP. Because of the precipitating antibody and the time of onset after exposure, many authors feel an Arthus reaction or type 3 antigen-antibody immune complex reaction is the mechanism of HP. Other reports favor a cell-mediated (type 4) immune response. These authors point to the early mononuclear infiltration of the lung and subsequent development of granulomas, as well as the presence of T cells in the bronchoalveolar lavage which produce lymphokines on exposure to pigeon antigen.[75] Other information favors a type 2 or cytotoxic reaction as the immune mechanism of HP because the walls of the small bronchioles contain HP antigen, antibody, and complement in the absence of vasculitis; the vasculitis would be expected if a type 3 reaction were invoked.[76]

The clinical history is probably the most important factor in the diagnosis and should include a detailed environmental history, including hobbies (family members as well), exposure to various humidification systems in the home, workplace, and even the car.[77,78] It is only by identifying and avoiding the etiologic agent that subsequent restrictive disease can be prevented. The finding of precipitating antibodies to agents of HP is suggestive of the diagnosis only if associated with a typical clinical picture, since exposed healthy populations also have such findings. Inhalation challenge using possible culpable antigens with development of acute symptoms, decreased lung volumes, and diffusing capacity postinhalation is helpful but potentially dangerous.[79] Assessing pulmonary function before and after an actual workplace exposure can be very revealing. Bronchoalveolar lavage can be diagnostic by yielding foamy macrophages and/or T cells that produce lymphokines on specific antigen exposure among symptomatic patients with HP and may prove to be a useful diagnostic procedure.[70]

Treatment consists of removal of the offending antigen by ceasing exposure through changing occupations or hobbies and/or the administration of corticosteroids. The presence of the acute syndrome usually warrants the use of steroids for periods of up to a week. When irreversible fibrosis develops, only symptomatic treatment is possible.

References

1. Becklake MR: Asbestos-related diseases of the lungs and other organs: Their epidemiology and implications for clinical practice. Am Rev Respir Dis 1976;114:187–227.
2. Meiklejohn: The origin of the term "Pneumonokoniosis." Br J Ind Med 1960;17:155–160.
3. Cooke WE: Pulmonary asbestosis. Br Med J 1927; 2:1024.
4. Epler GR, Carrington CD, Gaensler EA: Crackles (rales) and interstitial pulmonary disease. Chest 1978;73:331.
5. Parkes WR: Asbestos-related disorders. Br J Dis Chest 1973;67:261.
6. Regan GM, Tagg B, Thomson ML: Subjective assessment and objective measurement of finger-clubbing. Lancet 1967;1:530.
7. Ashcroft T: Epidemiological and quantitative relationships between mesothelioma and asbestos on Tyneside. J Clin Pathol 1973;26:832.
8. Turner-Warwick M, Parkes R: Circulating Rheumatoid and anti-nuclear factors in asbestos workers. Br Med J 1970;3:492.
9. Merchant JA, Klouda PT, Soutar CA, et al: The HL-A system in asbestos workers. Br Med J 1975; 1:189.
10. Fournier-Massey G, Becklake MR: Pulmonary function profiles in Quebec asbestos workers. Bull Physiopathol Respir (Nancy) 1975;11:429.
11. Weill H: Diagnosis of asbestos-related disease. Chest 1987;91:802–803.
12. Murphy RL, Gaensler EA, Redding RA, et al: Low exposure to asbestos: Gas exchange in ship pipe coverers and controls. Arch Environ Health 1972; 25:253.
13. Holt PF, Mills J, Young DK: Experimental asbestosis in a guinea pig. J Pathol Bacteriol 1966;92: 185–195.
14. Begin R, Masse S, Bureau MA: Morphologic features and function of the airways in early asbestosis in the sheep model. Am Rev Respir Dis 1982; 126:870–887.
15. Churg A: Asbestos fiber content of the lungs in patients with and without asbestos airway disease. Am Rev Respir Dis 1983;127:470–473.
16. Jodoin G, Gibbs GW, Macklem PT, et al: Early effects of asbestos exposure on lung function. Am Rev Respir Dis 1971;104:525–535.
17. Ostrow D, Cherniak RM: Resistance to airflow in patients with diffuse interstitial lung disease. Am Rev Respir Dis 1973;108:205.
18. Gibson GJ, Prede NB: Lung distensibility: The static pressure volume curve of the lungs and its clinical assessment. Br J Dis Chest 1976;7:143–184.
19. Begin R, Cantin A, Berthiaume Y, et al: Airway function in life time non-smoking older asbestos workers. Am J Med 1983;75:631–638.

20. Regan GM: The relative importance of clinical, radiological and pulmonary function variables in evaluating asbestosis and chronic obstructive airway disease in asbestos workers. Clin Sci 1971; 41:569.
21. Gaensler EA, Carringon CB, Coutu RE, et al: Pathological, physiological, and radiological correlations in the pneumoconioses. Ann NY Acad Sci 1972;200:574.
22. Jones NL: Exercise testing in pulmonary evaluation: rationale, methods, and the normal respiratory response to exercise. N Engl J Med 1975; 293:541–544.
23. Epler GR, McLoud TC, Gaensler EA, et al: Normal chest roentgenograms on chronic diffuse infiltrative lung disease. N Engl J Med 1978;298: 934–939.
24. Epler GR, McLoud TC, Gaensler EA: Prevalance and incidence of benign asbestos pleural effusion in a working population. JAMA 1982;247:617–622.
25. Hillerdal G: Non-malignant asbestos pleural disease. Thorax 1981;36:669–675.
26. Gaensler EA, Kaplan AI: Asbestos pleural effusion. Ann Intern Med 1971;74:178.
27. Anderson HA, Selikoff IJ: Pleural reactions to environmental agents. 1978;37:2496–2500.
28. Wright PH, Hanson A, Kreel L, et al: Respiratory function changes after asbestos pleurisy. Thorax 1980;35:31–36.
29. Miller A, Teirstein AS, Selikoff IJ: Ventilatory failure due to asbestos pleurisy. Am J Med 1983; 75:911–919.
30. Enterline P, De Coufle P, Henderson V: Respiratory cancer in relation to occupational exposures among retired asbestos workers. Br J Ind Med 1973;30:162–166.
31. Hammond EC, Selikoff IJ, Seidman H: Asbestos exposure, cigarette smoking and death rates. Ann NY Acad Sci 1979;330:473–490.
31a. Reeves AL: The carcinogenic effect of inhaled asbestos fibre. Ann Clin Lab Sci 1976;6:549.
32. Chahinian AP: Treatment of diffuse malignant mesothelioma, A review. Mt Sinai J Med 1978; 45:54.
33. Stumphius J: Epidemiology of mesothelioma on Walcheren Island. Br J Ind Med 1971;28:59.
34. Oels HC, Harrison EG, Carr DT, et al: Diffuse malignant mesothelioma of the pleura: A review of thirty-seven cases. Chest 1971;60:564.
35. Porter GN, Cheek JM: Pleural mesothelioma, review of tumor histogenesis and report of twelve cases. Thorac Cardiovas Surg 1968;56:869.
36. Eisenstadt HB: Benign asbestos pleurisy. JAMA 1965;192:195–201.
37. Parkes WR: Occupational lung disorders, ed 2. Diseases due to free silica. London, Butterworths, 1982 pp 134–170.
38. Banks DE, Morring KL, Boehlecke BA, et al: Silicosis in silica flour workers. Am Rev Respir Dis 1981;124:445–450.
39. Jones RN, Turner-Warwick M, Ziskind M, et al: High prevalence of antinuclear antibodies in sandblasters' silicosis. Am Rev Respir Dis 1976;113: 393–395.
40. Buechner HA, Ansari A: Acute silico-proteinosis: A new pathologic variant of acute silicosis in sandblasters, characterized by histologic features resembling alveolar proteinosis. Dis Chest 1969; 55:274–284.
41. Hailey WC, Brown M, Buechner HA, et al: Silicomycobacterial disease in sandblasters. Am Rev Respir Dis 1974;100:115–125.
42. Wolinsky E: Tuberculosis, in Baum GL, Wolinsky E (eds): Textbook of Pulmonary Diseases, ed 3. Boston, Little Brown & Co, 1983 p 533.
43. Wolinsky E: Other mycobacterial diseases, in Baum GL, Wolinsky E (eds): Textbook of Pulmonary Diseases, ed 3. Boston, Little Brown & Co, 1983 p 575.
44. Gross P, Westrick ML, McNerney JM: Tuberculosilicosis: A study of its synergistic mechanisms. J Occup Med 1960;2:571–575.
45. Caplan A: Certain unusual radiologic appearances in the chest of coal-miners suffering from rheumatoid arthritis. Thorax 1953;8:29–39.
46. Chatgidakis CB, Theron CP: Rheumatoid pneumoconiosis (Caplans syndrome): A discussion of the disease and a report of a case in a European Witwatersrand gold miner. Arch Environ Health 1961; 2:397–408.
47. Kleinerman J, Merchant JA: Occupational lung diseases: Silicosis, coal-workers pneumoconiosis and miscellaneous pneumoconioses, in Baum GL, Wolinsky E (eds): Textbook of Pulmonary Diseases, ed 3. Boston, Little Brown & Co, 1983 pp 473–768.
48. Morgan WKC: Industrial bronchitis. Br J Ind Med 1978;35:285–291.
49. Kleinerman J, Merchant JA: Occupational lung diseases, asbestos-, talc-, and beryllium-related respiratory diseases, in Baum GL, Wolinsky E (eds): Textbook of Pulmonary Diseases, ed 3. Boston, Little Brown & Co, 1983 pp 769–788.
50. Karkinen-Jaaskelainen M, Maatta K, Pasila M, et al: Pulmonary berylliosis: Report on a fatal case. Br J Dis Chest 1982;76:290–297.
51. Parkes WR: Occupational Lung Disorders, ed 2. Silicates and lung disease. London, Butterworths, 1982 pp 233–332.
52. Gamble JF, Fellner W, Dimeo MJ: An epidemio-

logic study of a group of talc workers. Am Rev Respir Dis 1979;119:741–753.

53. Kleinfeld M, Messite J, Shapiro J, et al: Lung function in talc workers: A comparative physiologic study of workers exposed to fibrous and granular talc dusts. Arch Environ Health 1964;9:559–566.
54. Kleinfeld M, Messite J, Kooyman O, et al: Pulmonary ventilatory function in talcosis of lung. Dis Chest 1964;46:592–598.
55. Hasan FM, Kazemi H: Chronic beryllium disease: A continuing epidemiological hazard. Chest 1974; 65:289–293.
56. Kanarek DJ, Wainer RA, Chamberlain RI, et al: Respiratory illness in a population exposed to beryllium. Am Rev Respir Dis 1975;108:1295–1302.
57. Hazard JB: Pathologic changes of beryllium disease: The acute disease. AMA Arch Ind Health 1959;19:179.
58. Sterner JH, Eisenbud M: Epidemiology of beryllium intoxication. AMA Arch Ind Hyg Occup Med 1951;4:123.
59. Epsteine PE, Dauber JH, Rossman MD, et al: Bronchoalveolar lavage in a patient with chronic berylliosis: Evidence for hypersensitivity pneumonitis. Ann Intern Med 1982;97:213–216.
60. Sprince NL, Kazemi H, Hardy H: Current (1975) problem of differentiating between beryllium disease and sarcoidosis. Ann NY Acad Sci 1975;29: 654.
61. Andrews JL, Kazemi H, Hardy H: Patterns of lung dysfunction on chronic beryllium disease. Am Rev Respir Dis 1969;100:791.
62. Deodhar SD, Barna B, Van Ordstrand HS: A study of the immunologic aspects of chronic berylliosis. Chest 1973;63:309–313.
63. Williams WJ, Williams WR: The value of beryllium lymphocyte transformation tests in chronic beryllium disease and in potentially exposed workers. Thorax 1983;38:41–44.
64. Williams WR, Williams WJ: Comparison of lymphocyte transformation and macrophage migration inhibition tests in the detection of beryllium hypersensitivity. J Clin Pathol 1982;35:684–687.
65. Dinda P, Chatterjee SS, Riding WD: Pulmonary function studies in bird breeders' lung. Thorax 1969;24:374–378.
66. Schlueter DP, Fink JN, Sosman AJ: Pulmonary function in pigeon breeders disease: A hypersensitivity pneumonitis. Ann Intern Med 1969;70: 457–470.
67. McCormick JR, Thral RS, Ward PA, et al: Serum angiotensin-converting enzyme levels in patients with pigeon breeders disease. Chest 1981;80:431–433.
68. Fink JN, Schlueter DP, Sosman AJ, et al: Clinical survey of pigeon breeders. Chest 1972;62:277–281.
69. Hargreave FE, Pepys J: Allergic respiratory reactions in bird fanciers provoked by allergan inhalation provocation tests: Relation to clinical features and allergic mechanisms. J Allergy Clin Immunol 1972;50:157–173.
70. Patterson R, Wang JLF, Fink JN, et al: IgA and IgG antibody activities of serum and bronchoalveolar fluid from symptomatic and asymptomatic pigeon breeders. Am Rev Respir Dis 1979;120:1113–1118.
71. Barbee RA, Calois Q, Dickie HA, et al: The long-term prognosis in farmer's lung. Am Rev Respir Dis 1968;97:223–231.
72. Schuyler MR, Thigpen TP, Salvaggio JE: Local pulmonary immunity in pigeon breeder's disease. Ann Intern Med 1978;88:355–358.
73. Berrens L: Enzymes in pigeon droppings of possible relevance to pigeon breeders' disease. Clin Exp Immunol 1971;9:393.
74. Marx JJ, Flaherty DK: Alternate pathway activation of compliment by antigens associated with hypersensitivity pneumonitis. Abstracted, J Allergy Clin Immunol 1975;55:71.
75. Rankin J, Kobayashi M, Barbee RA, et al: Pulmonary granulomatoses due to inhaled organic antigens. Med Clin North Am 1967;51:459–482.
76. Schlueter DP: Infiltrative lung disease hypersensitivity pneumonitis. J Allergy Clin Immunol 1982; 70:50–55.
77. Fink JN, Banaszak EF, Thirede WH, et al: Interstitial pneumonitis due to hypersensitivity to an organism contaminating a heating system. Ann Intern Med 1971;74:80–83.
78. Kumar P, Marier R, Leech SH: Hypersensitivity pneumonitis due to contamination of a car air conditioner. Letter to the Editor. N Engl J Med 1981;305:1531–1532.
79. Burge PS: Problems in the diagnosis of occupational asthma. Br J Dis Chest 1987;81:105–115.

4

Radiological Features of Asbestosis

Albert Solomon and Gerhard K. Sluis-Cremer

Asbestos is a physical paradox, being both fibrous and crystalline. Asbestos minerals belong to two groups, the amphiboles and the serpentines. Serpentine in certain localities assumes a fibrous structure known as chrysotile asbestos, which is the principal commercial type.[1]

In the amphibole group of asbestos there are six minerals, and five of them are fibrous, including crocidolite, amosite, anthophyllite, tremolite, and actinolite. The latter three are not extensively mined, but may be etiologic agents when diseases ascribed to asbestos exposure occur in localities where other asbestos minerals are neither used nor present. In practice, radiologic changes occur following exposure to chrysotile (white asbestos), crocidolite (blue asbestos), or amosite (brown asbestos).

Russia, Canada, South Africa, and the United States are the major producers of asbestos, most of the commercially important chrysotile asbestos being mined and milled in Canada and Southern Africa.[2] Other regions where chrysotile is mined include Russia, China, and, to a lesser extent, Italy, Cyprus, and the United States.[3] Crocidolite is exclusive to South Africa, whereas anthophyllite comes mainly from Finland.[2] Exposure to asbestos dust may result from mining, milling, or in the sorting of the rock.

Asbestos is mined by both surface (ie, open cast) and deep-mining methods; mining operations include drilling and blasting, often generating large amounts of dust.[4] Asbestos rock is sorted prior to milling and in the process of cobbing crocidolite, the rock is hammered to free the asbestos. Chrysotile is generally freed from serpentine rock, in which it is embedded, during open-cast mining. The related amphibole rock contains amounts of quartz, and therefore asbestosis and silicosis may occur concomitantly on exposure.[5]

Use of Asbestos

Asbestos has a unique combination of qualities, such as tensile strength, fibrous structure, imperviousness to water, and resistance to chemical action and decay. Additional invaluable properties include fire resistance and poor conduction of heat and sound, thus accounting for its ubiquitous and commercial use as evidenced by an estimated world production in 1974 of 5 million tons.[6] More than 90% of the asbestos used in the United States is chrysotile.[7]

World War II created an unprecedented demand for asbestos products, with more than 3,000 uses for asbestos products having been documented. As a result, many cases of asbestosis and the effects of previous asbestos exposure have been recognized recently.

The Asbestos Risk

Following legislation, the working environment is now more strictly controlled, thus reducing the hazards of the mining, milling, transport and manufacture of asbestos products. However, working conditions more than two decades ago did not offer the same protection in handling asbestos or its manufactured products. Consequently, medical scientists now have the task of investigating the injurious results produced by the inhalation of asbestos dust many years after exposure.

Asbestos previously used in the building industry now creates problems of exposure in the demolition of buildings and in the disposal of asbestos waste, for asbestos is practically indestructable, and because it is very dry, the proportion of respirable fiber is high, especially during the removal of old insulation.[8] Extensive use of asbestos in ship building produced a hazard at virtually every level of construction.[9]

Unexpected sources of exposure to inhalation of asbestos fiber have come to light in furnace and kiln workers. Protective asbestos textile clothing and unlined fire-fighting asbestos helmets, extensively used during World War II, and the flash barrier guarding high-tension electrical switch gear used by mining electricians[10] resulted in asbestos-fiber inhalation.

Persons engaged in the handling of asbestos or asbestos products in primary or secondary occupations are also at risk, and the use of asbestos-contaminated material in homes constitutes a latent source of exposure. It is unlikely, however, that inhalation of minute concentrations of asbestos fibers are a danger to health.

Clearance Mechanism in the Lung

Mucociliary clearance, together with secretions containing mucus, prevents environmental pollution of the airways and lungs. Fibers coated with mucus in the upper airways are propelled toward the oropharynx by beating cilia, which constitute a mucociliary escalator that enables some of the fibers in the conducting airways to be eliminated. In this way the majority of fibers are rapidly and efficiently cleared after inhalation.

Inert fibers tend to be eliminated mainly by the bronchial route, whereas alveolar fibers, ie, those deposited distal to the ciliated airways, are usually phagocytosed by alveolar macrophages, which engulf the fibers and then migrate to the mucociliary escalator, from where they are eliminated. Fibers that find their way into the interstitial lung space are removed by macrophages via tissue fluid to lymphatics and regional lymph nodes. By injuring or killing the alveolar macrophage, silica and asbestos may cause the release of proteolytic enzymes, which set up inflammatory changes that lead to pulmonary fibrosis, a prolonged or slow phase of fiber clearance continuing for many months or even years.[11]

Pathology

The parietal pleura is almost invariably thickened in asbestosis. The affected lungs in well-established asbestosis may, however, become encased in a thick and often calcified pleural layer of dense hyaline fibrous tissue. Isolated white raised plaques of noncalcified or calcified dense hyalinized fibrous tissue are frequently found on the parietal pleura in the absence of any obvious lung damage in persons who were exposed to asbestos many years previously. These parietal pleural areas of thickening are more often localized posteriorly adjacent to rib rather than intercostally, but are also found in the lower anterior and lateral chest and on the upper aponeurotic surfaces of the diaphragm.[12] The lesions are bilateral and may be a few millimeters to 1-cm thick; although irregularly shaped, they are circumscribed with a convex surface, possibly together with small multinodular plaques. Large lesions have an irregular distribution on the inner surface of the rib cage, but may enlarge and fuse to form an extensive diffuse shield-like plaque. Irregular dystrophic calcification is often present. Microscopically, the raised lesions consist of collagen fibers with hyaline changes, are avascular and acellular, and contain a few spindle-shaped fibroblasts (Fig. 4.1). Some of these plaques show "pseudoelastic" tissue staining, possibly due to changes in the collagen composition. Asbestos bodies are not detected in the lung tissue in about half the cases with plaque formation.

It is not clear how these small asbestos fragments reach the parietal pleura, or if they are in fact responsible for the formation of these plaques; a possible route suggested by von Hayek[13] is via the tracheobronchial lymph nodes. The fibers enter the anterior mediastinal lymph channels and then, moving against the normal lymph flow, finally find their way into the intercostal lymphatics, which run along the upper and lower margins of the intercostal space on the pleural surface. Alternatively, fibers that have lodged in the periphery of

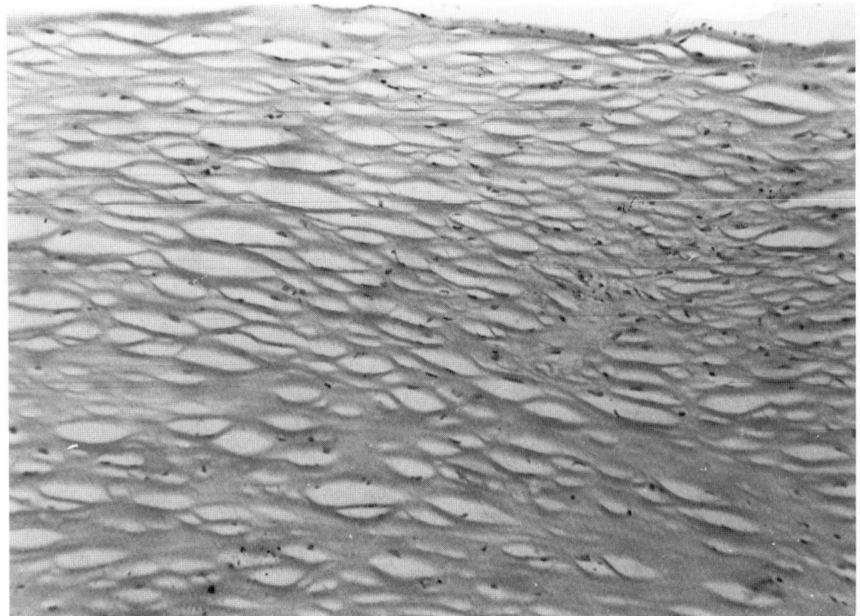

Figure 4.1. Photomicrograph demonstrating acellular thickened pleura.

the lung may penetrate to reach the pleural surface (Fig. 4.2). Asbestos-related pleural reactions, in addition to diffuse pleural fibrosis and plaque formation, include pleural effusions, often hemorrhagic.[12]

The fibrotic changes that occur in the lung result from the inhaled asbestos bodies found in the alveolar spaces (Fig. 4.3). Initially, a patchy obliterative bronchiolitis develops and later spreads distally into the alveolar ducts, atria, and alveolar walls.[14] Alveolar wall fibrosis occurs, as well as a desquamative alveolitis, which becomes organized by connective tissue.[15] The fibrosis is usually spread evenly through both lower lungs at the pleural margins. As the fibrosis increases in severity, the changes become more pronounced (Fig. 4.4); the resulting extensive fibrosis causes the interlobar septa to become thick and fibrosed. With progressive fibrosis, the small arteries and arterioles undergo mural thickening owing to muscle hypertrophy and subintimal thickening, possibly resulting in pulmonary hypertension, right ventricular hypertrophy, and finally cor pulmonale with heart failure.[16]

Massive fibrotic lesions occurring in asbestos miners appears to be due to the combined presence of silica particles and asbestos fibers and are probably related to the quartz content in the mined asbestos rock[5]; solid upper lobe fibrotic lesions are apparently related to tuberculous infections.[3] Large opacities also occur with chrysotile, where no silica contaminant is implicated (Fig. 4.5).

The Chest Radiograph

Despite the advent of modern imaging techniques, a good quality chest radiograph remains basic to the investigation of asbestosis. Regular monitoring of workers and epidemiological surveys are beyond the practical scope of newer methods such as computed tomography (CT), but are invaluable for solving contentious and problematic interpretations of pleural and parenchymal pathology. Certainly the chest and abdominal assessment of mesotheliomas has been made easier by CT. Since bilateral pleural thickening among asbestos-exposed workers is an indication of significant asbestos exposures, and the diagnostic accuracy is significantly increased by identifying pleural thickening with oblique views, it has been suggested that the incorporation of these views routinely in screening asbestos-

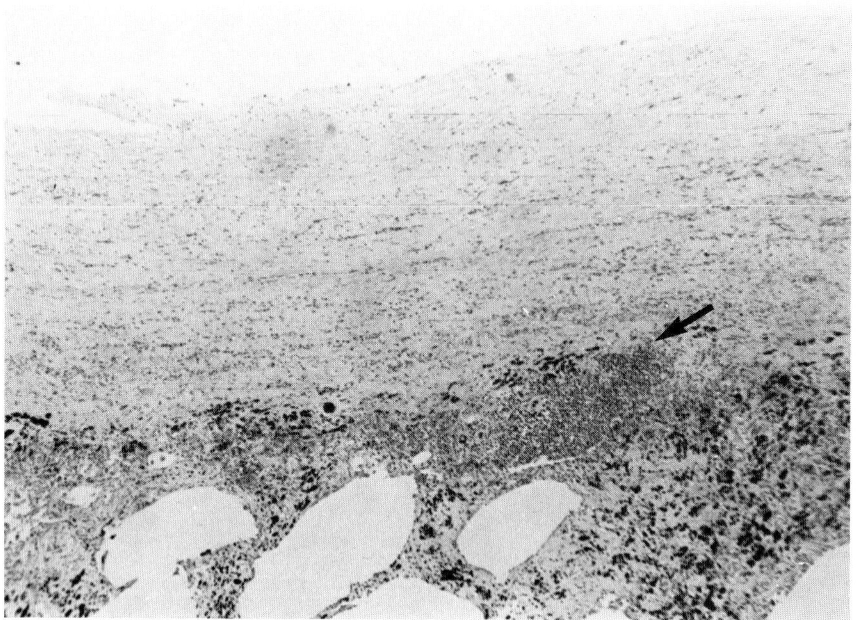

Figure 4.2. Well-marked visceral pleural thickening. *Arrow* indicates border of underlying lung parenchyma.

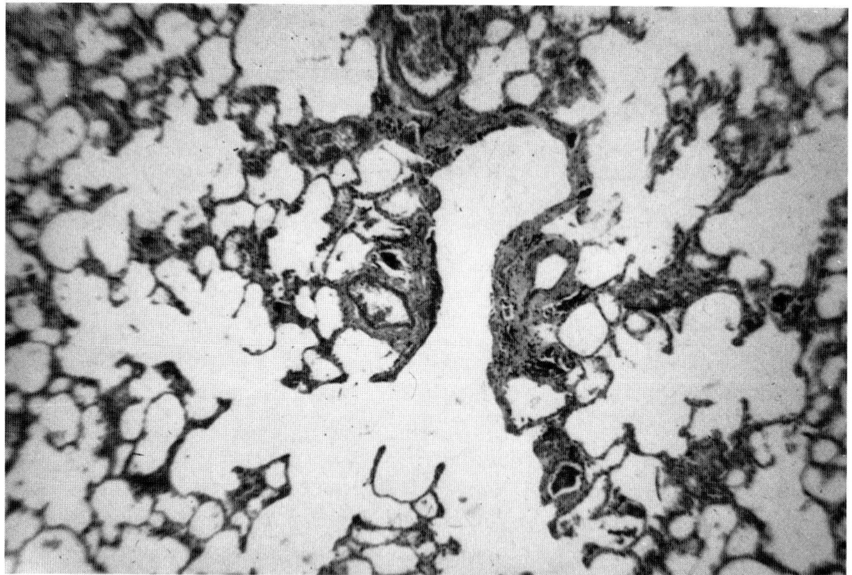

Figure 4.3. Slight asbestosis with fibrosis around the respiratory bronchioles.

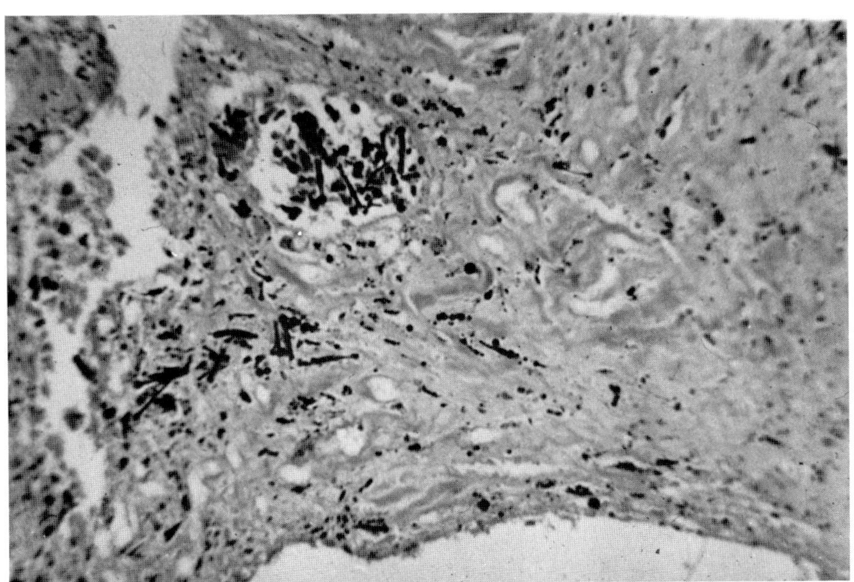

Figure 4.4. Marked asbestosis with numerous asbestos bodies.

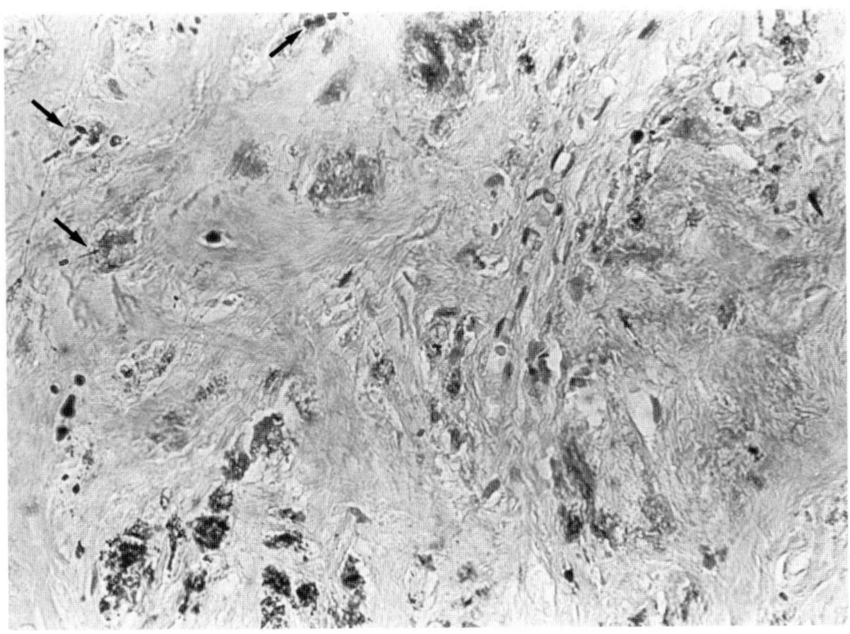

Figure 4.5. Section of massive fibrosis with asbestos bodies (*arrows*).

exposed individuals is justified[17] (Figs. 4.6 and 4.7).

The chest radiograph is essential in the asbestos industry initially as part of the preemployment investigation to identify preexisting diseases and later as the point of reference to which subsequent radiographs can be compared. The intervals between successive radiographs should be determined by the industrial health care worker. Obviously, workers at considerable risk in the mining or handling of asbestos products will require at least yearly radiographs of the chest. Where excellent precautionary methods are established, a repeat radiograph may not be necessary in the under-40-year-old worker for at least 5 years after the initial film. With advancing years and continued exposure, more frequent chest radiographs become necessary, preferably annually. The current practice for worker surveillance is a chest radiograph at yearly intervals, which is routinely employed as one of several indices of response to inhaled dust. Satisfactory surveys of large numbers of workers engaged in the handling of asbestos materials can be managed at the working site with a well-equipped mobile x-ray van that is capable of taking standard full-sized radiographs and dry developing on the spot.[18]

Confusing Companion Shadows on the Chest Radiograph

The serratus anterior is a large curved quadrilateral muscle that lies on the side of the chest and the medial wall of the axilla. The fleshy muscle insertions and the fat surrounding the muscle slips are commonly seen on the posteroanterior chest radiograph (particularly when the muscle is well developed) and may be partly superimposed on the lateral margin of the lung, seen as a companion line from the third rib to just above the costophrenic sulcus. It is most probably caused by the bulky posterior margin of the serratus anterior where it leaves the chest wall to approach the scapula. The medial border is clearly retained and fades laterally into the soft tissue. Identifying this companion shadow avoids overdiagnosing uncalcified pleural or extrapleural manifestations of asbestos exposure.[19]

Occasionally a rib fracture with an organized overlying subpleural hematoma gives rise to a pleural opacity that could be mistaken for a plaque associated with asbestos dust inhalation. Peripheral soft-tissue changes adjacent to the costal margin between the second and sixth rib are composed mostly of fatty tissue between the rib and the parietal pleura.[20] The extrapleural fat may be mistaken for pleural disease.

Pleural Manifestations Associated With Asbestos Dust Exposure

Radiologically the pleural effusions associated with asbestos dust exposure are most often small and may not be associated with pleural plaques or calcification. The initial pleural reaction or serositis may produce a lamellar pleural effusion that escapes detection. The smaller pleural effusion may fill the costophrenic sulcus and track upward in the lateral axillary pleural space with a shallow concave medial margin as is usually found in other exudative or transudative effusions. Organization of a significant volume of free pleural fluid gives rise to a convex margin (Fig. 4.8).

The effusions, unilateral or bilateral, can persist for some months and even for as long as a year. Occasionally there is a belated recurrence of the effusion on the same or opposite side of the chest. A blunted costophrenic angle is a consequence and probably a residue for most asbestotic pleural effusions and as such is an important marker for past effusions. In approximately half the cases, diffuse pleural thickening accompanies asbestos-related pleural effusions[21] (Fig. 4.9).

Pleural Thickening: Fibrosis

Pleural reaction in asbestos-exposed individuals is a nonspecific response that occurs in a variety of other conditions, eg, viral or pyogenic inflammations, trauma, embolism, and following irradiation. Pleural thickening occurs with such frequency in asbestos-exposed persons as to warrant its inclusion in the International Labor Organization (ILO) classification of 1980.[22] Thickening of the pleural

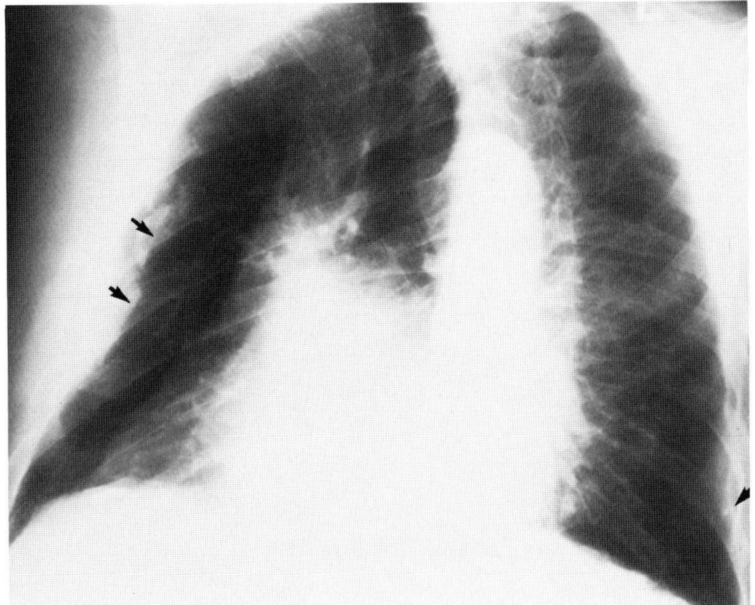

Figure 4.6. A 40° left anterior oblique chest radiograph demonstrating a problematic pleural change. The right pleura has calcified pleural plaques (*arrows*). The left pleural stripe has a normal convex bulge; additionally there is slight blurring of the stripe medially with a small spot of calcification (*arrow*), ie, a plaque is present.
Worked in asbestos mine for 14 years.

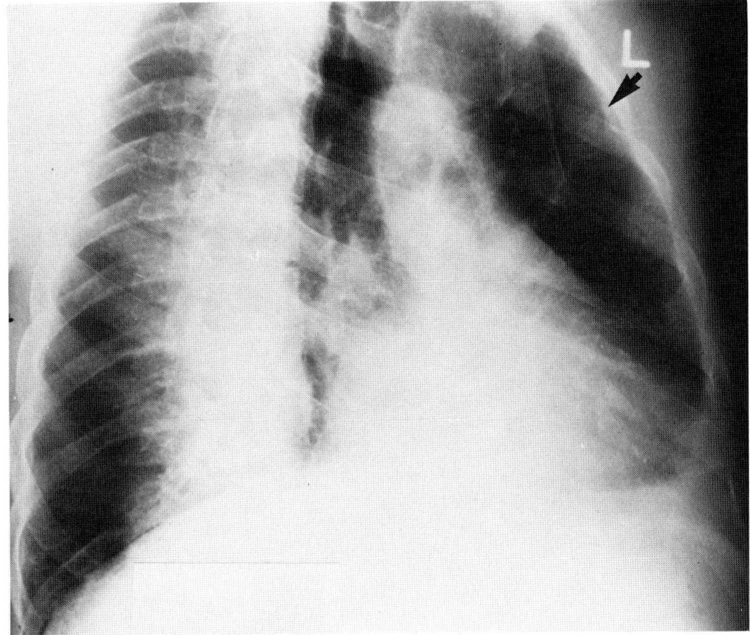

Figure 4.7. A 40° right anterior oblique chest radiograph demonstrating a problematic pleural change. The right pleural stripe is normal. The normal pleural stripe can assume a medial convex bulge, without thickening. On the left, however, there is a localized pleural plaque (*arrowhead*). The pleura has become thickened with an irregular flat medial border. The left costophrenic angle is obliterated, a nonspecific sign that also occurs in exposure to asbestos and can follow an asbestos pleural effusion.
Asbestos worker with 38 years' exposure; he also had slight reduction of carbon monoxide diffusion.

A

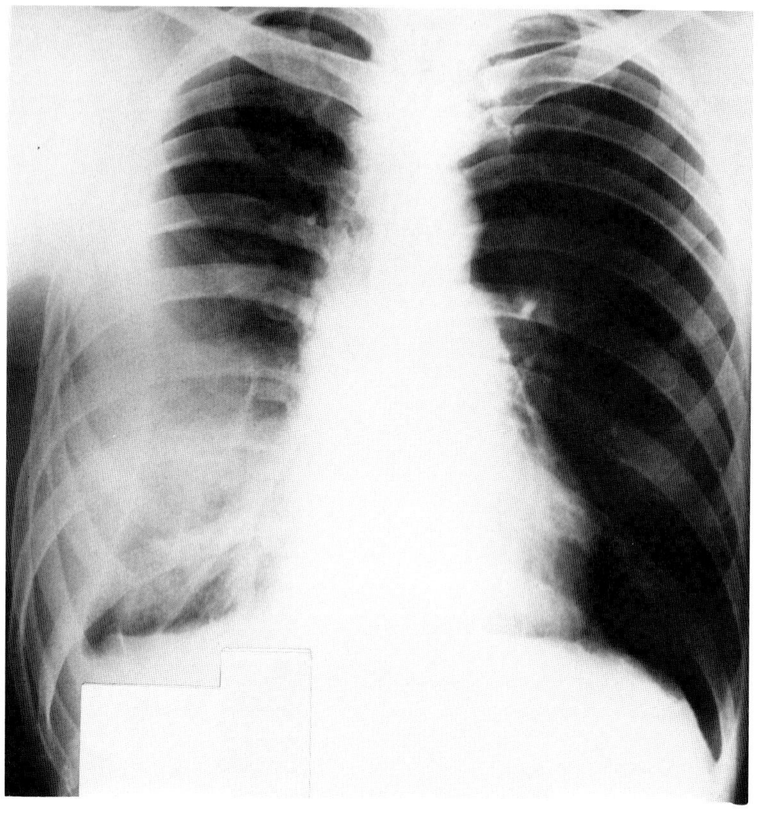

B

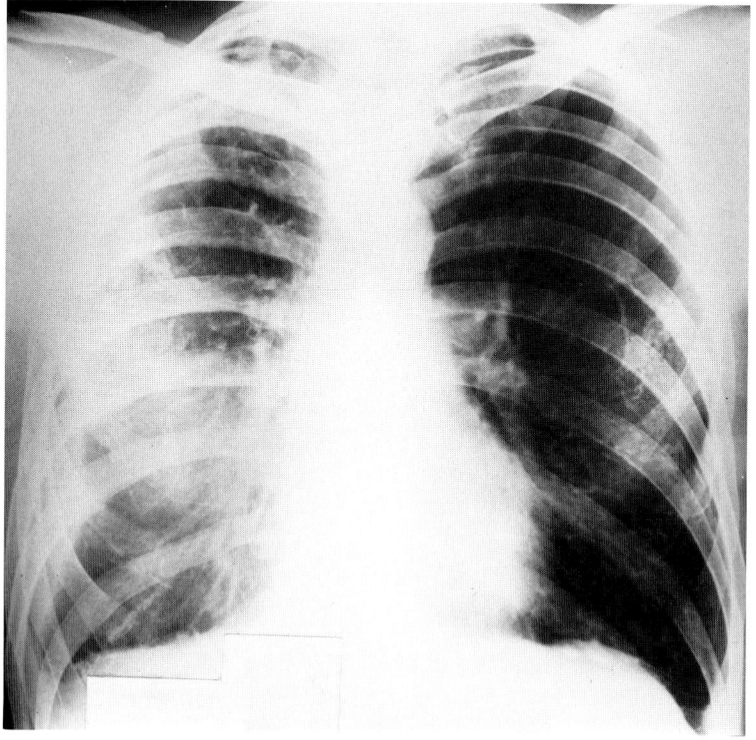

Figure 4.8

Figure 4.9. Diffuse pleural abnormality. Diffuse bilateral pleural opacification with obliteration of the costophrenic sulci and blurring of the cardiac outline. Pleural effusions occur both early and late after asbestos exposure. Known high-asbestos exposure starting 16 years previously.

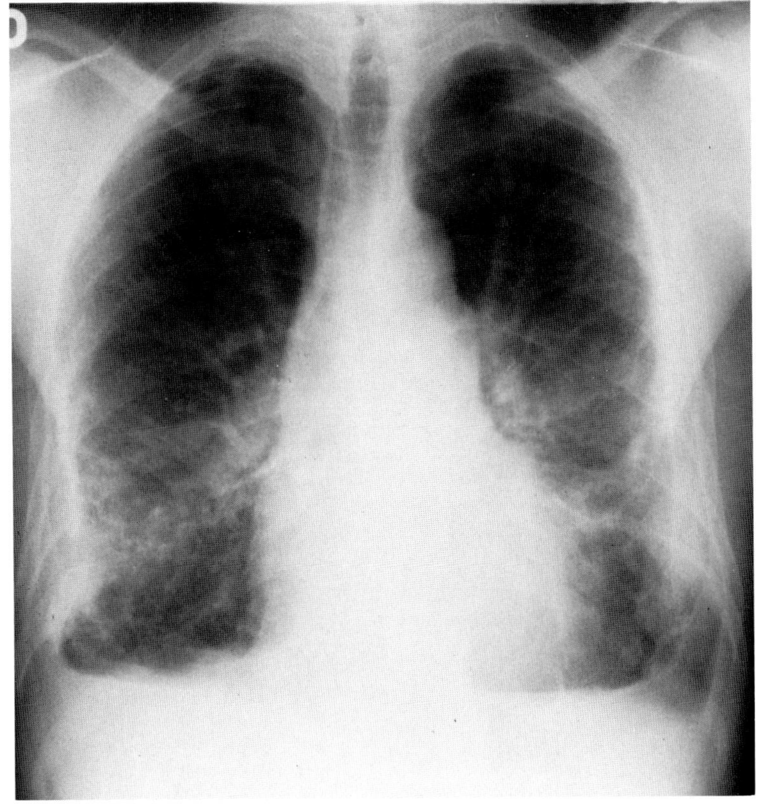

Figure 4.8. Belated pleural effusion. **A**. Encapsulated right pleural effusion with faint calcified plaques on the left. Five years later the effusion organized into pleural thickening with calcification. Calcified plaques indicate the first exposure was at least 15 years previously; recommenced work with asbestos in 1958; acute pleural effusion in 1965. On aspiration, blood-stained pleural fluid. Neither tubercule nor malignant cells found. **B**. Extensive bilateral pleural plaque formation and calcification implicating asbestos as the cause of the previous effusion. The fluid previously in the right main interlobar fissure (**A**) subsequently organized: the anterior end has thickened and calcified (**B**).
Exposure to asbestos: 9 years, 1958–1967. Encapsulated effusion 1965; minimal aspiration (8 ml of straw-colored fluid).

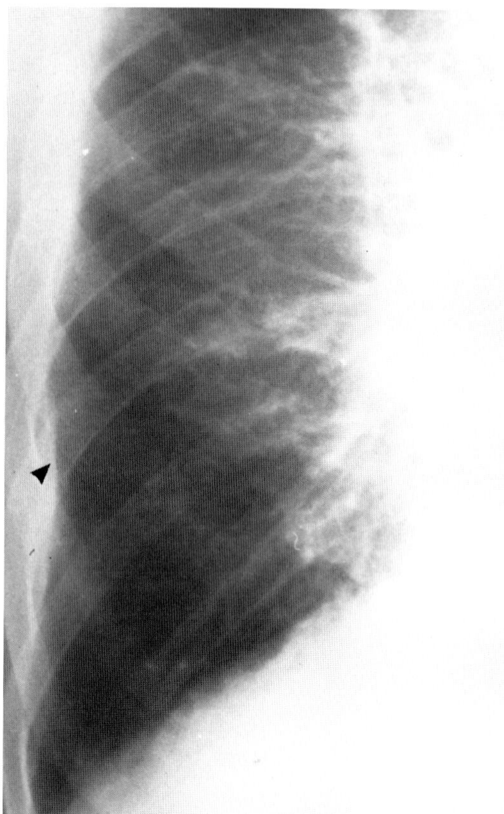

Figure 4.10. Pleural plaque (lamellar plaque). A peripheral lamellar pleural plaque can be due to asbestos, if all other causes are excluded, and can be seen if sufficiently thick and tangential to the x-ray beam. Using high kilovoltage, hyaline plaques are well demonstrated, but calcification may be obscured. Asbestos exposure for 2 years, 20 years previously.

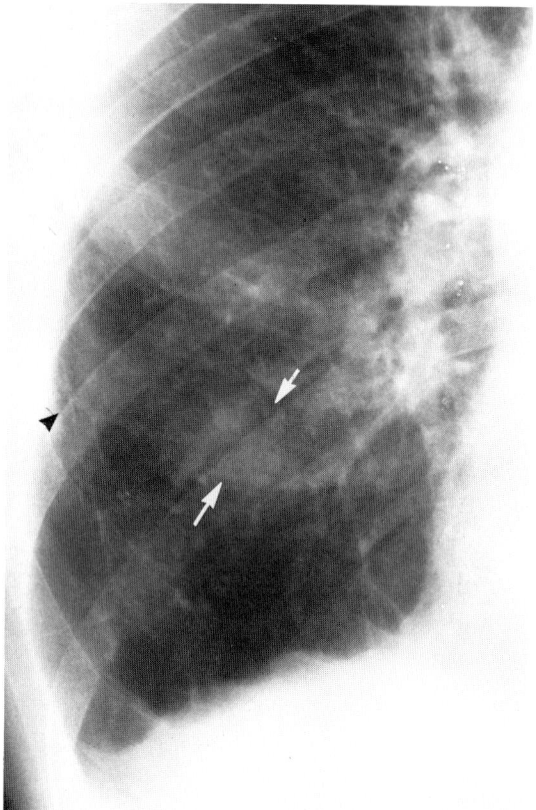

Figure 4.11. Noncalcified pleural plaques. Magnified view: an axillary lamellar plaque, outline of a noncalcified plaque obscured by the anterior end of a rib. Diaphragmatic pleural tags present. Asbestos exposure starting 12 years previously.

line, which is usually applied to the chest wall, may extend for some distance up to the posterior and lateral thoracic cage. A pleural line up to 2 mm in thickness might be described as suspect[23]; one that exceeds 2 mm is considered pathologic.

An en face view of pleural thickening presents a structureless lesion with a vague veiling effect; on close examination an edge is sometimes visible. Bilateral or even occasionally unilateral thoracic pleural opacification may be seen in asbestos-exposed individuals.[24] No portion of the pleural surface, visceral or parietal, is immune to fibrotic thickening.[4] Pleural changes are most frequently observed in the lower chest regions[25] (Fig. 4.10). As a general rule, progressive pleural fibrosis is seen without accompanying calcific changes and can be diagnosed as resulting from asbestos exposure only with a confirmatory history, other causes having been excluded.[2] The pleural thickening is as a rule bilateral and symmetrical, sometimes accompanied by costophrenic sulcus obliteration.[26]

In some instances the pleural change has developed following an effusion, with progression to thickening over a few years[21] and often coexists with underlying pulmonary fibrosis.[26] It appears that men with diffuse pleural abnormalities have more symptoms and signs and lower lung function values than those without pleural abnormalities.[27] Diffuse pleural fibrosis may produce extremely severe pulmonary restrictions and result in cor pulmonale and death.[28] Differentiation between diffuse pleural thickening and the circumscribed

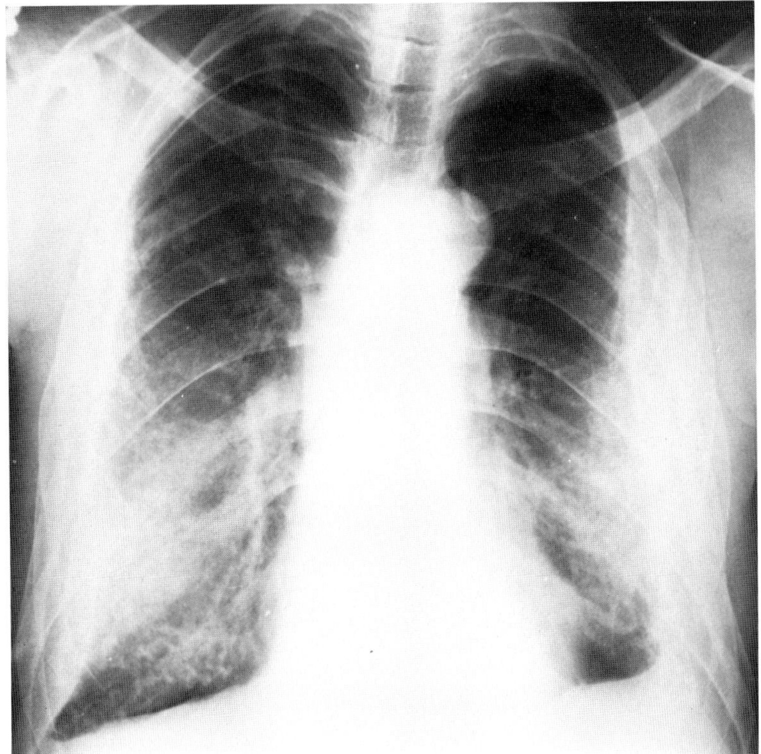

Figure 4.12. Gross bilateral pleural thickening and calcification–encasement of both lungs. Extensive pleural thickening and symmetrical calcification with distortion of left hemidiaphragm. Both costophrenic angles obliterated. Right hemidiaphragm flat and straightened. No parenchymal asbestosis visible through pleural shadowing. Asbestos exposure years previously suggesting the asbestos-induced effusions were hemorrhagic; they are commonly asymptomatic. Hemorrhagic effusions are likely to calcify early. Tuberculosis, trauma, and empyema were excluded.
Sawing asbestos cement pipes, 1969–1974.

plaque necessitates the use of the oblique chest radiograph[29] and possibly a CT scan.

The ILO classification of radiographs includes the recording of pleural thickening, which is graded according to width and extent along the lateral thoracic cage. Pleural thickening of less than 3 mm in width should be considered as low grade. Unless the thickening progresses and increases in width, it could be nonpathological (Fig. 4.11).

Localized pleural streaks can converge to a point on the lateral midthoracic wall. A pleuropericardial distortion of the clear cardiac outline is also occasionally noted. These pleural streaks are indicative of localized, possibly isolated pleural reactions and fibrosis following on an exudative pleuritis. A midzonal longitudinal density of pleural thickening, can occur as a remnant of exudative pleurisy.[30]

Diffuse Fibrotic Pleural Calcification

Thickened pleura from any cause, such as empyema, tuberculosis, or hemothorax, may become calcified. A period of 2 years is usually the minimum required for such calcification. On the other hand, calcification of the pleura in silicate exposure is usually associated with plaque formation and occurs 20 years after the initial exposure.[31]

The more extensive pleural calcifications possibly reflect diffuse pleural fibrosis with subsequent calcification rather than extensive and diffuse plaque formation. Anterior and posterior mediastinal pleural reflections and the paravertebral pleural line rarely calcify diffusely and encase the whole lung[25] (Fig. 4.12).

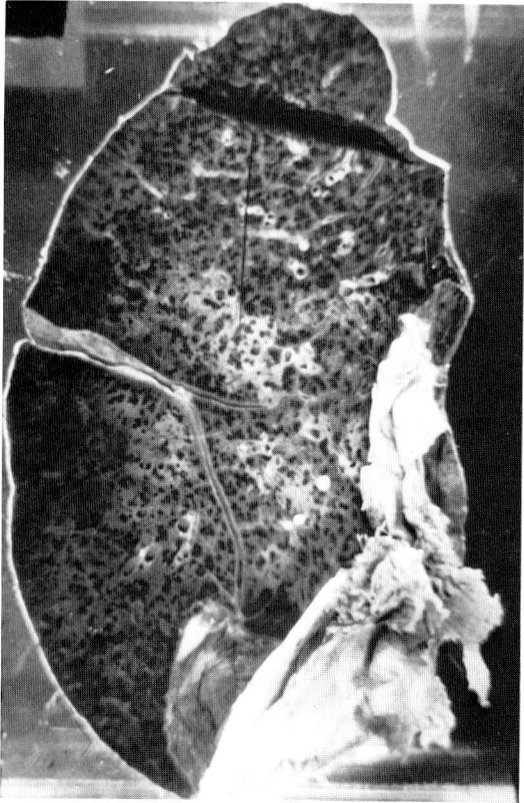

Figure 4.13. Lung section demonstrates thickened visceral pleura (including interlobar fissure). Note extensive plaque (lower right) present on the diaphragm.

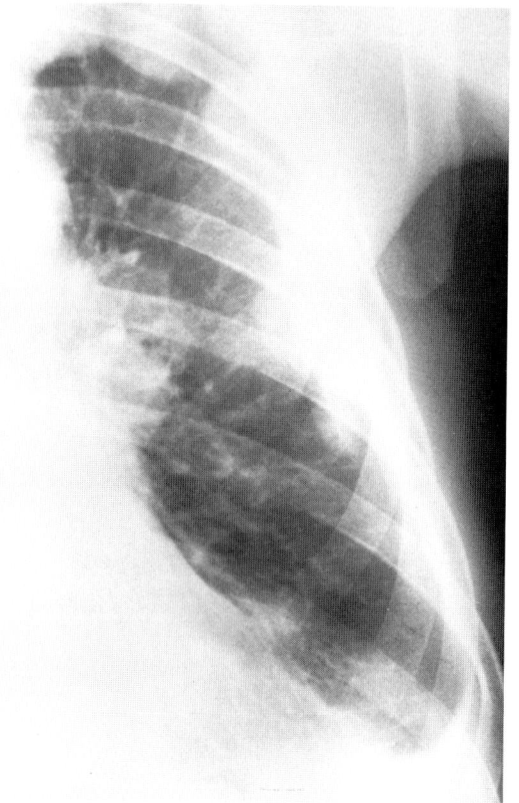

Figure 4.14. Enlarged radiograph (asymptomatic person). Large plaques indistinguishable from mesothelioma. Asbestos exposure more than 15 years previously. Regular x-ray monitoring over some years showed no change.

Hyaline and Calcified Pleural Plaque Associated With Asbestos Dust Exposure

Plaques are distinct from fibrous pleural thickening. In the consensus of most observers, plaques are commonly found along the external aspect of the parietal pleura. In recent years radiological attention has additionally been directed to the occurrence of major and minor interlobar pleural changes reflecting either visceral pleural fibrosis or plaque formation[10] (Fig. 4.13).

Plaques are recognized as well-circumscribed, elevated areas usually of an irregular shape, with a smooth convex surface. They are often bilateral, best demonstrated over the lower lung fields, close to the lateral thoracic rib margin (Fig. 4.14). If looked for carefully, plaques may be found on the aponeurotic surface of the diaphagm, where they produce slight mound-like irregularities on the usually smooth dome-like diaphragmatic contour.[32] Dystrophic calcifications occur in the degenerative areas of collagen and when sufficiently dense, permit easier recognition of the plaque.[1] Bilateral pleural plaques are associated with exposure to all types of asbestos.[2] Whether calcified or not, these pleural plaques are symptomless and are not considered responsible for lung function impairment.[33] They may occur on their own, but workers with these changes are more likely to develop progressive parenchymal fibrosis than those without.[34]

Plaques may be difficult to demonstrate radiologically until they are of sufficient thicknesses, ie, greater than 3 mm, or manifest visible areas of calcification.[35] Many plaques are detected only at autopsy. Plaques may be seen as ill-defined low-density opacities, round or elliptical in shape, more often visible in the lower zones. Occasionally, the outline of the plaque is contiguous with an adjacent rib and difficult to define. The oblique chest film is invaluable in this situation, allowing visibility of the plaque in many instances. Seen en face, a pleural plaque is a poorly defined opacity resulting from the x-ray beam striking the pleural surface perpendicularly. Interdigitating muscle shadows, extrapleural fat, or the companion pleural line should not be confused with plaque formation.

The more lateral and peripheral plaque is recognized as a vertical lamellar pleural thickening with a convex medial margin between the sixth and ninth ribs.[36] Oblique chest views, sonography, or CT are all useful means for plaque demonstration. The plaque size can be variable, sometimes being no larger than 1 to 2 cm. The bigger plaques have a surprisingly large area, easily defined when extensively calcified (Fig. 4.15).

Calcification of Hyaline Pleural Plaques

Calcification in a pleural plaque usually occurs more than 20 years after the initial exposure to asbestos.[37] The longer the time lapse after the initial exposure, the greater the incidence of calcified plaques. The presence of calcified pleural plaques serves as an endemic marker of environmental exposure.[38] Pleural calcification occurs, not unexpectedly, more frequently in older people.[32] However, calcified plaques and intrapulmonary fibrosis often do not coexist.[39] Calcification in an area of localized pleural thickening or opacification constitutes certain evidence of the presence of a pleural plaque[31] (Fig. 4.16).

Hyaline plaques calcify from the base, becoming more densely calcified with the passage of time. Any portion of the pleura may undergo calcification. Plaque formation is frequently noted on the diaphragm. Calcified plaques are seen along the lateral chest wall and paravertebral gutters, but are more frequently visualized in the lower zones.[24] The process of calcification need not be uniform. Accordingly, the calcified area visible on the chest radiograph does not always define the true extent of a plaque. Irregular calcification in hyaline plaques produces many unexpected radiological patterns (Fig. 4.17). The calcifications are often of variable shape, some being linear and only a few centimeters in size. Occasionally a massive diffuse encuirass deposit results. Straight linear calcification, oval, ring-like, or leaf-shaped outlines may be formed. Plaques are usually bilateral, tending to have a symmetrical distribution. However, the demonstration of low-grade sparse calcification is dependent on a good quality radiograph. Routine radiography reveals only about 15% of plaques. Significantly more plaques are found at autopsy than are detected radiologically,[40] as a proportion of plaques found postmortem or at thoracotomy are not sufficiently radiopaque to be identified on the standard radiograph.

The Visceral Pleura in Asbestos-Exposed Individuals

The visceral or pulmonary pleura is a serous membrane that covers the surface of the lungs and lines the fissure between the lobes. On chest radiographs the fissures are seen as white hair-line shadows, and their average thickness is about 0.2 mm. Abnormal thickening of the major and minor fissures is easily assessed in chest roentgenograms. Posteroanterior, lateral, and oblique chest projections will produce an accurate image of the oblique and horizontal visceral pleural changes. The observation of thickened or calcified pleural fissures or plaques is the only radiographic method of diagnosing involvement of visceral pleura. It is not possible to identify or separate the visceral pleura covering the rest of the lung surface from the adjacent parietal pleura on a normal chest film.

Visceral pleural changes may be the sole radiological evidence of asbestos exposure, or they may exist in conjunction with parietal pleural, or in association with parenchymal asbestosis[41] (Fig. 4.18). The most extensive pleural and parenchymal x-ray abnormalities occur in those heavily and continuously exposed to asbestos. It is not surprising, therefore, to find interlobar pleural reactions in such patients. In South African miners

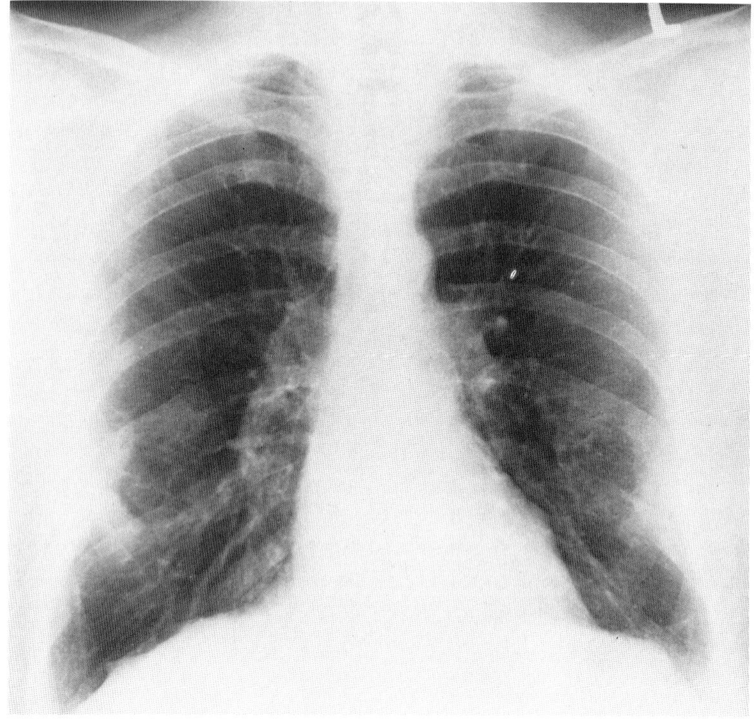

A

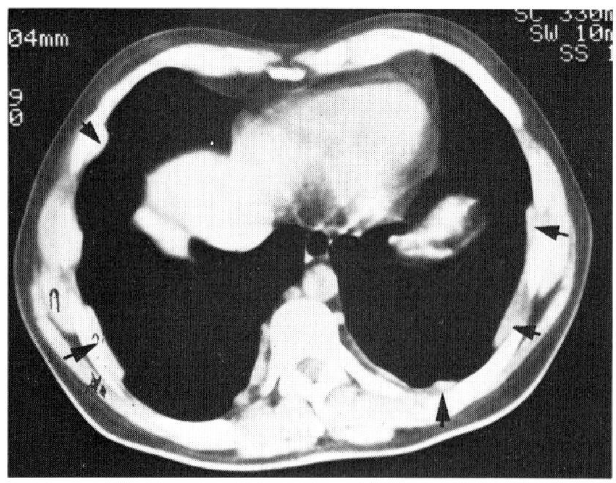

B

Figure 4.15. Chest x-ray and CT demonstration of noncalcified plaques. **A**. Bilateral symmetrical basal and peripheral plaques on chest x-ray film. **B**. CT left anterior plaque (*arrows*). A CT slice following chest examination shows anterior and posterior pleural plaques (*arrows*), including paravertebral plaques (central white area = heart and diaphragm).

thickened fissures increase in prevalence from about 2% in men who have worked with asbestos 7 years or less, to 25% in those with more than 15 years of exposure. Other asbestos-associated pleural or parenchymal abnormalities may occur in 69% of those men with thickened fissures who have been exposed to asbestos dust inhalation. The presence of a thickened fissure as an isolated abnormality is also related to the duration of asbestos exposure. Examination of serial films of asbestos miners who have thickened fissures as an isolated abnormality suggests that the fissures thicken slowly and progressively.[41]

Visceral pleural plaque formation is most convincingly demonstrated by finding calcification present in an area of pleural thickening. Local interlobar pleural thickening and distortion can represent plaque formation in minor or major fissures.[10] A CT scan of the thorax can define and verify fissural plaque formation and accurately

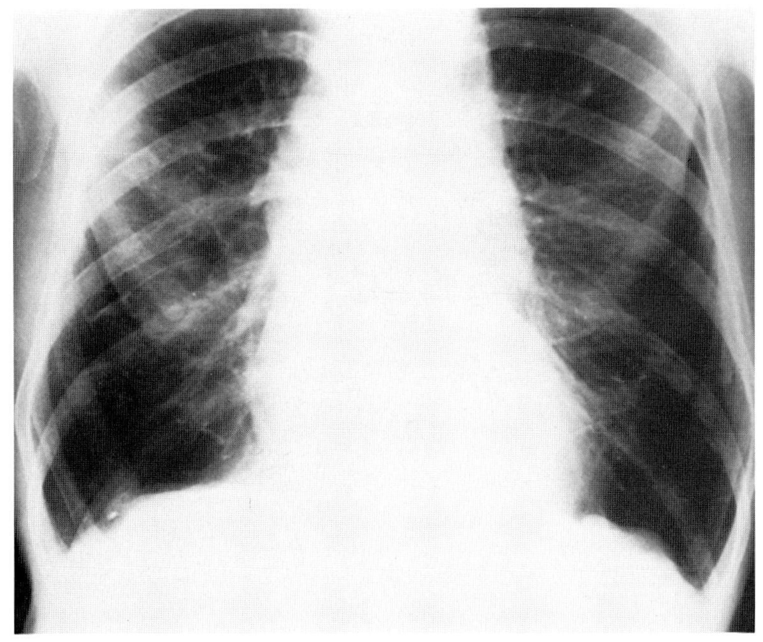

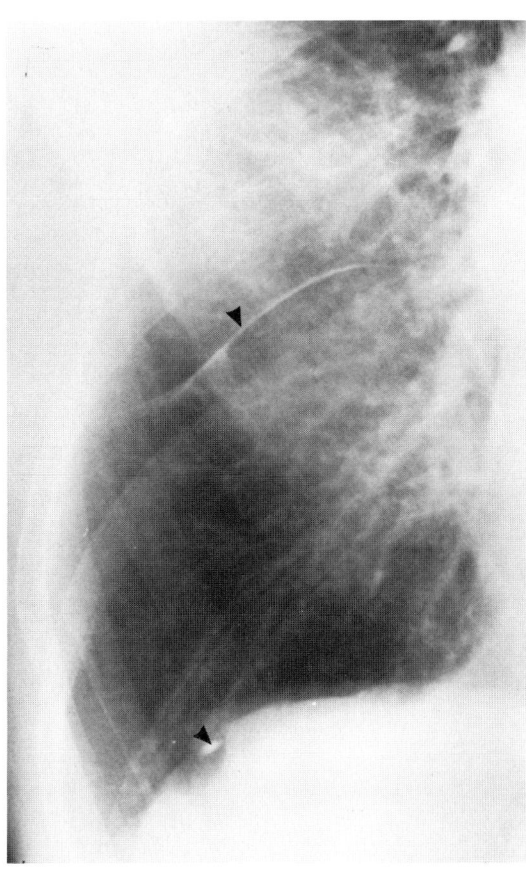

Figure 4.16. Calcified and noncalcified pleural and diaphragmatic plaques with interlobar fissural thickening in the absence of radiologically detectable lung asbestosis. **A**. Variable en face and lamellar plaques in both upper and lower thoracic regions. The left cardiac border is peaked and irregular. The irregularity of the diaphragm indicates plaque formation. **B**. Thickened right interlobar fissure and partially calcified diaphragmatic plaque. The thickened lesser fissure is a pleural manifestation of exposure to asbestos.
Two years exposure, 40 years previously.

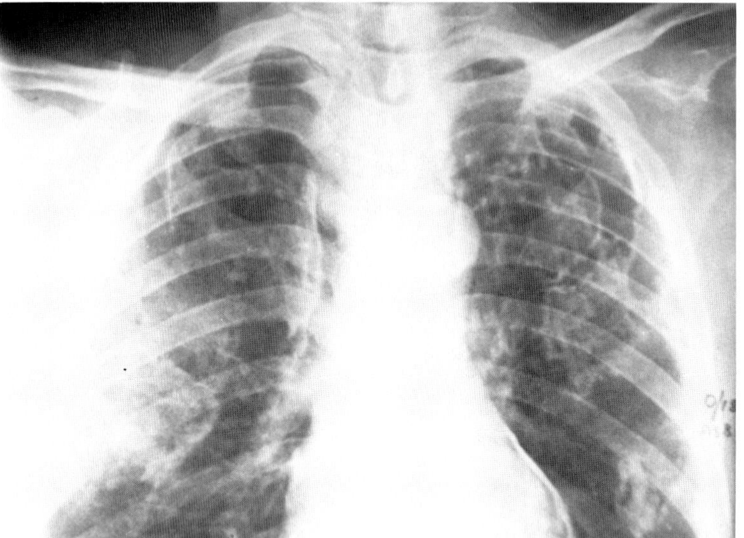

Figure 4.17. Diffuse and extensive pleural calcifications. Extensive areas of calcification of pleura adjacent to the mediastinum, heart, and diaphragm, as well as thoracic wall. Calcified pleural plaques are usually parietal, but can be visceral, as shown at autopsy.

Six years' asbestos exposure, 45 years previously. Asbestos service, 1926–1932. X-ray examination, 1977.

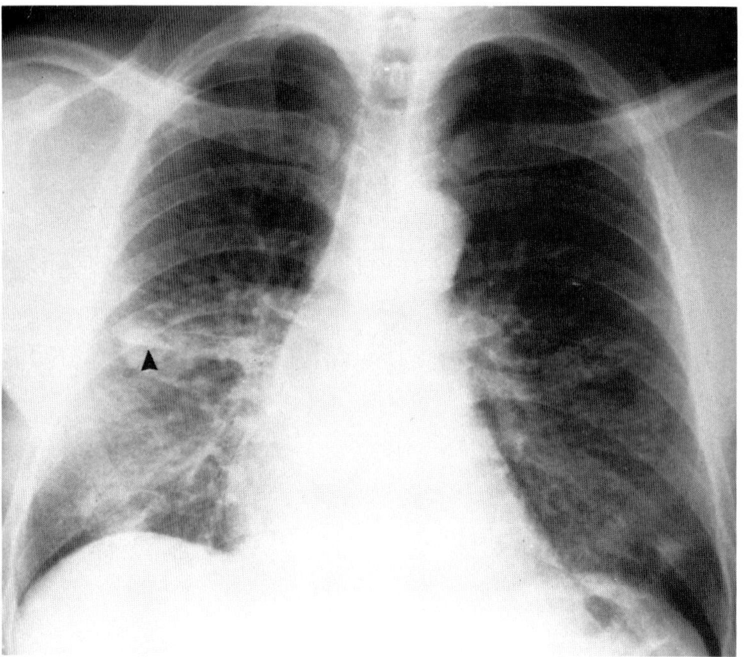

Figure 4.18. Coarse parenchymal fibrosis with right interlobar visceral plaque. Radiograph shows a mixture of t/u irregular opacities. The right midzone irregularities are under 1 cm and not a conglomerate massive opacity, and does not necessarily imply a more severe form of asbestosis than occurs with smaller size opacities. The right interlobar fissure demonstrates a noncalcified visceral plaque. Asbestos exposure in high dust atmosphere, 9 years.

detect and identify the calcium content of such plaques.

The Diaphragm in Asbestosis

The parietal diaphragmatic pleura covers that part of the thoracic portion of the diaphragm that lies lateral to the base of the pericardium; however, a strip of the thoracic surface of the diaphragm, adjoining its costal attachment, is free from the parietal pleura, except posteromedially. The pleura, covering the aponeurotic surface of the diagphragm itself, cannot be easily separated from the underlying membraneous portion.[42]

The diaphragm consists of a peripheral muscular portion, taking its fleshy fibers from the sternocostal and vertebral body structures. The central aponeurotic or membraneous portion of the diaphragm is covered by and closely applied to the parietal pleura. It is not surprising, therefore, to find hyaline and calcified pleural plaques predominantly in the central area of the diaphragmatic cupola.

Diaphragmatic plaque formation may be overlooked initially. Subtle diaphragmatic parietal pleural irregularities herald the formation of the plaque. These may be either a localized area of straightening or a small, convex, upward protuberant projection on the diaphragmatic cupola. Occasionally, a well-formed irregular protuberance becomes visible. These noncalcified plaques are only recognized about 15 years after the initial exposure to asbestos dust. More than one plaque may be found on the dome of the diaphragm and they are often bilateral and symmetrical. A single calcified diaphragmatic plaque is often the only manifestation of previous asbestos exposure and indicates that initial exposure occurred at least 20 years previously.[43] It is unusual to see these calcific plaques on the diaphragm peripherally, ie, in the region of the muscle bundles[44] (Fig. 4.19)

Straightening of the midportion of the diaphragm is a result of plaques on the tendinous area.[45] This central diaphragmatic change precedes the calcification that may be revealed by later radiographs.[46]

Lobular Atelectasis and Its Association With Asbestos-Induced Pleural Disease (Pseudotumor)

Peripheral infolding of the lung, ie, rounded atelectasis caused by associated parietal and visceral pleural thickening, produces a pseudotumor that may simulate a pleural or parenchymal neoplasm.[47] There are, however, distinctive radiologic features that permit differentiation of this pseudotumor from the other pleural or parenchymal changes associated with asbestosis (Fig. 4.20).

The lobular atelectatic pseudotumor, when fully formed, can be demonstrated on the chest radiograph as a rounded subpleural opacity, with a diameter of 2 to 7 cm at the lung base. A distinctive feature is the arcuate course of the corresponding pulmonary vessels and bronchi, providing a "comet-tail" as they converge toward the region of the atelectatic lung. Pleural thickening is invariably present, with the greatest diameter of the pleural thickening being adjacent to the mass. The acute angle between the mass and the adjacent pleura is indicative of the intraparenchymal location of the pseudotumor. There is usually aerated lung tissue between the diaphragm and the associated rounded atelectasis. Thickening of the interlobar fissure with infolding of the pleural surface is part of the process.[48] The full extent of the pseudotumor is most effectively shown by a CT scan. Extensive pleural thickening is often accompanied by an adjacent pleural plaque. The lesion is usually a static process and accelerated progression of the changes requires further investigation[49] (Fig. 4.21).

The radiologic features offer little controversy; however, the etiologic sequence is speculative. An acceptable theory suggests that a shrinking fibrous plaque or scar in the pleura can cause intussusception of the inner layers of the pleura into the lung and collapse of the lung caught between the plaited pleura. The bronchi and blood vessels supplying the area of collapse are retracted toward the lesion and pulled close together.[50] Continuing pleural thickening leads to increased atelectasis with the associated lung segment folded between the sheets of thickened pleura.[51]

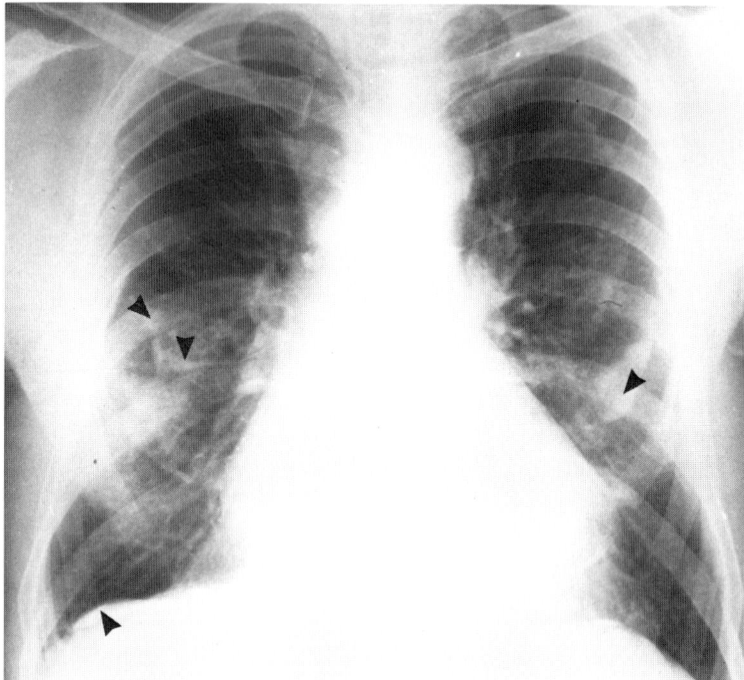

Figure 4.19. Diaphragmatic and pleural plaque calcification showing noncalcified and calcified plaques. Plaques can also occur in the interlobar fissure and later calcify (right minor fissure). Calcified plaques are also present peripherally, parallel to the underlying ribs (*arrowheads*), and there are bilateral diaphragmatic calcifications.
Asbestos exposure, 1937–1974. Soft and calcified plaques, 1967; extensive calcified plaques, 1974.
◁

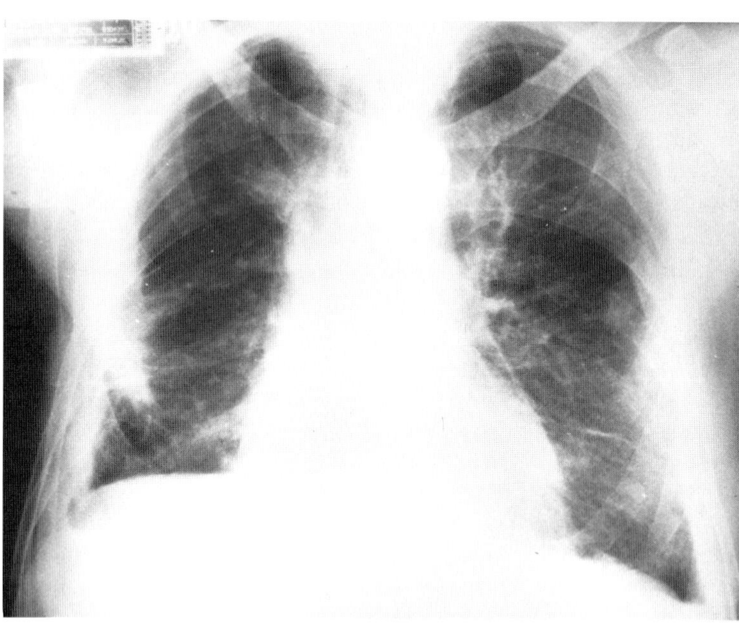

A

Figure 4.20. Problematic pleural thickening. **A**. Chest radiograph showing diffuse bilateral axillary pleural thickening with "pleural mass" on right. **B**. CT scan on same patient shows extensive right pleural thickening, posterior pleural plaque formation (*arrows*), and minimal left pleural thickening. Heart outline seen centrally behind the sternum. **C**. Same patient as in **B**. The CT cut at diaphragm level (heart outline and right diaphragm anteriorly) demonstrates extensive calcification of posterior pleura (*arrows*); not visible on chest radiograph.
Asbestos exposure, 1940–1975. Asymptomatic patient. No significant radiographic change over some years.

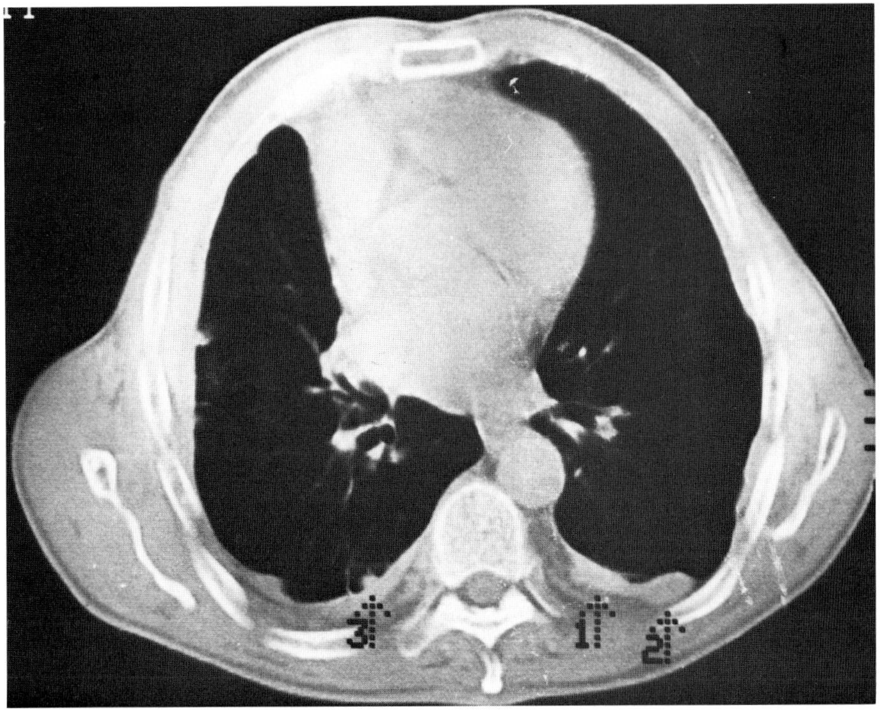

B

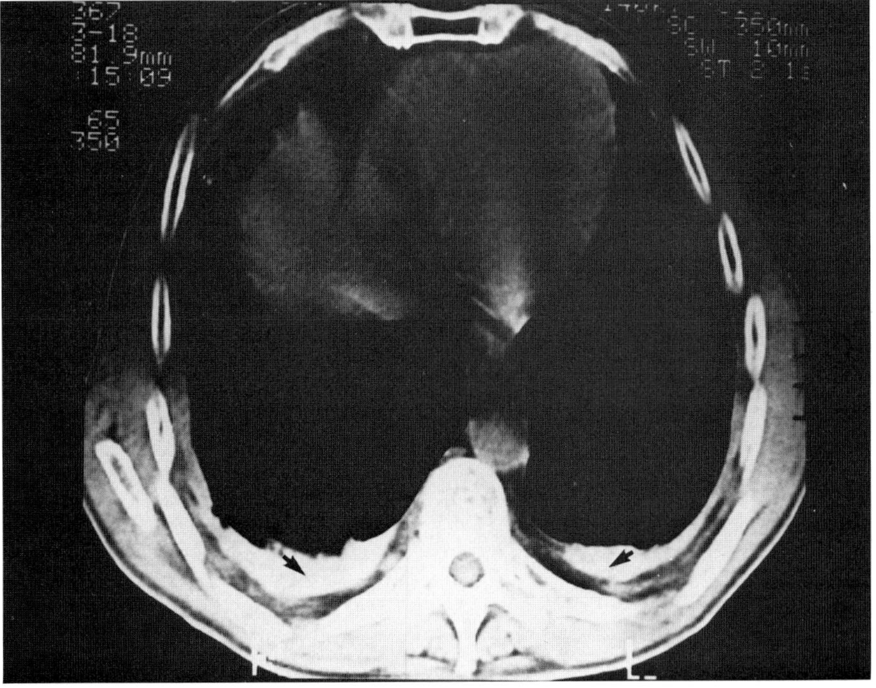

C

Figure 4.20

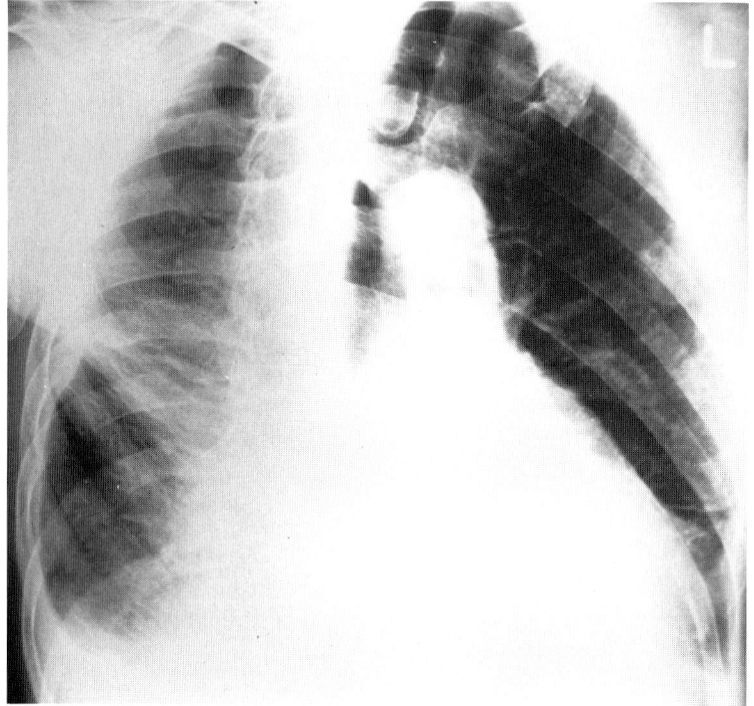

A

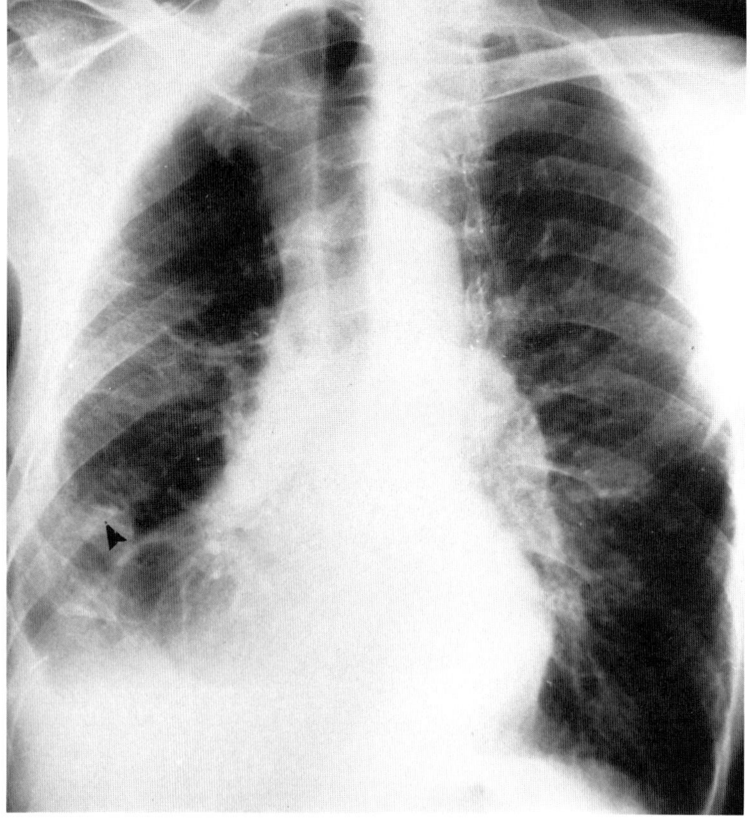

B

Figure 4.21

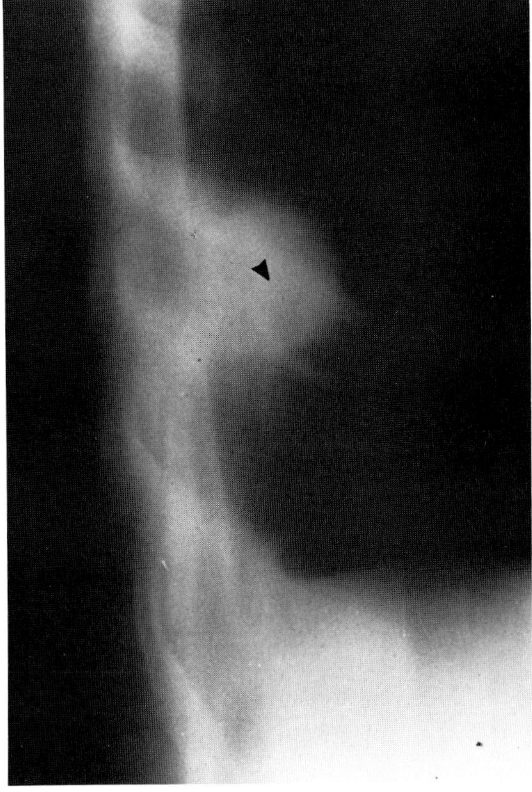

Figure 4.21. A pseudotumor due to lobular volume loss in asbestosis. **A**. (1980) Slight lower zone irregular opacities, diffuse midzone pleural fibrosis. **B**. (1982) Extensive right pleural thickening with associated organized fluid in the right costophrenic sulcus. **C**. The curved vascular leash on the medial aspect of the right lower zone opacity is shown on the tomographic cut. **B** and **C** show the progression to a round opacity with pleural, parenchymal, and vascular components. Asbestos exposure, 1950–1982.

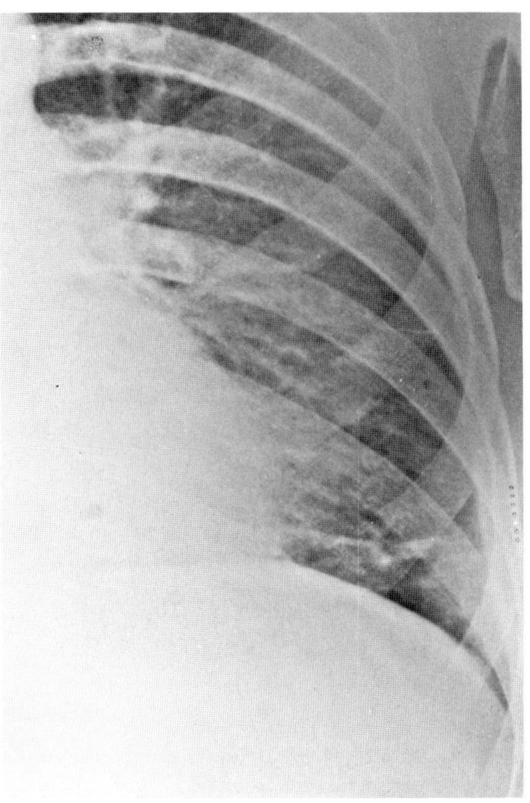

Figure 4.22. Bilateral early irregular opacities. Fine irregular opacities predominantly lower lung field (enlarged left lower lung field).

Radiologic Changes in Pulmonary Fibrosis

Early pathologic lung changes following asbestos dust inhalation are most difficult to assess; their interpretation is one of the most subjective matters in radiology. The earliest manifestations may be no more than an exaggeration of normal lung markings, readily simulated by a chest radiograph taken in poor inspiration, or by underexposing a normal chest x-ray film. The x-ray changes are bilateral, fairly symmetrical, and predominantly basal (Fig. 4.22)

Initially, vessel markings seem to extend more peripherally to the lung pleura than usual. However, the same appearance can be seen normally on a high kilovolt chest x-ray film. As the pulmonary fibrosis becomes established, a nodular disruption of the smaller vessels occurs. On occasion, a

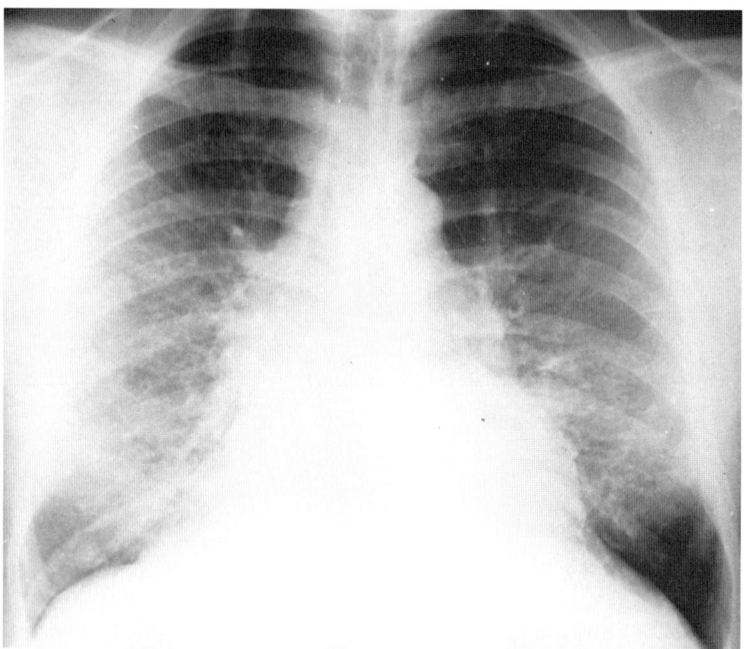

Figure 4.23. Moderate-sized irregular linear opacities. Bilateral basal symmetrical irregular opacities. The greater width of the irregular opacities does not necessarily represent a more severe form of disease. Basal fibrosis has produced upper lobe blood diversion. Asbestos exposure, 16 years; silica exposure, 6 years.

horizontal fine peripheral linear pattern (closely resembling Kerley B lines) is noted.[31] There is nothing specific about these early changes, and they are also seen in elderly patients, in patients with left ventricular or left auricular failure, fibrosing alveolitis, and in certain collagen lung disease, for example, that associated with scleroderma or rheumatoid disease. As the fibrosis progresses, the basal opacities coarsen, became more pronounced, and spread to involve more of the lungs, although usually remaining predominant in the lower zones (Fig. 4.23).

The ILO classification categorizes these opacities as regular or irregular "nodules," with measurements for recording the different sizes. The irregular opacities may assume a fine, medium, or coarse linear appearance. A ground glass veiling, sometimes seen on a chest film in a patient with asbestosis, is produced when the disease process in the lung parenchyma increases the density without the deposits being individually recognized.[6]

Regular rounded opacities on chest roentgenograms are not a common x-ray finding in asbestosis. They have been observed in some South African asbestos miners when the rock mined has a high silica content. This "silicotic" lung response probably accounts for the small rounded opacities occasionally noted on the chest film of asbestos miners[36] (Fig. 4.24).

Irregular basal opacities are seen in the chest radiograph in persons with significant asbestosis, but minor degrees of lung fibrosis are not necessarily manifested radiologically. The opacities can be linear or blotchy irregularities. The short linear basally disposed irregularities have been aptly likened to chalk or crayon lines of variable thickness. They are accordingly described as fine, medium, or coarse opacities (ie, s, t, u ILO classification). Approximate measurements have been used in their descriptive assessment.[27] However, as fibrosis of the lungs produces a variable pattern, these irregular lines can also be accompanied by irregular round opacities. The mixed lesions are referred to in most descriptions as a reticulonodular pattern, ie, irregular linear-nodular opacities. Reticulations conjure the picture of a fine lace-like network, which is seldom seen. The descriptive difficulties of these pleomorphic lung changes are compounded by the frequent superimposition of pleural opacification in asbestos-exposed individuals (Fig. 4.25).

The more advanced, less common pulmonary abnormalities include small ring-like opacities somewhere in the range of 5 to 7 mm, and often up

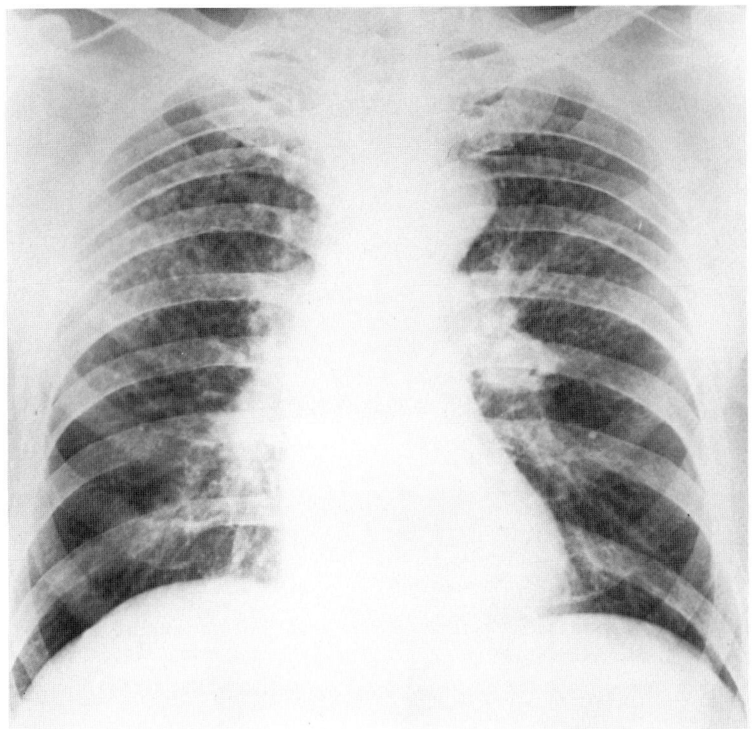

Figure 4.24. Regular upper zone opacities in asbestosis (± quartz). As South African amphibole rock contains quartz, asbestos and silicosis can occur together, or silica can alter recognized radiological patterns of asbestosis. Regular diffuse nodular opacities, massive opacities, and the unusual occurrence of upper zone asbestotic lung fibrosis can be seen in miners working the amphibole rock. Exposure to asbestos dust for one year, 27 years previously. Sputa negative for tuberculosis. Transbronchial lung biopsy of the right upper lobe showed confluent foci of fibrosis with ferruginous bodies and evidence of moderate asbestosis of alveoli.

to 10 mm. These changes have been referred to as a honeycomb pattern[52] (Fig. 4.26).

The heterogeneous appearance attributable to intrapulmonary lesions make a standardized classification of pulmonary asbestosis difficult. The separation and identification of the more coarse blotches or medium or thick lines is sometimes impossible. The new ILO classification allows a greater latitude for the coding of the different shapes of lung opacities on the chest radiograph by incorporating the concomitant use of symbols, ie, rounded or irregular. The predominant lesion would then be expressed with the initial symbol, eg, RI would suggest the presence of both rounded and irregular opacities, with more rounded than irregular opacities, as denoted by the initial symbol.[22]

Parenchymal x-ray changes due to asbestosis are sometimes aggravated by nonoccupational factors, such as cigarette smoking or exposure to other toxic agents. In fact, only 3% of nonsmokers had significant radiological interstitial changes in one investigated group, whereas changes of an interstitial nature in asbestos workers who smoked varied from 8% to 12%. This relationship seems most significant in the category of mild asbestos exposure, where nonsmokers sometimes have no abnormal radiographic manifestations.[53] By comparison, 19% of heavy smokers have significant "interstitial" x-ray changes. In the series studied, 22% of all smokers combined had significant interstitial x-ray abnormalities.[53] Several additional studies have corroborated that increased asbestos dust exposure and smoking caused a greater degree

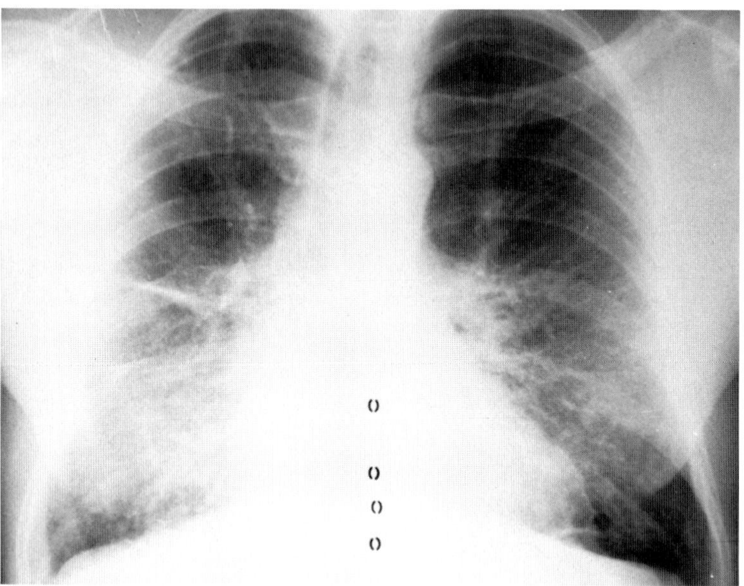

Figure 4.25. A ground glass appearance of both lower and middle zones; associated thickening of right interlobar fissure. The ground glass appearance is due to a combination of pleural and parenchymal disease. There is a combination of fine and medium irregular lung opacities; the veiling is due to the pleural thickening. Exposure to asbestos dust as a miner, 19 years.

of radiographic abnormalities.[54] Smoking appears to lower the threshold of asbestos exposure for production of pleural and interstitial disease, allowing these abnormalities to develop earlier than in nonsmokers. Individual susceptibility also influences both the initial appearance and the subsequent progression of asbestosis radiologically.[17] A significant number of asbestos-exposed workers with established radiological asbestosis-related changes demonstrate progression of the changes after removal from the source of exposure, whereas those workers with no radiographic asbestosis-related changes are much less likely to show radiological features of parenchymal opacities after removal from the asbestos exposure.[55] In smokers, x-ray alterations can manifest in less than 20 years after mild asbestos exposure.[54] Initially moderate, radiographic progression increases as the follow-up period is extended; the changes then only become recognizable when reviewed and compared over an interval of years. Rapid progression, ie, significant advancing x-ray changes when reviewed over 3 years, is less commonly encountered. Some patients with minimal but definite radiographic changes, in fact, show greater degrees of progression compared with those in the more advanced x-ray categories. However, x-ray progress is unpredictable, and many cases of asbestosis do not advance with uniform rapidity. The majority of patients with severe category asbestosis do not show significant radiographic progression over some years.[56]

Somewhat obversely, whatever the reason, increased parenchymal and pleural radiological abnormalities occur in a small proportion of men with no occupational asbestos exposure. This proportion increases with age and is probably significantly influenced by smoking habits. These increased lung markings on films that appear related to age and smoking habits may adversely affect readings in the older age group.[57]

The prevalence of pleural and parenchymal abnormality appears strongly related to the duration of asbestos exposure at work. The overall prevalence of abnormality in one series increased from 4% in men with exposure for 1 year, to 47.9% in men with more than 15 years of exposure. Overall, small irregular parenchymal opacities were found in 7.3% of the workers investigated; the prevalence of parenchymal abnormalities being

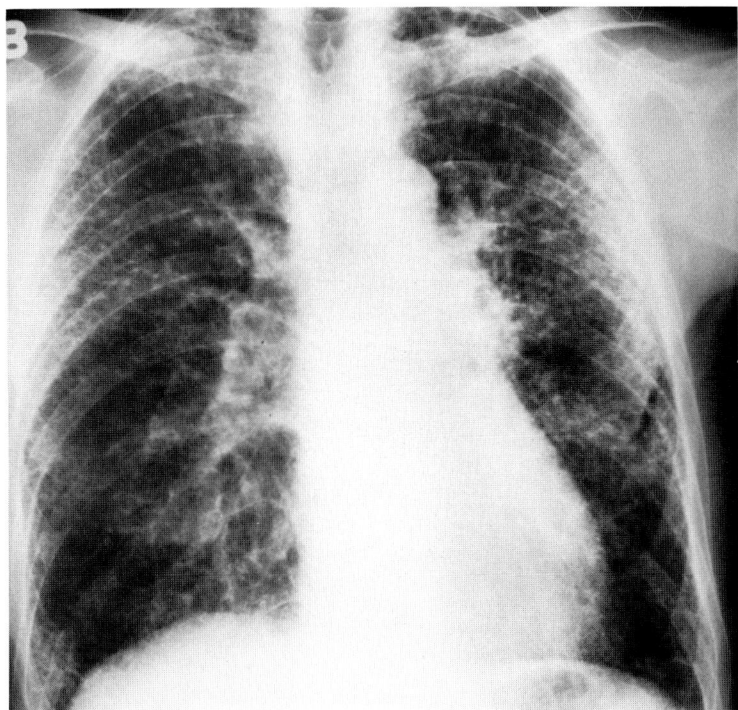

Figure 4.26. Diffuse reticulonodular shadows with honeycombing: Advanced radiological pattern of interstitial fibrotic lung disease. There is a diffuse "honeycomb" appearance involving both lungs, with a "shaggy" cardiac outline. Severe respiratory disability was present. Lung function tests showed a restrictive pattern with a compliance loss and a diffusion defect. A lung biopsy confirmed asbestos bodies in an end-stage lung with diffuse collagenization of the lung interstitium.

significantly predicted by fiber concentration. Abnormality on radiographs was, in general, also significantly associated with age. The younger workers, ie, up to the age of 40 years, had fewer parenchymal abnormalities than men over 40 years old. In this latter group, as many as 9% showed parenchymal opacities.[57]

Areas of dense fibrotic concentrations, ie, severe parenchymal fibrosis, have been described in asbestosis.[58] These areas are recognized as diffuse areas of parenchymal opacification. They are infrequent, but when noted, they are predominantly in the lower zones. Additionally, large, more homogenous opacities, although uncommon, are occasionally noted in chest radiographs of asbestos-exposed workers.[5] These areas of massive fibrosis, which by definition exceed 1 cm, present as circumscribed or ill-defined lesions (Fig. 4.27). They are nonsegmental and in asbestosis are found in both upper and lower zones of the lung.[59] They are invariably associated with diffuse pleural fibrosis,[60] often become very large, and can be multiple. Unlike the large opacities found on the chest x-ray films of gold or coal workers, they do not appear to migrate to the mediastinum. Cavitation has not been described with large opacities in asbestosis. Not unexpectedly, asbestos workers with radiological evidence of large opacities have a significant associated profusion of irregular opacities in the lungs correlating with their high dust exposure; these changes include fine and coarse parenchymal linear opacities of the lungs, as well as pleural lesions.[36] In one group of asbestos workers studied, histological examination of the massive opacities showed, in addition to the presence of asbestos fibers, hyaline and concentric fibrosis of the type associated with silicotic fibrosis. The high quartz content of the South African amphibole probably influences the appearance of these lesions. An infective element, as in massive

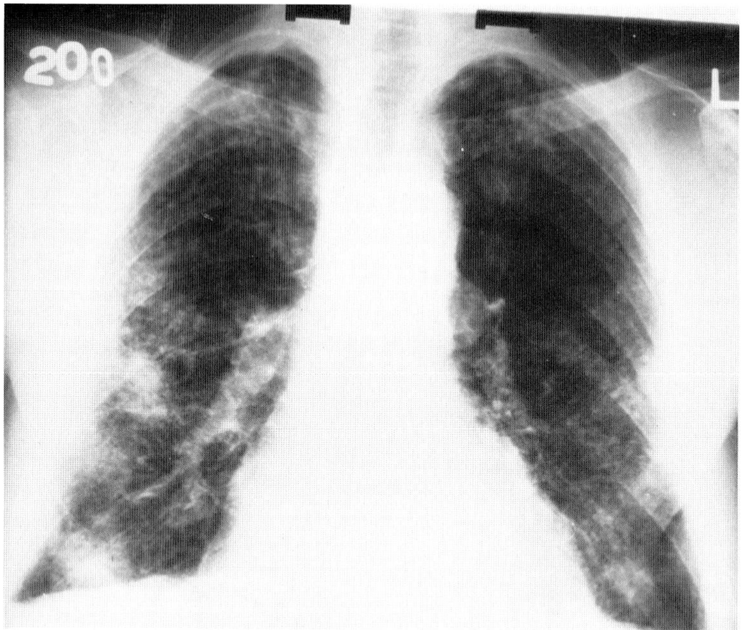

Figure 4.27. Extensive nodules with large basal opacities. Extensive diffuse nodular opacities involving all zones of both lungs, with massive opacities in the lower zones (changes influenced by asbestos and silica combination).
Asbestos exposure with added silica, 25 years.

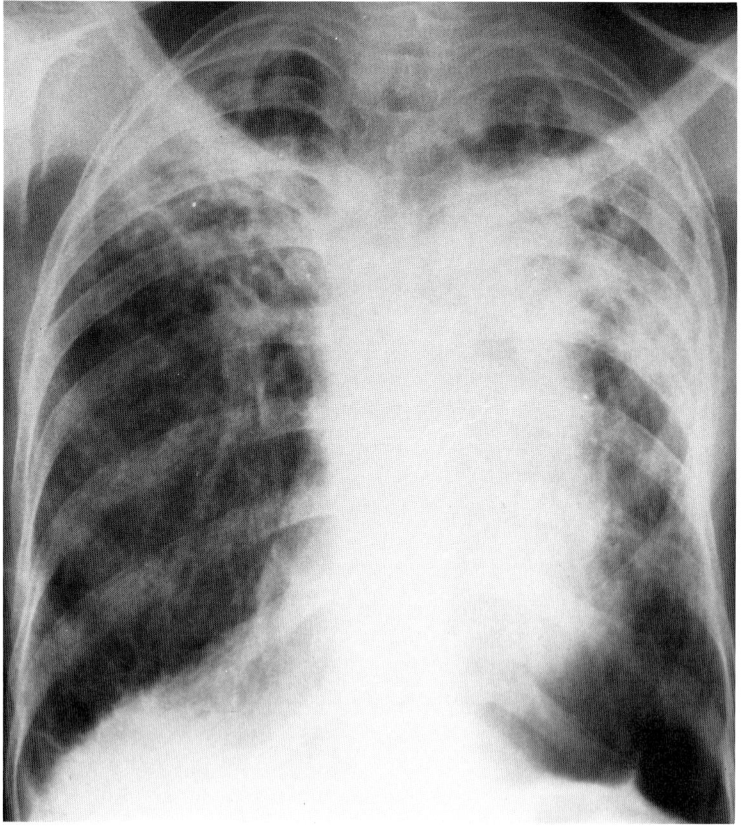

Figure 4.28. Massive opacities in asbestosis with associated silica exposure. Bilateral upper zone massive opacities after many years of asbestos exposure with silica dust inhalation. The massive opacities associated with silicosis are predominantly in the upper zones associated with marked fibrosis. The lower two thirds of the lungs demonstrate irregular opacities. At left base there is an area of hyperradiancy with diaphragmatic adhesions. Worked in an asbestos factory under bad conditions, then for 3 years in a gold mine, followed by 12 years of low asbestos dust exposure. Autopsy: No evidence of tuberculosis. The large masses consist of irregularly disposed collagenous tissue packed with asbestos bodies.

fibrosis of gold miners, might also play a role in the formation of massive opacities in asbestosis.[5] The concentration of inhaled fibers, as well as the duration of exposure, is the most likely factor in the production of the massive fibrosis. This is exemplified by four asbestos miners exposed to a high dust concentration over a prolonged period. Three of these suffered continuous exposure in excess of 10 years[5] (Fig. 4.28).

Advanced and florid roentgenographic evidence of pulmonary asbestosis has a definite pathologic correlation, ie, severe macroscopic evidence of asbestotic fibrosis being present at autopsy. Conversely, minor and sometimes moderate fibrosis of the lung at postmortem examination has no preceding radiographic evidence of abnormalities.[5]

Rheumatoid Pneumoconioses in Asbestosis

Rheumatoid pneumoconiosis[61] has certain characteristic radiological features. A number of rounded, usually almost peripheral lung nodules appear over a few months. Their size varies from 0.5 to approximately 5 cm, although generally they do not exceed 2 to 2.5 cm. They occasionally precede radiographic changes of pneumoconiosis or appear with minimal associated lung changes.[61] Some of these necrobiotic nodules additionally cavitate. These patients have rheumatoid arthritis, as manifested by rheumatoid factor in their serum. Radiographic features can antedate the clinical appearance of rheumatoid arthritis.[6] Despite the statement that the syndrome can be associated with asbestosis, its manifestation remains limited to isolated case reports.

Problems in the Radiological Diagnosis of Asbestosis

The presumptive diagnosis of asbestosis and asbestos-related pleural changes in the correct context, ie, in a person with a known exposure history, usually offers little difficulty. Problems, however, arise in those cases where basal "fibrotic" lesions of a different etiology are encountered. The radiologist is hard pressed in these situations to offer a diagnosis. Conversely, there will be occasions when a presumptive diagnosis of asbestosis will be incorrect despite the elicitation of an exposure history. Asbestosis possesses no pathognomic clinical or radiographic features.

Equal involvement of the lower lung zones by fibrosis with slow progression, associated pleural thickening, plaque formation, and costophrenic sulcus obliteration are features that favor the diagnosis of asbestosis. Basal lung abnormalities also result from other pathology, eg, scleroderma, rheumatoid disease, long-standing sarcoid disease, idiopathic or organic fibrosing alveolitis, lymphangitis carcinomatosis, and multiple neurofibromatosis.

Rapid progression of lung changes over months to 2 to 3 years should raise the possibility that the disease is not asbestosis. Upper zonal distribution of lesions or a honeycomb pattern is unusual in asbestosis. Certain connective tissue disease, eg, rheumatoid, can have an associated pleural effusion that may be unilateral. Constitutional symptoms and clinical manifestations unrelated to asbestosis require careful investigation to establish the final diagnosis. There will obviously be occasions where lung biopsy is necessary, eg, atypical x-ray features associated with abnormal progression or distribution of lung changes—constitutional symptoms and diseases or drugs that are known to simulate lung changes of asbestosis.

Incidence of Mesothelioma

Malignant mesothelioma remains a rare tumor with a variable incidence of 1 to 9 cases per million persons per year in the general population of the Western countries.[62] It sometimes follows a relatively brief but intense asbestos exposure. The proportion of cases attributable to asbestos exposure varies; it is greatest in the more highly industrialized communities. However, even in these communities no relationship with asbestos can be established in a proportion varying from 10% to 30% of the cases reported. Not all mesotheliomas are due to asbestos: eg, endemic mesothelioma in some areas of Turkey is believed to be due to a fibrous form of zeolite; in India it is due to vegetable fiber. Mesothelioma, when attributable to asbestos, usually has a latent period of 20 to 40 years or longer.[63]

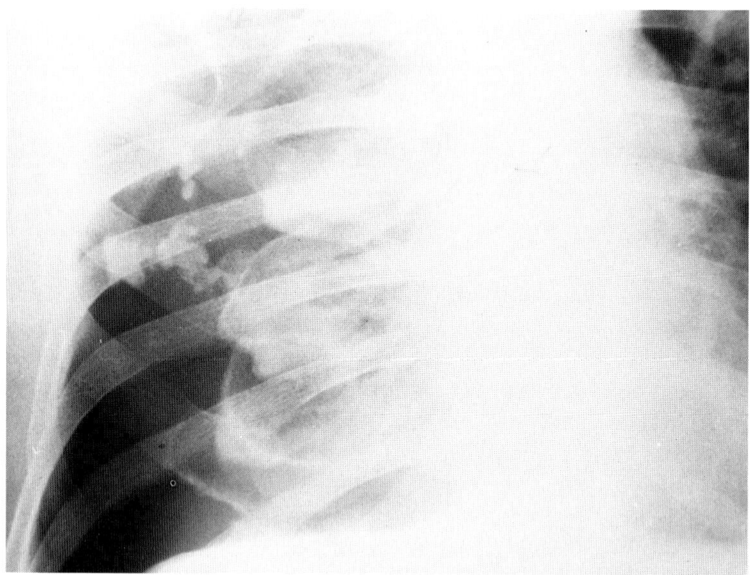

Figure 4.29. Mesothelioma with a spontaneous pneumothorax. Large pneumothorax with peripheral nodules of mesothelioma visible along the surface of the retracted lung representing multifocal lesions. Calcified parietal pleural plaques of previous asbestos exposure. The pleural space remains free of adhesions. A pleural effusion developed subsequently. Aspiration confirmed malignant serosal cells and a raised hyaluronic content of the pleural fluid.
Radiographer to a mobile x-ray unit for asbestos mines.

Presentation of Mesothelioma

More than half (56%) of a group of patients with mesothelioma presented with a large pleural effusion, and dyspnea was the principal complaint. An additional 16% had small effusions. Initially, patients with mesothelioma need not be very ill. Three of a group of 78 patients suffering from mesothelioma had recurrent effusions for more than 3 years before developing other symptoms. In an additional 49 cases, there were either no effusions or effusions too small to be a likely cause of dyspnea.[64] Pain in small effusions occurred in 79% of patients, whereas only 64% with large effusions complained of pain.

Pain is a common and frequent accompaniment of mesothelioma. Rather unusual presentations of pain and sometimes fever of about 2 months' duration preceding the tumor advent by 1 to 5 years have been recorded. Intermittent recurrent pleurisy as often as two to five times has also been described before other features develop. Unusually a mesothelioma presents with spontaneous pneumothorax[36] (Fig. 4.29). Abnormal chest x-ray findings preceded clinical symptoms by 3 to 4 months in 3% of Law et al's series.[64]

The tumor arises from either the parietal or visceral pleural surface. Malignant mesothelioma is an inexorable progressive tumor that encases the pleural surface and invades the adjacent structures of the mediastinum and chest wall (Fig. 4.30) and is often fairly extensive at initial presentation (Figs. 4.31 to 4.33).

Mesothelial extension can result in other complaints and clinical manifestations. These include dysphagia, superior vena caval obstruction, stridor, shoulder pain, a large contralateral effusion, troublesome ascites, abdominal pain, small-bowel obstruction, and supraventricular tachycardia.[64]

The tumor extension is at first intrathoracic, involving the mediastinum. Total encasement of the thoracic cage and mediastinum occurs with extension to the diaphragm, contralateral pleura, pericardium, and peritoneum. Distal metastases, though not common, are often disclosed at postmortem. These include lesions in the contralateral

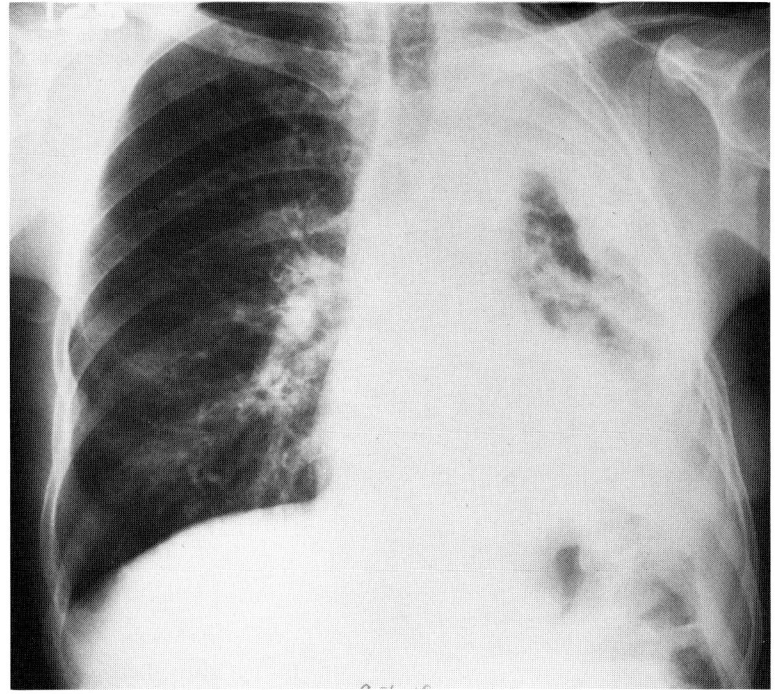

Figure 4.30. Lung and mediastinal encasement by malignant mesothelioma. Total encasement by tumor of left lung and mediastinum. The trachea is only slightly displaced, the mediastinum is fixed, and the left hemithorax shows volume loss. Asbestos exposure 24 years previously.

lung, liver, adrenal, kidney, and brain.[64] Local thoracic cage involvement with adjacent bony destruction can be overlooked if attention is not directed to the ribs and vertebrae.[65]

Radiological Features

The diagnosis of primary or metastatic pleural tumor requires a high index of suspicion in the patient with an obscure pleural effusion and chest pain. Pleural effusion can develop in all cases of mesothelioma, but has been variably reported as the initial presentation in 29% to 80% of cases.[66] The early mesothelial tumor implants, if very small, escape radiographic detection. Computed tomographic examination of the chest permits superlative demonstration of the underlying serosal growth. The induction of a pneumothorax is now a superfluous procedure. In the past it was often considered essential to profile the submerged tumor mass with an induced pneumothorax. However, CT is not always able to detect superficial diaphragmatic involvement.[67]

Significantly, no shift of the mediastinum occurs despite the presence of a large pleural effusion. This fixity is due to the encasement of the mediastinum causing loss of normal mediastinal movement (Fig. 4.30). The inability to expand the underlying lung results in a significant decrease in the volume of the affected thorax. Accompanying features include rib crowding, a scoliosis convex to the tumor side, and an elevated diaphragm. Bilateral pleural effusions are infrequent in mesothelioma. Their occurrence at initial presentation indicates bilateral disease and has been documented in 10% of cases[66,68] (Fig. 4.34).

Pleural thickening caused by the mesothelioma is initially diffuse, occurring unilaterally in 40% to 65% of cases, but stud-like pleural protrusions may manifest themselves early. Unfortunately, they can escape detection or be confused with plaque formation. A diffuse thick serosal encasement of the lung surface indicates a late manifestation of the malignant mesothelioma. This rind-like pleural tumorous thickening has a lobulated or crenated margin and can encase the entire peripheral chest wall and mediastinum, extending to the

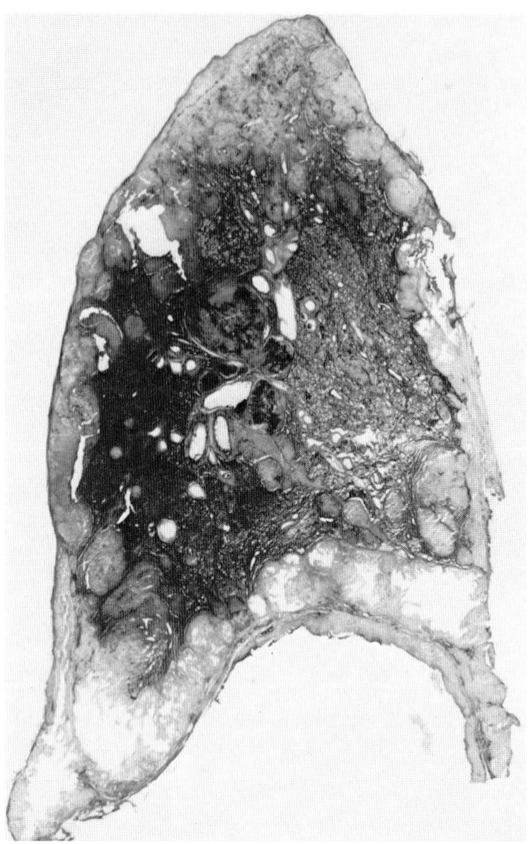

Figure 4.31. Malignant mesothelioma of the pleura encasing the lung with minimal extension into the interlobar fissure.

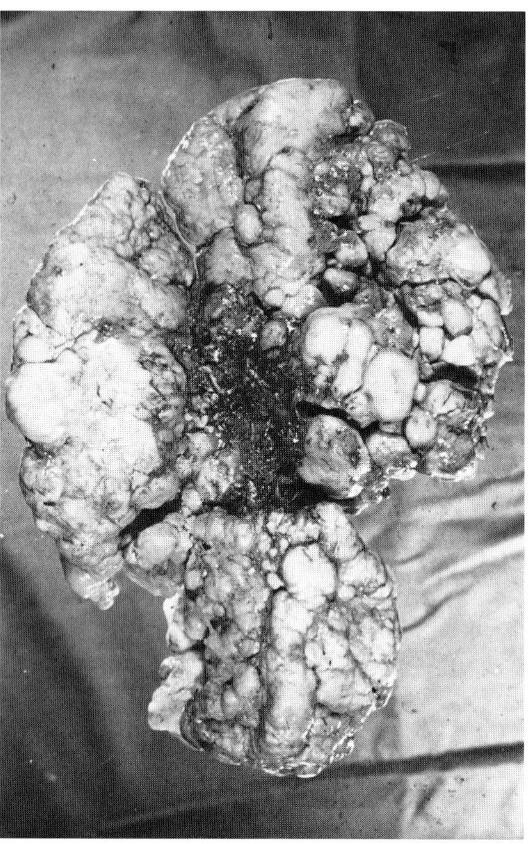

Figure 4.33. A florid mesothelioma with extensive lung encasement resulting in almost total compression of the lung.

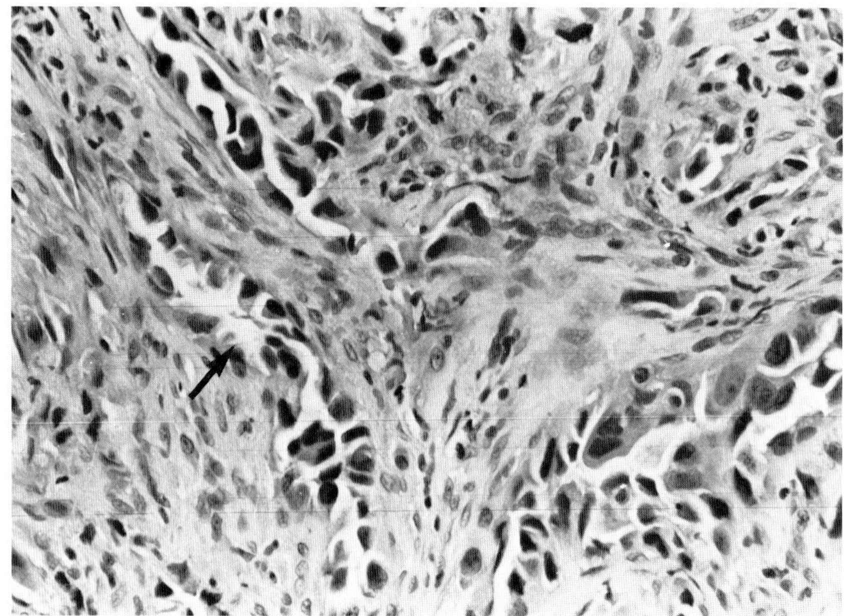

Figure 4.32. Photomicrograph. Mesothelioma clefts lined by atypical malignant cells (*arrows*).

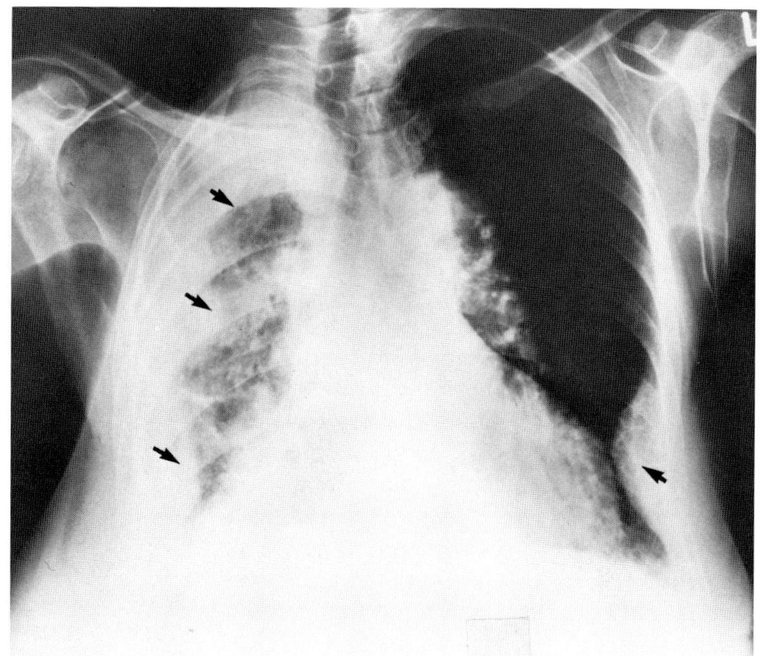

Figure 4.34. Bilateral pleural mesothelioma. The right hemithorax is encased by a mesothelioma with fixity of the mediastinum and associated hemithoracic volume reduction. The left basal pleural mass was also a mesothelioma. Asbestos exposure 40 years previously.

diaphragm. The lobular pleural thickening in some instances is most marked at the lung bases. If the patient survives long enough, the tumor with extension through the diaphragm results in bowel displacement and fixation. Gastrointestinal or even ureteric obstruction can then result. Contiguous invasion and obstruction produces superior or inferior vena caval syndromes; pericardial involvement with distortion of the cardiac outline, shape, or size; or esophageal encirclement with obstruction. Routine radiologic assessment requires venography to show caval obstruction, echocardiography to demonstrate the pericardial involvement, barium contrast studies to elucidate the esophageal and gastrointestinal status, and an intravenous pyelogram to demonstrate the renal situation,[35,66] whereas CT study offer the possibility of a comprehensive demonstration of the spread of the tumor in the thorax and below the diaphragm.[69]

The Tumor Silhouette

In the absence of a pleural effusion, the large tumor mass is easily visible and is unlike the disk-like change of a pleural plaque. The crenulated margin is sometimes only detected in profile, a lateral chest radiograph being necessary to demonstrate the edge of the growth silhouetted above the diaphragm. Multiple discrete masses are, however, more common than a single tumor.[68] The distinct feature of these masses is their large size, which often exceeds 5 cm when first detected.[66] Even in the presence of a large pleural effusion, the mesothelioma, like the "tip of the iceberg" (Fig. 4.33), might be seen protruding through the associated fluid.

Soft-tissue tumor invasion, ie, subcutaneous extension, is frequent at previous aspiration sites or following thoracotomy. The spread of the tumor subcutaneously is less common as a spontaneous phenomenon.[64]

Lung Nodules

Satellite lung lesions can result from direct spread or permeation of the lymphatics in septa or around the blood vessels and bronchi. Their presence is noted in 4% to 15% of cases.[66] Computed tomography separates lung lesions from pleural masses. The interfissural "parenchymal mass" is, in fact, sometimes the mesothelial growth taking origin from the visceral pleural surface. Alternatively, the primary pleural tumor often extends into an interlobar fissure.[70]

Hilar Lymphadenopathy

Extension of the disease along the mediastinal pleural reflection gives rise to hilar prominence simulating lymph node involvement. The latter is less frequent than tumor encasement of the hilum, occurring in only 12% to 26% of cases.[66]

Bony Thoracic Involvement

Tumor pressure can result in periosteal reaction initially and finally in rib destruction. Bony involvement in mesothelioma is variably reported in 2% to 20% of cases. In the undiagnosed patient, it is difficult to separate the peripheral mass and associated rib destruction from a malignant peripheral primary or secondary lung cancer or a neoplasm arising in a rib, nerve sheath, fascia of the intercostal muscles, or other thoracic structures. Pleural metastases have resulted from breast carcinoma, lymphoms, thymus, stomach, adrenal, thyroid, and pancreatic malignancies; 95% of pleural tumors are, in fact, metastatic; only 5% of malignant pleural tumors are primary.[71]

Associated Changes Indicating Asbestos Exposure in Mesothelioma

Accompanying signs of asbestosis have been described in one third of the cases of mesothelioma. The pleural plaques and lung changes are often obscured on the side of the tumor. However, it is possible that the occasional calcified plaque is engulfed by the progress of the serosal growth and escapes detection. The parenchyma or pleura in the opposite lung is usually only moderately involved.[72]

The severity of asbestosis does not appear to influence the development of mesothelioma, a minimal exposure to asbestos dust years before the development of a mesothelioma being the usual history. There is, however, a dose-response relationship in the development of mesothelioma.[73]

Diagnosis of mesothelioma during life is dependent upon securing an adequate sample of tissue at pleural biopsy. This may necessitate thoracoscopy or even thoracotomy; even so, this may fail to produce evidence of malignancy. Pleural fluid cytology, while possibly revealing malignant cells, does not finalize the diagnosis. Elevated concentration of hyalouronic acid in the pleural fluid is not specific for either mesothelioma or malignancy.[74]

Asbestos and Lung Cancer

Radiological detection of early lung cancer remains a constant challenge. The mosaic of radiologic changes in asbestosis confuses the problem of early recognition of the associated lung neoplasm. Nevertheless, the synergistic effect of cigarette smoking and asbestos exposure in producing lung cancer is well established.[2] There appears to be an eightfold excess risk for lung cancer deaths in asbestos-exposed workers who do not smoke; but this risk is greatly increased in those workers who smoke. A dose response exists, with lung cancer being markedly more common in groups who are more heavily exposed to inhalation of asbestos dust[75] (Fig. 4.35)

Radiology

Lung cancer in asbestosis often closely resembles a circumscribed peripheral pleural mass, much like the presentation of mesothelioma. Despite the well-documented radiologic changes associated with pulmonary cancer, differentiation from mesothelioma is often not possible. Hilar lymph node enlargement, distant metastases, bony secondaries with a small lung lesion, and the character of the lung opacity—ie, smooth outline or peripheral lymphangitic extension from the opacity—are more in keeping with a primary lung cancer than a primary serosal tumor.[35]

Other Asbestos-Related Malignancies

An excess of gastrointestinal malignancies other than peritoneal mesothelioma possibly occurs in asbestos-exposed individuals. Attention has also been drawn to the possibility that asbestos workers carry an increased risk for cancer of the larynx. There may be a multitude of synergistic factors that interact to produce laryngeal cancer.

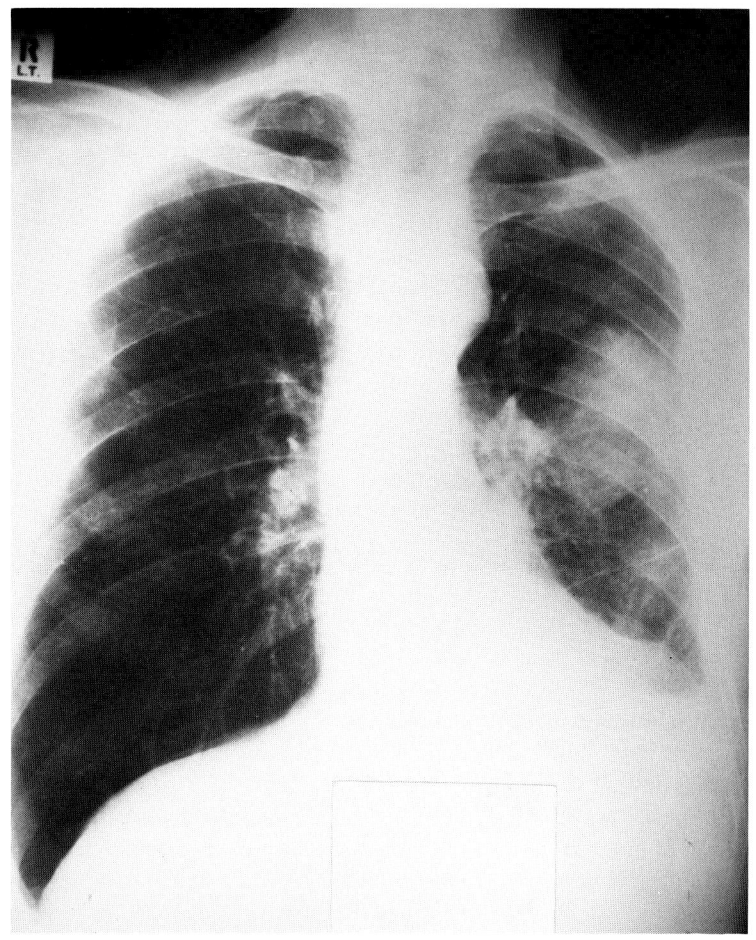

Figure 4.35. Asbestos and carcinoma. Large mass in the left lung with associated "malignant" pleural effusion (proved to be a carcinoma).
Asbestos exposure in excess of 15 years; regular cigarette smoker.

Computed Tomography—Assessment of Pulmonary Abestosis and Mesothelioma of the Lungs and Abdomen

Regular surveillance of people working with, or exposed to, asbestos is conveniently and economically managed by annual chest radiographs. Large-scale surveys of asbestos-exposed workers remain heavily reliant on the practical use of chest films.

Subpleural fat pads are sometimes erroneously mistaken for noncalcified pleural plaques. Generally, these fat pads are larger and more extensive in obese subjects; however, even thin patients can develop extensive pleural fat deposits.

Fat deposits arising from the surfaces of the ribs and hanging over the adjacent intercostal muscles tend to concentrate at the level of the midthoracic wall (in the region of the fourth to eighth ribs), between the anterior axillary line and the angle of ribs posteriorly. Small lobules of mobile fat also occur within the visceral pleura along the interlobar fissures. Computed tomography is convincingly able to distinguish these fat pads from pleural plaques by their low attenuation. Moreover, when pleural plaques occur in areas of subpleural fat deposition, the CT scan will demonstrate the plaque on the surface of the fat collection.[76]

The greatest problem in diagnosing early pleural abnormalities lies in distinguishing pleural from normal companion shadows. Abnormal pleura is easily recognized on CT scans (Fig. 4.36).

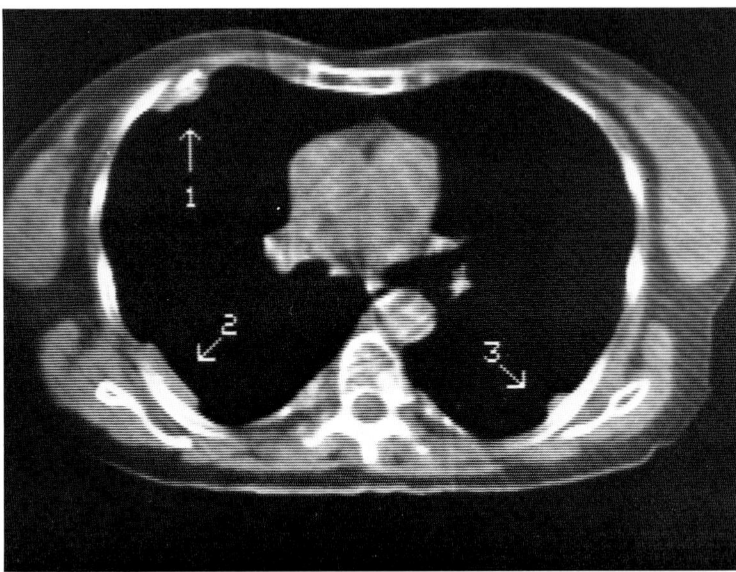

Figure 4.36. CT in the assessment of pleural plaques. CT has a contributory role in areas of diagnostic dispute. Multiple uncalcified symmetrical posterior plaques (*arrows 2 and 3*) and calcified anterior plaque (*arrow 1*).

The extent and circumferential nature of pleural changes are more reliably assessed by CT scans than by chest films.[77] The thickened pleura is visible adjacent to the underlying ribs. The asbestotic plaques are usually of uniform density, unless calcified, and can easily be seen as a local protuberance of soft tissue adjacent to the ribs. With adjustment of the window setting, the area can be "highlighted" on CT. Calcification is not always dense enough to be recognized on a plain radiograph, whereas CT is more sensitive in this regard.

Computed Tomography in Lung Fibrosis

The CT scan demonstrates underlying parenchymal lung changes despite extensive associated pleural disease (Fig. 4.37). Computed tomography has an important role to offer in cases of contentions legislation where compensation and liability in asebestos-exposed individuals arise.

The assessment of interlobar fissues by CT is somewhat limited. This is because only a small portion of the fissure is demonstrated, as the body plane is cut axially on CT, whereas the entire fissure can be seen when cut tangentially on a plain chest radiograph. Nevertheless, thickened fissures and plaque formation in a fissure are demonstrable using high resolution CT.

High-resolution CT can demonstrate both asbestos-related pleural disease and parenchymal abnormalities consistent with asbestosis; but this method may have limitations in assessing diffuse pleural thickening.[78] High-resolution CT should be used to complement the clinical and radiological assessment of subjects that have had asbestos exposure and is not meant to be the initial investigative procedure.

The diagnosis of interstitial lung disease on CT can confidently be made by demonstrating thickened septal and intralobular lines, nondependent lines or dense bands not related to the vessels,[79] subpleural curvilinear densities, and honeycombing. Some of these changes may be obscured or induced by gravity-dependent density,[78-80] in which case the patient may have to be scanned in the prone (nondependent) position to demonstrate the persistence of the structural abnormalities of the interstitium.[78-80]

Computed tomography complements the clinical and radiological assessment of patients who have had asbestos exposure and can resolve contentious abnormalities seen on the chest radiograph. The chest radiograph, however, provides a cost-effective, reliable, and easily available examination of

Figure 4.37. Early interstitial fibrotic change of asbestosis demonstrated by CT. CT scan at diaphragm level (large white areas) showing bilateral early irregular linear lung infiltrates (*arrows 3 and 4*) not visible on chest radiograph. Note the associated extensive pleural thickening (*arrows 1 and 2*).

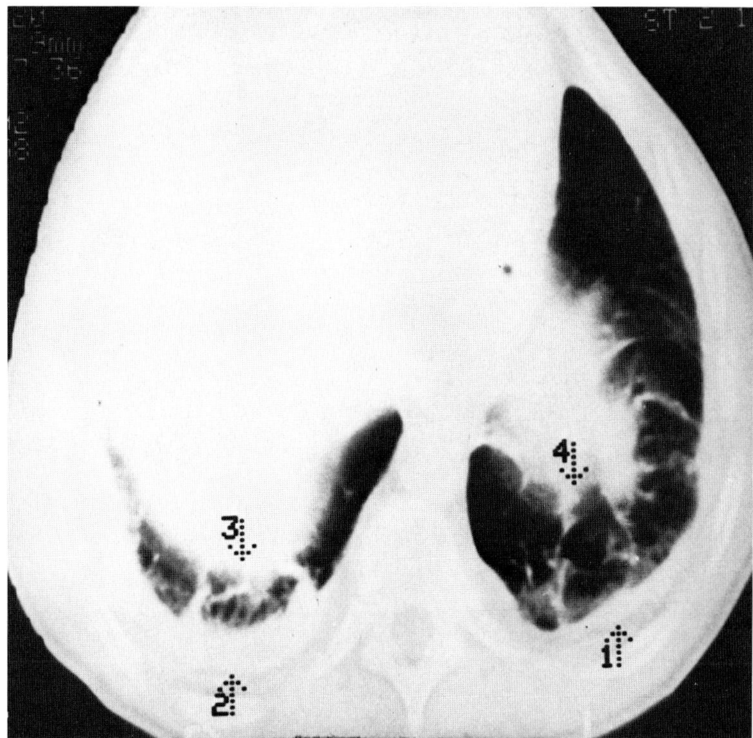

the patient at risk, as well as efficient monitoring of the progress and changing pattern of parenchymal disease.

Computed Tomography in Mesothelioma

The chest radiograph in mesothelioma is not able to offer the same assessment as the CT examination. The unique three-dimensional ability of CT produces a more complete display of the disease, showing the extent of mediastinal, pericardial, chest wall, and transdiaphragmatic invasion. The disclosure of pericardial involvement, of subcarinal and retrotracheal masses, and of the spread of tumor through the hemidiaphragm with invasion of the liver, bowel, and retroperitoneal structures are now within the radiologist's capability using CT,[81] but cannot be assessed on the chest radiograph. A large pleural effusion on a chest radiograph interferes with the demonstration of either contiguous or disseminated extension of the disease.

Serial CT is now used to monitor therapy, providing an objective indication of tumor growth and reliably demonstrating the anatomic structures involved in the evolution of the tumor. With serial scans during treatment, tumor regression or growth can be measured, even when the patient's clinical status and plain films appear stable[69] (Figs. 4.38 and 4.39).

Computed Tomography in Peritoneal Mesothelioma

Primary peritoneal mesothelioma, while decidedly uncommon, is occasionally reported. They appear to be related to more prolonged and heavy asbestos exposure than is usual with pleural mesotheliomas.[82] Patients with peritoneal mesothelioma often complain of abdominal pain and increasing

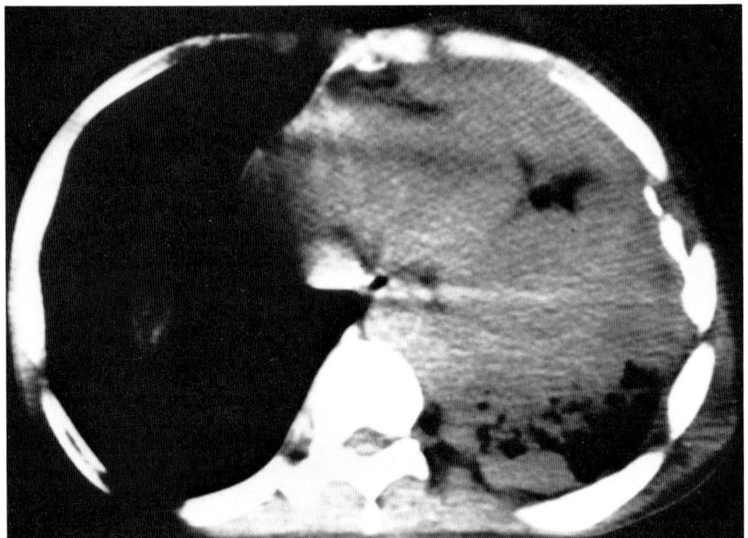

Figure 4.38. CT scan with a mesothelioma mass in the retrocrural region, and rib erosion of the left chest. The mesothelioma has spread over the diaphragm and through the aortic haitus with retroperitoneal invasion.

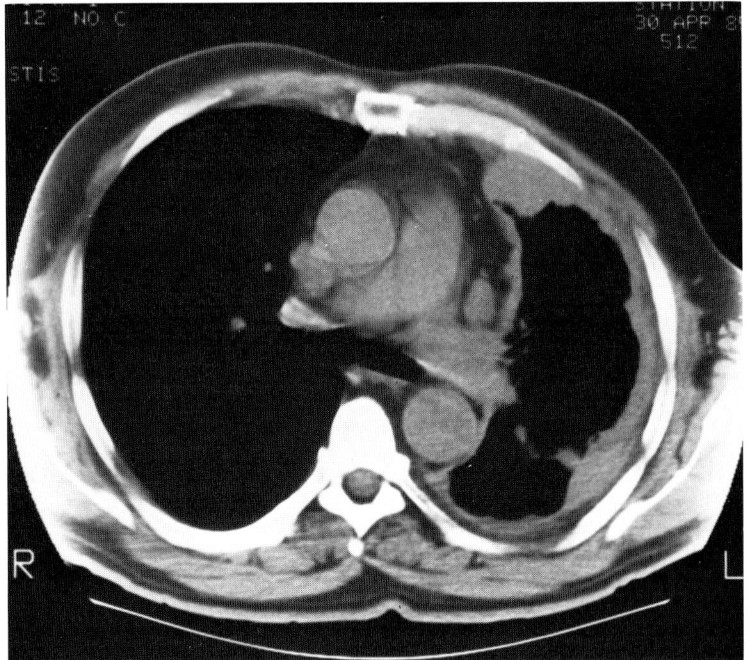

Figure 4.39. CT scan with mesothelioma mass and interlobar fissure invasion. Mesothelioma encasing the left hemithorax with associated volume loss and interlobar tumor extension. The malignancy has also extended into the anterior chest wall.

girth. Ascites and an abdominal mass are usually found at presentation. The serosal tumor spreads in a sheet-like manner over the peritoneal abdominal surface, but localized tumor masses or nodularities also occur. These changes are difficult to differentiate from gastrointestinal carcinomas, lymphomas, and diffuse carcinomatosis.

The CT evaluation of the abdomen reveals the true extent and nature of the tumor spread. Ascites is usually found; however, this does not obscure the associated soft-tissue masses. There may be sheet-like thickening of the entire mesentery. Fusion of the thickened peritoneum and omentum gives rise to a soft-tissue density between the bowel and the anterior abdominal wall. Soft-tissue thickening of the leaves of the mesentery gives rise to a stellate-like appearance of the rigid pleated mesentery.

The findings on CT of thickened peritoneum, ascites, pleated rigidity of the mesentery, and omental involvement suggest peritoneal mesothelioma[82] but are more usual with metastatic tumors.

References

1. Parkes WR: Asbestos related disorders. Br J Dis Chest 1973;67:261–300.
2. Becklake MR: State of the art: Asbestos related diseases of the lung and other organs; their epidemiology and implications for clinical practice. Am Rev Resp Dis 1976;114:187–227.
3. Parkes WR: Occupational Lung Disorders, ed. 2. Chapter: Silicates and Lung Disease. London, Butterworth, 1982, pp 233–332.
4. Morgan WKC, Seaton A: Occupational Lung Diseases. Chapter 9: Asbestosis. Philadelphia, WB Saunders Co, 1975, pp 124–148.
5. Solomon A, Goldstein B, Webster I, et al: Massive fibrosis in asbestosis. Envir Res 1971;4:430–439.
6. Fraser RG, Pare JAP: Diagnosis of Diseases of the Chest. The Pneumoconioses and Chemically Induced Lung Diseases. Philadelphia, WB Saunders Co, 1979, pp 1475–1570.
7. Casey KR, Rom WN, Moatamed F: Asbestos related diseases. Clin Chest Med 1981;2:179–201.
8. Harries PG: Experience with asbestos disease and its control in Great Britain's naval dockyards. Envir Res 1976;11:261–267.
9. Felton JP: Radiographic search for asbestos-related disease in naval ship-yard. Ann NY Acad Sci 1979;330:341–352.
10. Solomon A, Sluis-Cremer GK, Goldstein M: Visceral pleural plaque formation in asbestosis. Envir Res 1978;19:258–264.
11. Newhouse MT, Bienestock J: Respiratory tract defence mechanism. In Baum GL, Wolinsky E (eds): Textbook of Pulmonary Disease, ed 3. Boston, Little Brown & Co, 1983, pp 3–24.
12. Spencer H: Pathology of the Lung, vol 1, ed 3. Oxford, Pergamon Press, 1977, p 426.
13. Von Hayek M: The Human Lung. Krahl VE (trans). New York, Hafner, 1960.
14. Hourihane DOB, McCaughey WTE: Pathological aspect of asbestosis. Postgrad Med J 1966;42:613–622.
15. Webster I: The pathogenesis of asbestosis. Pneumoconiosis. Proceedings of the International Conference, Johannesburg, Shapiro HA (ed). Cape Town, Oxford University Press, 1969, pp 117–119.
16. Kleinerman J: Textbook of Pulmonary Diseases. Baum GL, Wolinsky E (eds). Boston, Little Brown & Co, Chapter 38, 1983, p 773.
17. Baker EL, Greene R: Incremental value of oblique chest radiographs in the diagnosis of asbestos-induced pleural disease. Am J Ind Dis 1982;3:17–22.
18. Solomon A: Industrial Shadows, Inaugural Lecture. Johannesburg. Witwatersrand University Press, 1977, pp 1–19.
19. Gilmartin D: The serratus anterior muscle on chest radiographs. Radiology 1979;131:629–635.
20. Gluck MC, Twigg HL, Ball MF, et al: Shadows bordering the lung on radiographs of normal and obese persons. Thorax 1972;27:232–238.
21. Epler GR, McLoud TC, Gaensler EA: Prevalence and incidence of benign asbestos pleural effusion in a working population. JAMA 1982;247:617–622.
22. ILO 1980 International Classification of Pneumoconioses.
23. Greene R, Boggis C, Jantsch H: Asbestos-related pleural thickening: Effect of threshold criteria on interpretation. Radiology 1984;152:569–573.
24. Solomon A: The radiology of asbestosis. S Afr Med J 1969;43:847–851.
25. Solomon A, Sluis-Cremer GK, Glyn-Thomas R, et al: Calcified plaques on mediastinal pleural reflections associated with asbestos dust exposure. Am J Ind Med 1984;6:53–57.
26. Hillerdal G: Non-malignant asbestos pleural diseases. Thorax 1981;36:669–675.
27. Harries PG: The effects and control of diseases associated with exposure to asbestos in a naval dockyard. MD Thesis, London, 1970.
28. Miller A, Tierstern AS, Selikoff IJ: Ventilatory failure due to asbestos pleurisy. AM J Med 1983; 65(6):911–919.
29. Brityon MG: Asbestos pleural diseases. Br J Dis Chest 1982;76:1–10.
30. Mattson SB: Monosymptomatic exudative pleurisy in persons exposed to asbestos dust. Scand J Respir Dis 1975;56:263–272.
31. Fletcher DE, Edge JR: The early radiologic changes in pulmonary and pleural asbestosis. Clin Radiol 1970;21:355–365.
32. Rous V, Studney J: Aetiology of pleural plaques. Thorax 1970;25:270–284.
33. Lumley KPS: Physiological changes in asbestos pleural disease, in Watton WH (ed): Inhaled particles IV. Oxford and New York, Pergamon Press, 1977, p 781.

34. Sheer G: Asbestos associated disease in employees of a Devon port dockyard. Ann NY Acad Sci 1979; 300:281–288.
35. Solomon A: The radiology of asbestos-related disease with special reference to diffuse mesothelioma. Semin Oncol 1981;8:290–301.
36. Solomon A: Radiology of asbestosis. Proceedings of the International Conference, Johannesburg, 1969. Shapiro HA (ed). London, Cape Town Oxford University Press, 1970, pp 243–247.
37. Selikoff IJ: The occurrence of pleural calcification among asbestos insulation workers. Ann NY Acad Sci 1965;132:351–367.
38. Sluis-Cremer GK, du Toit RSJ: Asbestos-related radiological changes in residents of South African amphibole asbestos mining fields and the fibre counts to which they may have been exposed, in Wagner JC (ed): Biological Effects of Mineral Fibres, vol 2, 1980, pp 559–563.
39. Andersen HA, Selikoff IJ: Pleural reactions to environmental agents. Fed Proc 1978;37:2496–2500.
40. Hourihane DOB, Lessof L, Richardson PC: Hyaline and calcified pleural plaques as an index of exposure to asbestos. A study of radiological and pathological features of 100 cases, with a consideration of epidemiology. Br J Med 1966;1:1069–1074.
41. Solomon A, Irwig LM, Sluis-Cremer GK, et al: Thickening of pulmonary interlobar fissures: exposure-response relationship in crocidolite and amosite miners. Br J Ind Med 1979;36:195–198.
42. Cunningham's Textbook of Anatomy, ed 12. Romanes GJ (ed). Oxford, Oxford University Press, 1981, p 514.
43. Sargent EN, Jacobson G, Wilkinson EE: Diaphragmatic pleural calcification following short occupational exposure to asbestos. AJR 1972;115:473–478.
44. Meurmann L: Asbestos bodies and pleural plaques in a Finnish series of autopsy cases. Act Pathol Microbiol Immunol Scand [Suppl] 1966, p 181.
45. Roberts WC, Ferrans VJ: Pure collagen plaques on the diaphragm and pleura. Chest 1972;61:357–360.
46. Hirsch A, Di Menza L, Dorbon F, et al: Diaphragmatic straightness in 302 asbestos-exposed patients: Biological effects of mineral fibres, vol 2. Wagner JC (ed). IARC Sci Publ 1980;30:523–526.
47. Dernevik L, Gatzinsky P, Hultman E, et al: Shrinking pleuritis with atelectasis. Thorax 1982;37: 252–258.
48. Mintzer RA, Gore RM, Vogelzang RL, et al: Rounded atelectasis and its association with asbestos-induced pleural disease. Radiology 1981; 139:567–570.
49. Tylen U, Nilsson U: Computed tomography in pulmonary pseudotumors and their relation to asbestos exposure. J Comput Assist Tomogr 1982;6(2): 229–237.
50. Case records of the Massachusetts General Hospital. N Engl J Med 1983;308(24):1466–1472.
51. Mintzer RA, Cugell DW: The association of asbestos-induced pleural disease and round atelectasis. Chest 1982;81:457–460.
52. Soutar GA, Simon G, Turner-Warwick M: The radiology of asbestos-induced disease of the lungs. Br J Dis Chest 1974;68:235–252.
53. Polakoff PL, Horn BR, Schere OR: Prevalence of radiographic abnormalities among Northern California shipyard workers. Ann NY Acad Sci 1979;330:333–339.
54. Pearle JL: Smoking and duration of asbestos exposure in the production of functional and roentgenographic abnormalities in shipyard workers. J Occup Med 1982;24:37–40.
55. Becklake MR, Liddell FDK, Manfreda J, et al: Radiological changes after withdrawing from asbestos exposure. Br J Ind Med 1979;36:23–28.
56. Gregor A, Parkes RW, du Bois R, et al: Radiographic progression of asbestosis. Preliminary report. Ann NY Acad Sci 1979;330:147–156.
57. Irwig LM, du Toit RSJ, Sluis-Cremer GK, et al: Risk of asbestosis in Crocidolite and Amosite mines in South Africa. Ann NY Acad Sci 1979;330:35–52.
58. Hurwitz M: Roentgenologic aspects of asbestosis. AJR 1961;85:256–262.
59. Hillerdal G: Asbestos exposure and upper lobe involvement. AJR 1982;139:1163–1166.
60. Green RA, Dimcheff DG: Massive bilateral upper lobe fibrosis secondary to asbestos exposure. Chest 1974;65:52–55.
61. Telleson WG: Rheumatoid pneumoconiosis (Caplan's syndrome) in an asbestos worker. Thorax 1961;16:372–377.
62. McDonald JC, McDonald AD: Epidemiology of mesothelioma from estimated incidence. Prev Med 1977;6:42–46.
63. Medical Advisory Panel to the Asbestos International Association: Criteria for the diagnosis of asbestosis and considerations in the attribution of lung cancer and mesothelioma to asbestos exposure. Int Arch Occup Environ Health 1982;49:357–361.
64. Law MR, Hodson ME, Turner Warwick M: Malignant mesothelioma of the pleura: clinical aspects and symptomatic treatment. Eur J Respir Dis 1984;65:162–168.
65. Steiner RM, Cooper RW, Brodovsky H: Rib destruction: a neglected finding in malignant mesothelioma. Clin Radiol 1982;33:61–65.
66. Wechsler RJ, Rao VM, Steiner RM: The radiology of malignant mesothelioma. CRC Crit Rev Diag Imaging 1984;20:283–310.

67. Law MR, Gregor A, Husband JE, et al: Computed tomography in the assessment of malignant mesothelioma of the pleura. Clin Radiol 1982;33:67–70.
68. Solomon A: Radiological features of diffuse mesothelioma. Proceedings of the International Conference, Johannesburg, 1969. Edited by H.A. Shapiro. London, Cape Town Oxford University Press, 1970, pp 261–265.
69. Mirvis S, Dutcher JP, Haney PJ, et al: CT of malignant pleural mesotheliomata. AJR 1983;140:665–670.
70. Solomon A: A comparative study of mesothelioma and asbestosis using computed tomography and conventional chest radiography. Letter to the Editor, Radiology 1983;148:316.
71. Theros EG, Feigin DS: Pleural tumors and pulmonary tumors. Semin Roentgenol 1977;12:239–247.
72. Solomon A: Radiological features of diffuse mesothelioma. Environ Res 1970;3:330–335.
73. Newhouse MT, Berry G: Predictions of mortality from mesothelial tumors in asbestos factory workers. Br J Ind Med 1976;33:147–151.
74. Castor CW, Naylor B: Acid mucopolysaccharide composition of serous effusions. Cancer 1967;20: 462-466.
75. Newhouse MT: Epidemiology of asbestos related tumors. Semin Oncol 1981;8:250–257.
76. Sargent EN, Boswell WD, Ralls PW, et al: Subpleural fat pads in patients exposed to asbestos: Distinction from non-calcified pleural plaques. Radiology 1984;152:273–277.
77. Kreel L: Computed tomography of the thorax. Radiol Clin North Am 1978;16:575–584.
78. Aberle DR, Gamsu G, Ray CS, et al: Asbestos-related pleural and parenchymal fibrosis, detection with high-resolution CT. Radiology 1988;166:729–734.
79. Bergin CJ, Muller NL: CT of interstitial lung disease. A diagnostic approach. AJR 1987;148: 8–15.
80. Friedman AC, Fiel SB, Fisher MS, et al: Asbestos-related pleural disease and asbestosis. A comparison of CT and chest radiography AJR 1988;150:269–275.
81. Alexander E, Clark RA, Celley DP, et al: CT of malignant pleural mesothelioma. AJR 1981;137: 287-291.
82. Whitley NO, Brenner DE, Antman KH, et al: CT of peritoneal mesothelioma: analysis of eight cases. AJR 1982;138:531–535.

5

The Radiographic Features of Coal Workers' Pneumoconiosis

W.K.C. Morgan

Introduction

The inhalation of coal mine dust may lead, under certain circumstances, to three distinct conditions, namely, coal workers' pneumoconiosis (CWP), silicosis, and industrial bronchitis.[1] Silicosis is uncommon in coal miners and usually results from the aerosolization of sand that is applied to the rails or tracks in order to provide traction for the electric or diesel locomotives that are used in the United States to haul coal from the face to the portal. Occasionally silicosis may occur in coal miners, specifically "hard headers" and "roof bolters." In these jobs the drills used by the miners traverse the coal seam and enter strata of rock lying above or below the coal seam. Many of these strata contain significant concentrations of free silica. Industrial bronchitis affects the airways and is a nonspecific response that results from the prolonged inhalation either of inert dusts or irritant gases, eg, sulfur dioxide.[2,3] Coal workers' pneumoconiosis is the condition that develops following prolonged inhalation of coal dust and is best defined as the deposition of coal mine dust in the lung parenchyma and the tissue's reaction to its presence.

Clearly it is possible for limited quantities of coal dust to be deposited in the lungs without producing a tissue response. The alveolar deposition of coal and other dusts leads to an outpouring of macrophages into the alveolar spaces. The macrophage ingests the dust particles and may migrate with its ingested particles to the terminal bronchiole, from where it is carried to the nasopharynx by the mucociliary escalator, and then either coughed up and expelled or swallowed. Alternatively, the macrophage may migrate into the interstitium and hence find its way into the lymphatics and lymph nodes where the foreign particles are deposited. Only when the lungs' defenses are overwhelmed with the result that particles accumulate in the parenchyma and thereby lead to the development of a pathological response, eg, fibrosis, alveolar proteinosis, can disease be said to be present. When the accumulation of dust particles in the lung and elsewhere in the respiratory tract is not associated with symptoms, decreased lung function, or an effect on life expectancy, it cannot be regarded as a disease in the true sense of the word. It is vitally important to distinguish between a physiological or adaptive response and an adverse health effect. Whereas the former constitutes a normal response to situations that occur frequently in everyday life and hence is part and parcel of the body's defense mechanisms, a health effect is associated with the transient or permanent development of symptoms, pulmonary impairment, or permanent pathological changes. The brief inhalation of particles or of a low concentration of an irritant gas may temporarily increase the airways resistance, but for the most part, unless the concentration is very high or prolonged, no symptoms result. As such, this type of response is best regarded as physiological or adaptive. Were the concentrations of the inhaled agents sufficiently high so as to lead to symptoms, this would constitute an adverse health effect. In the same context, asbestosis is clearly a disease, since it not only affects longevity, but may also lead to profound physiological impairment when severe. Other conditions such as stannosis, baritosis, and

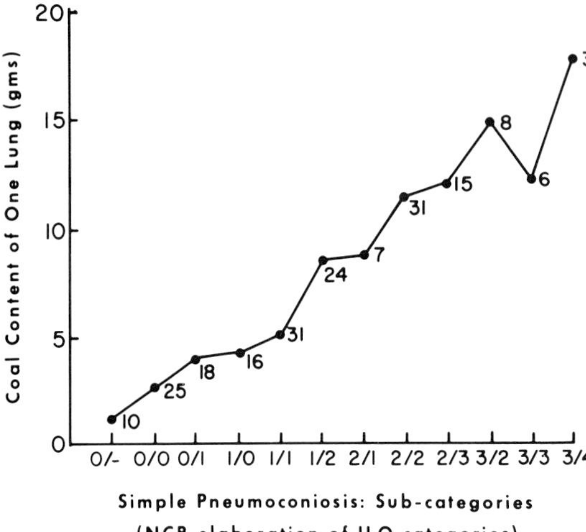

Figure 5.1. Relationship between coal content (grams) in one lung and radiographic category in life. The digit appearing against each point on the graph refers to the number of lungs analyzed. (Data supplied by the Safety in Mines Research Establishment, Sheffield, England.)

welders' siderosis do not lead to demonstrable pulmonary impairment or symptoms and since they have no effect on life expectancy, they can hardly be regarded as diseases, despite the presence of dramatic radiological abnormalities.

The importance and usefulness of chest radiographs in the pneumoconioses depends on the relationship between the extent and profusion of opacities present in the chest radiograph and the weight of retained lung dust.[4] The correlation between radiographic category and dust retention is especially reliable in coal workers' pneumoconiosis,[5] and numerous studies have shown that there is a straight line relationship between the coal dust content of the lungs and the Liddell elaboration of the International Labour Office (ILO) classification (Fig. 5.1).[6] The same is also true for asbestosis and silicosis; however, the correlation between the mineral content of the lungs and the radiographic category in these conditions tends to be less precise.

The exact pathological process and factors that produce the radiographic opacities that characterize pneumoconioses remain to some extent a mystery, and this is particularly true of coal workers' pneumoconiosis. It is clear that the atomic number of the element or elements deposited in the lungs is of great importance in the radiographic development of the small opacities that characterize pneumoconioses.[7] The higher the atomic number of the element inhaled, the less the weight of the element necessary to induce radiological abnormalities. Thus, tin and iron oxides, the agents responsible for the development of stannosis and siderosis, usually lead to dense radiopaque shadows. With coal, the factors influencing the development of the radiographic changes have not all been identified. Thus, the application of coal dust to the skin in considerable quantities fails to produce shadows on the chest radiograph. This led many to suppose that it was the accompanying fibrosis that was responsible for the development of the small radiological opacities. This is clearly not the case, since we now know that in most instances coal dust is almost entirely nonfibrogenic, and even in radiographic categories 2 and 3 the extent of the collagenous fibrosis is relatively minor, at least when compared with most other pneumoconioses.[7]

Studies from the Safety and Mines Research Establishment of Britain have shown that the mineral content of coal dust and, in particular, the content of mica, kaolinite, and to a lesser extent iron, are more closely associated with the development of radiographic abnormalities than is the presence of fibrosis. In a minority of coal miners the silica content of the coal mine dust appears to be important not only in inducing radiographic evidence of the condition, but also in influencing its progression.[8] It is stressed, however, that both coal and carbon in the complete absence of silica may lead to radiographic changes and that in the vast majority of coal miners, silica plays little role in the development of the radiological features of CWP.

Radiographic Features

Coal workers' pneumoconosis occurs in simple and complicated forms.[9] The definition and characteristics of simple and complicated disease are given in Chapter 2, which also describes the ILO classification. Simple CWP is a response to dust alone, whereas complicated CWP or progressive massive fibrosis (PMF), as it is often known, is a complex reaction to dust plus some other factor or factors as yet unknown. Simple CWP does not progress in the

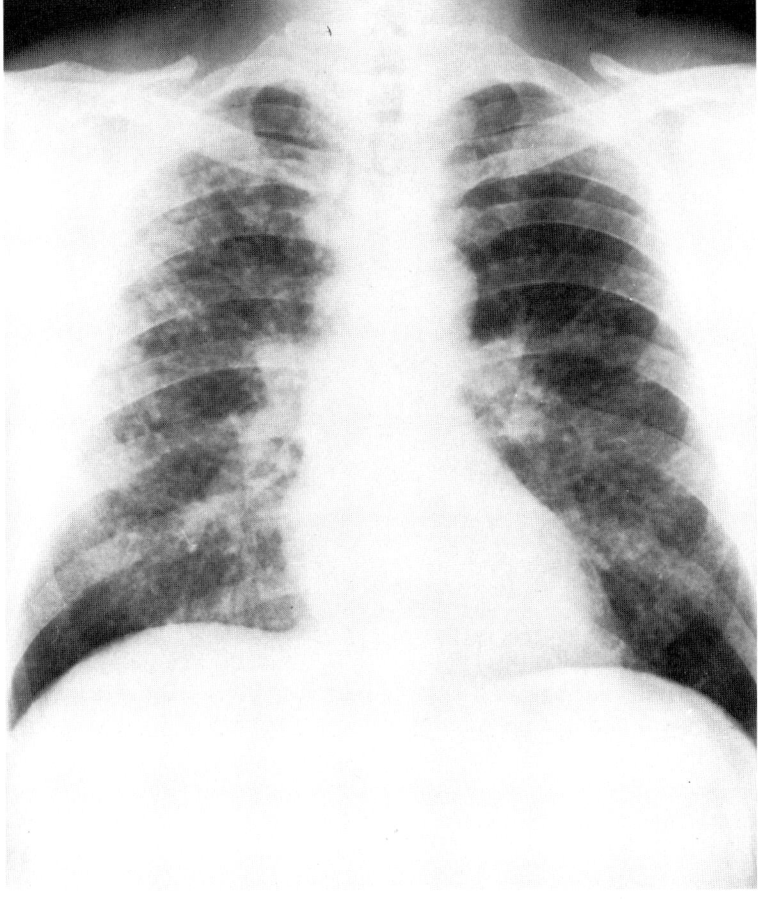

Figure 5.2. Radiograph of a subject with category 2/2 simple CWP with micronodular and nodular opacities (q/r).

absence of further dust exposure, and seldom, if ever, regresses. In contrast, PMF may develop after exposure has ceased and may progress in the absence of further exposure. A preexisting high dust burden, ie, category 2 or 3 simple CWP, is necessary for the development of PMF. Although in PMF the large opacities may increase in size in the absence of further exposure, the background profusion of small rounded opacities either remains unchanged or occasionally apparently decreases as a result of the conglomerate opacities enlarging and then retracting, thereby causing compensatory overdistension in the remainder of the lung. Hence the number of small opacities per unit volume of lung decreases as the remainder of the lung that is not involved by the conglomerate mass slowly increases in size and undergoes compensatory overdistension.

Small Regular or Rounded Opacities (p, q, and r)

Simple CWP is characterized by the development of small rounded or regular opacities throughout the lungs. The upper zones are first involved, and as the disease progresses, the opacities appear in the midzones and later spread to the whole of the lungs. Even so, the profusion remains greatest in the apical regions (Fig. 5.2).

All types of small rounded opacity, namely, p, q, and r, may be seen in the chest radiographs of coal miners; q opacities are by far the most common. The p or punctate opacity occurs less frequently and is associated with a minor reduction in the diffusing capacity. This has led some investigators to claim that the p type of opacity occurs in miners whose lungs are more emphysematous than those

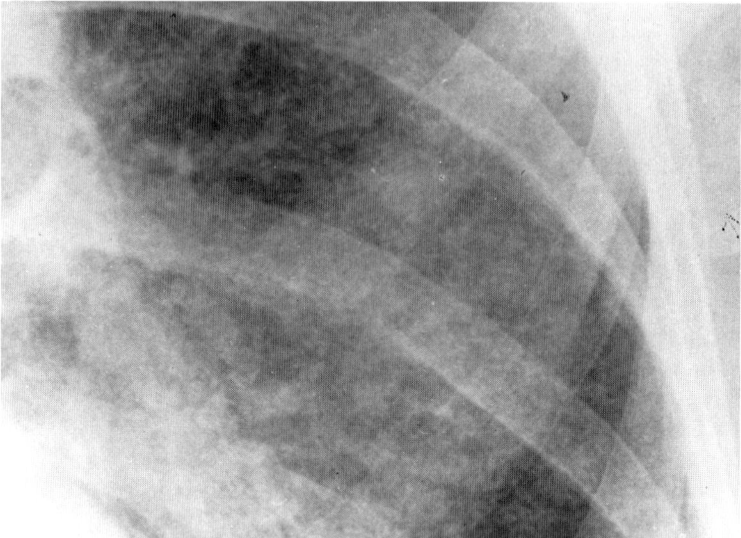

Figure 5.3. Magnified view of subject with category 3/3 simple pneumoconiosis. The opacities in this instance are of the punctate variety (p/p).

of miners with q and r opacities. Various detailed pulmonary function studies have been carried out to confirm this impression and show that there is minor loss of lung recoil and physiological evidence of emphysema. There is little doubt that miners with the p type of opacities have more emphysema[10] (Fig. 5.3), although it is not associated with obstruction, and in addition have larger airspaces.[11] The emphysema is associated with a slight reduction in the elastic recoil of the lungs, which in turn leads to greater abnormalities of gas distribution than are found in miners with q and r types of opacities[12,13] (Figs. 5.4 to 5.7).

The r type of opacity is relatively uncommon in coal miners unless they have been exposed to high concentrations of silica. The lungs in which r opacities are present usually show the typical histological features of silicosis. The r type of opacity is usually found in roof bolters, hard headers, and

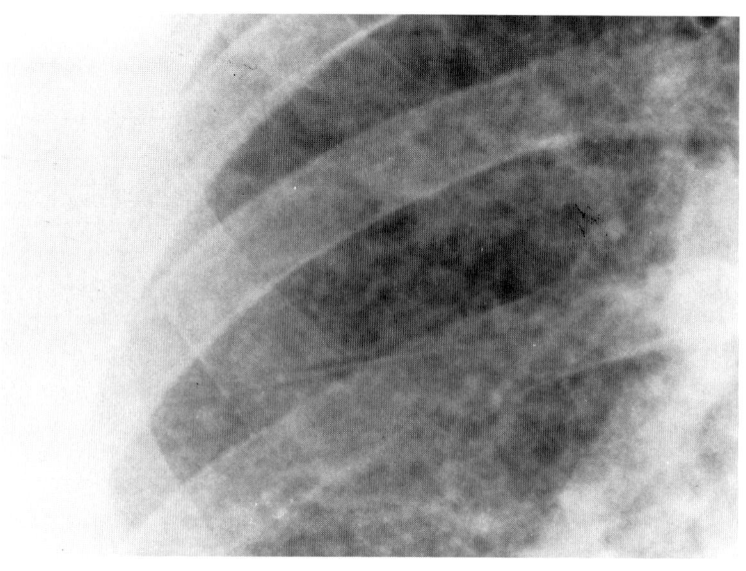

Figure 5.4. Magnified view of a subject with category 3/3 simple pneumoconiosis. The opacities in this instance are of the micronodular variety (q/q).

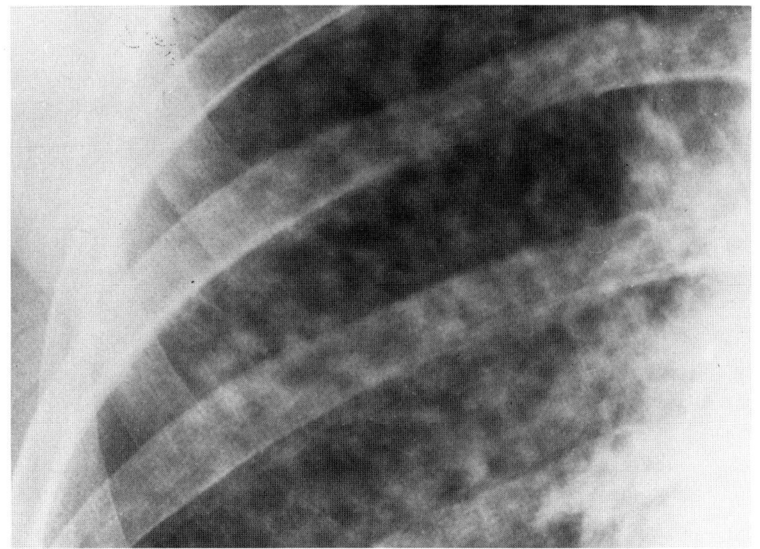

Figure 5.5. Magnified view of a subject with category 3/3 simple pneumoconiosis. The opacities in this instance are of the nodular variety (r/r).

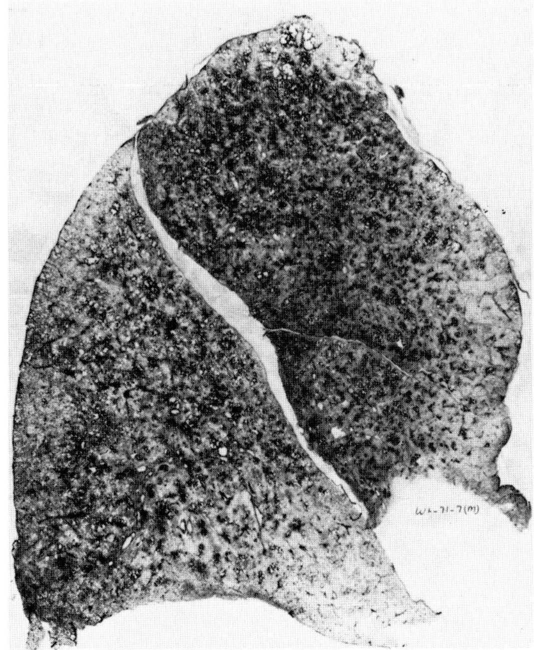

Figure 5.6. Whole-lung section in the inflated state of a subject with simple CWP. Note the black stellar-shaped aggregates of coal usually referred to as macules. There are also a few small emphysematous bullae at the apex. The subject died from nonrespiratory causes.

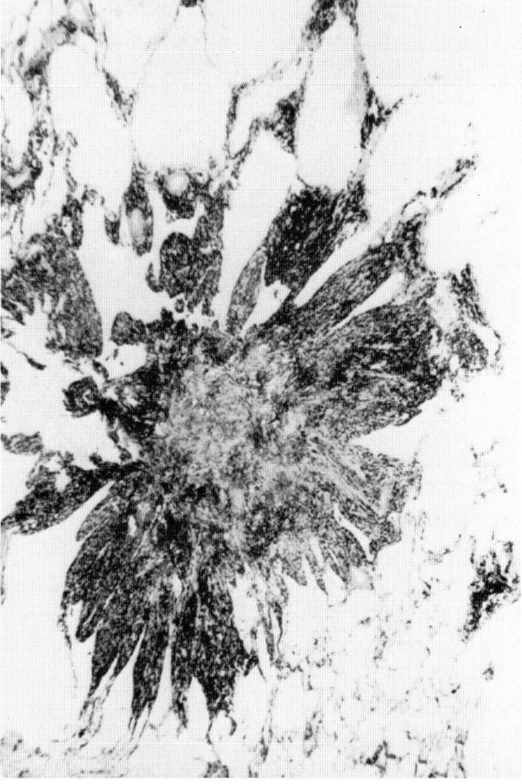

Figure 5.7. Showing a macule situated in the center of a lobule with a little collagenous fibrosis in its center. There are numerous dust-laden macrophages around the periphery.

motormen, all of whom have been exposed to silica during life.

Irregular Small Opacities (s, t, and u)

In a nonoccupationally exposed population, profuse irregular small opacities usually denote the presence of pulmonary fibrosis. In mining diseases of occupational origin, their presence is strong evidence in favor of exposure to asbestos and the typical fibrosis induced by this condition. This is certainly true when the lesions are profuse, namely, categories 2 or 3. Confusion, however, does arise in distinguishing asbestosis from other nonoccupational causes of diffuse fibrosis such as fibrosing alveolitis and scleroderma, since the radiographic appearances may be indistinguishable.

Over the past 10 years it has become apparent that scanty irregular opacities occur fairly frequently in both occupationally and nonoccupationally exposed groups.[14–19] Studies from South Wales described their occurrence in the radiographs of disabled coal miners.[15,16] The investigators from South Wales attributed their presence to a number of factors, including exposure to dust, cigarette smoking, and age. It has been suggested that coal workers whose radiographs have irregular opacities have a combination of both emphysema and interstitial fibrosis and that the fibrosis is far more marked than those with rounded opacities.[17] In a group of 357 coal workers who were referred to the Cardiff Pneumoconiosis Medical Panel, Cockroft et al. reported a reduction in the diffusing capacity and in Krogh's constant, but no effect on total lung capacity.[18] The forced expiratory volume in 1 second (FEV_1) and forced vital capacity (FVC) were decreased to the same extent. Residual volume (RV) on the other hand was found to be increased, a fact that should suggest loss of elastic recoil or small airways obstruction.[17] The authors were unable to reconcile the decrease in FEV_1 and FVC, which they attribute to fibrosis, with the increment in RV, which they attributed to emphysema. Clearly, either emphysema or fibrosis has to predominate, and if one were to assume that the former has the greater effect, then the FEV_1 should be reduced, the residual volume increased, and the FVC should remain relatively unchanged unless the increase in RV is severe. Were fibrosis to predominate, all volumes should be decreased. In the Musk study, irregular opacities were found in older and taller men and were associated with a lower diffusing capacity.[17] However, the FEV_1 and FVC were similar in those men with and without irregular opacities.

Most of these studies relating the presence of irregular opacities to lung function are replete with sophisticated statistical analyses and manipulations. Nevertheless their conclusions remain suspect. First, in almost every instance the population study has been selected from disability claimants and as such cannot be regarded as representative of coal miners as a whole. Second, for the most part the smoking history has been inadequate, and in many instances all the information available in this connection has been a simple statement to the fact that the man is either a smoker, a nonsmoker, or an exsmoker. In a few instances current cigarette consumption was quantitated, but little if any attempt was made to quantitate lifelong consumption in pack/years.

Similarly, in the multiple regression analyses, smoking is treated as an unchanging variable analogous to height or sex. This is clearly erroneous in that whereas height and sex are immutable or almost so, the effects of cigarette smoking are cumulative, and hence should be treated in exactly the same fashion as dust exposure and age. Increasing age is associated with increasing dust exposure and also to increasing effects from cigarette smoking; therefore to treat dust exposure, but not pack/years, as a continuous variable is unacceptable.

There is now ample evidence to indicate that cigarette smoking in the absence of dust exposure often leads to the development of scanty irregular opacities.[14,19] Similarly, it is apparent that such opacities may occur in numerous dusty occupations, most of which are unassociated with the development of emphysema, eg, exposure to manmade fibers, silica, and asbestos.[22,23] The longer the exposure to dust, the more likely are such opacities to be seen in the chest radiograph. However, considering that they occur in occupational settings that may lead to fibrotic diseases of the lungs (eg, asbestosis and silicosis) in which emphysema is characteristically absent, it is illogical to assume that the presence of such irregular opacities is in any way related to emphysema.

The classic studies of Auerbach provide an explanation for the presence of such opacities in smokers, and it is probable that the irregular opacities represent alveolar and peribronchiolar fibrosis and not emphysema.[20,21] Thus the majority of informed opinion believes that irregular opacities are unrelated to parenchymal dust deposition, except in the case of asbestosis, and reflect pathological changes induced by cigarette smoking or possibly, in a few instances, to peribronchial fibrosis related to bronchiolitis in the smaller conducting airways that has been induced by long-continued dust exposure.[22,23]

Large Opacities

Any opacity greater than 1 cm in diameter and pneumoconiotic in origin is, by definition, complicated pneumoconiosis or, as it is often known PMF.[9] Large opacities of nonpneumoconiotic origin, eg, those due to tuberculosis, lung cancer, or sarcoidosis, are automatically excluded. In some diseases, particularly tuberculosis, the radiographic distinction between PMF and the other conditions is often impossible, with the result that other studies are necessary to distinguish the two conditions.

Complicated pneumoconiosis or PMF is subdivided into stages A, B, and C according to the extent of the large opacities.[9] Stage A is defined as a large opacity between 1 and 5 cm in diameter, or if two or more such opacities are present, their combined diameter should not exceed 5 cm. When the opacity is greater than 5 cm in diameter but less than one third of a lung field, stage B is present. Here again, several large opacities may be present, but, provided they do not occupy more than a third of one lung field, this still constitutes stage or category B. When the opacity or opacities have a combined area greater than one third of one lung field, then stage C is present (Fig. 5.9).

Progressive massive fibrosis usually occurs on a background of category 2 or 3 simple pneumoconiosis, with the initial lesion most often developing in the posterior segment of one or the other upper lobe or in the superior segment of the lower lobe, that is, at the same sites that cavitary tuberculosis usually develops.[7] As the mass becomes larger, it tends to migrate toward the hilum, leaving an overinflated lobe behind it. Large opacities may be well-defined or ill-defined. A lack of precise definition, especially in the early stages, is more common in CWP than it is in silicosis. Although included in the earlier ILO classifications, the terms well-defined and ill-defined do not appear in the 1980 classification.

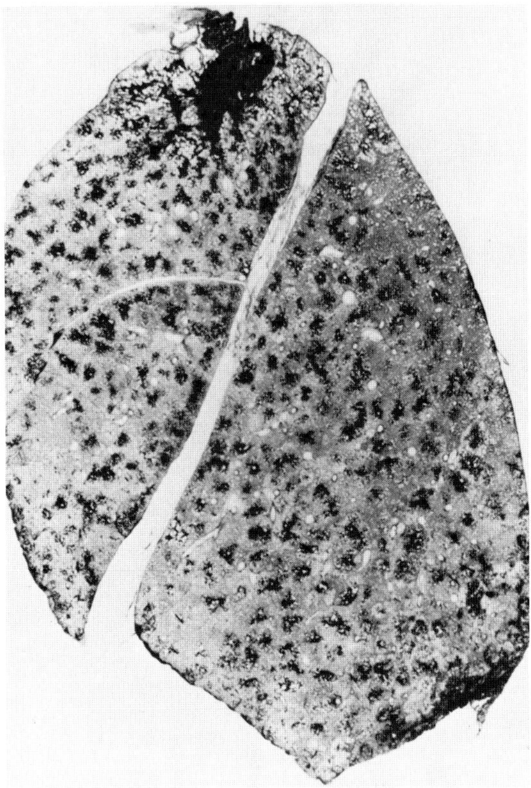

Figure 5.8. Large lung section of a subject with complicated pneumoconiosis. An early lesion is present at the apex and appears as an irregular black lesion. Elsewhere, typical large macules of simple CWP can be seen. Some of them show central translucencies, namely, focal emphysema.

Progressive massive fibrosis may appear after exposure to coal dust has ceased, provided the initial dust burden has been severe enough, and may also progress in the absence of further dust exposure. There are those who feel that occasionally this occurs in the background 0 or 1,[24] but it is rare, and under such circumstances, there may be an alternative explanation for the development of a large opacity, eg, tuberculosis. The attack rate for PMF varies but for miners with category 2 or more, it appears to be around 5% to 8% over a 5-year period.[24]

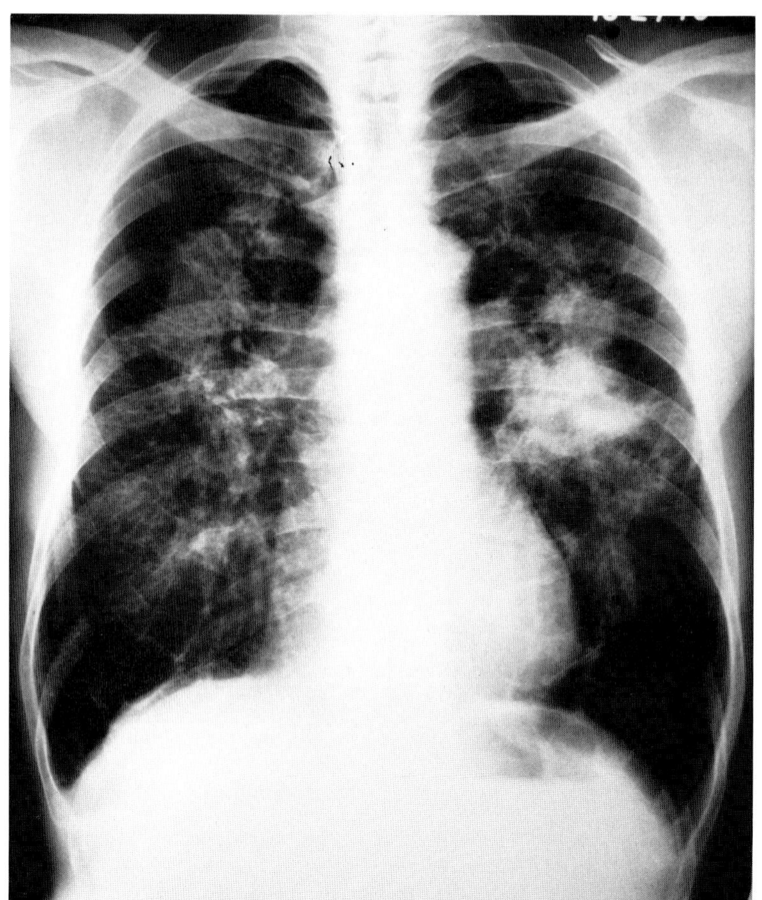

Figure 5.9. Complicated CWP or PMF, stage C. Note basal overdistension. Subject had combined restrictive and obstructive impairment.

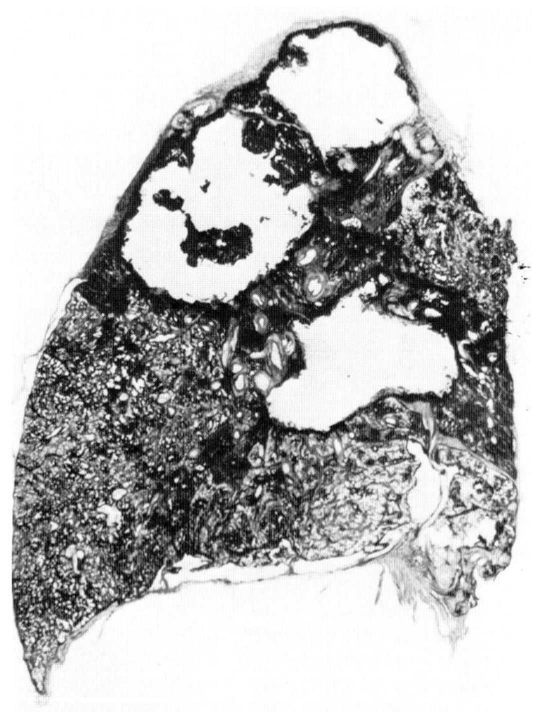

Figure 5.10. Whole-lung section of a subject with stage C complicated CWP. The conglomerate masses have cavitated owing to ischemic necrosis. At a later date, atypical mycobacteria (*M. kansasii*) were isolated from the subject's sputum. He died from cor pulmonale.

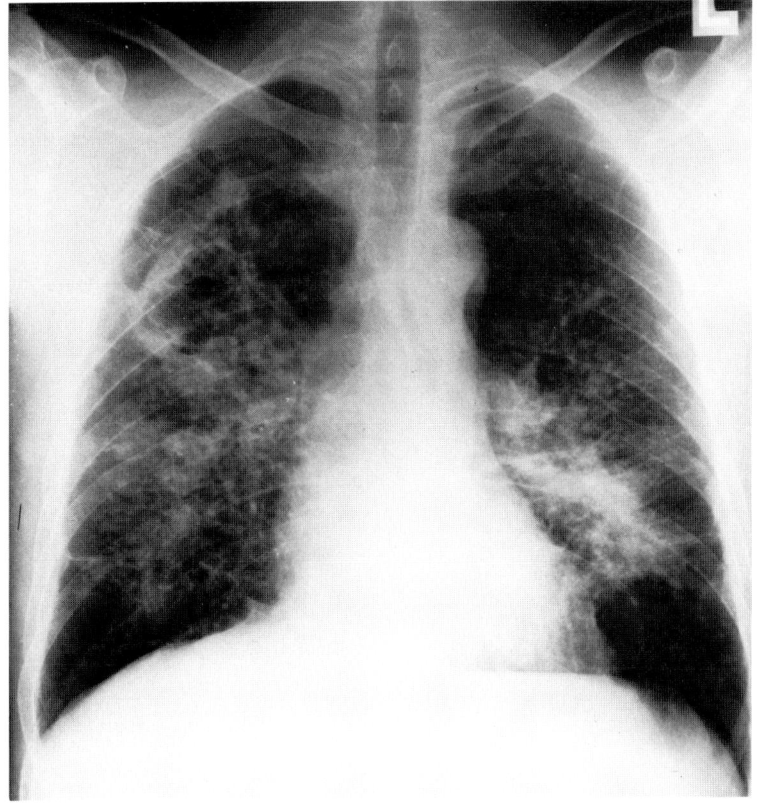

Figure 5.11. Complicated CWP, category C. The right upper lobe mass has undergone ischemic necrosis. This subject of Polish origin worked for only four years in a Belgian coal mine during the war. (Courtesy of Dr. D. Ahmad)

It must also be remembered that PMF is not necessarily massive or progressive, and in some subjects the lesion often appears and grows slowly for several years and then increases no further in size. In general, the older the man is at the time the massive lesion appears, the less likely he is to develop severe impairment. Should PMF develop before the age of 40, progression is the rule and disabling impairment occurs far more commonly (Fig. 5.9).

The large opacities that are seen in conglomerate silicosis are formed by the aggregation of the small nodules that characterize the simple form of the disease. In contrast, in complicated CWP the conglomerate mass tends to be more amorphous and less well-defined. Whole lung sections show that in complicated CWP the individual nodules have coalesced and can no longer be distinguished. The conglomerate mass appears as a black, poorly defined lesion, often with liquefaction at its center. Progressive massive fibrosis characteristically encroaches on, and eventually destroys, both the adjacent blood vessels and the airways. As the mass increases in size, the vessels and airways are incorporated into the conglomerate lesion, but sometimes microscopic remnants are discernible on section.[24] The pulmonary blood supply adjacent to and around the mass is also compromised and in a few instances is completely obliterated by the surrounding emphysematous changes. Progressive massive fibrosis may cavitate either as a result of ischemic necrosis or infection. The latter is usually due to *Mycobacterium tuberculosis* or atypical mycobacteria; rarely other organisms may be responsible[24] (Fig. 5.10).

Patients with stage A and many with early stage B complicated pneumoconiosis have no lung function abnormalities. However, as the disease progresses from B to C, shortness of breath and cough usually develop. Occasionally, the mass will cavitate and then the patient may cough up large volumes of black sputum, so-called melanoptysis (Fig. 5.11). Pulmonary function measurements in late stage B and stage C PMF show decreased lung volumes, a reduced diffusing capacity, and

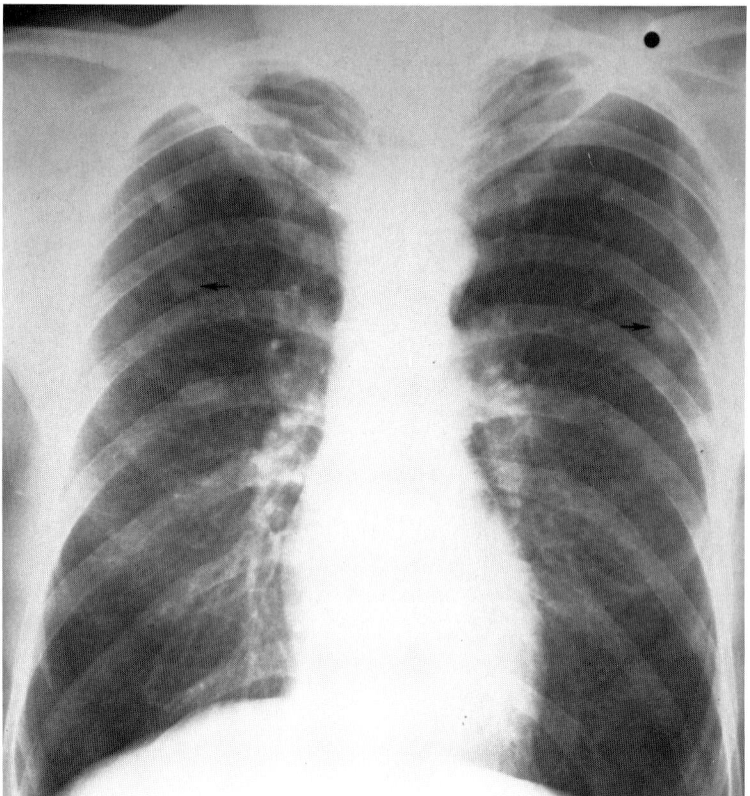

Figure 5.12. Posterior anterior view of a subject with Caplan's syndrome. Small rounded nodules can be seen in the periphery of the lungs. The subject's serum was positive for rheumatoid factor and antinuclear activity. Note also that there is no background of simple CWP.

pulmonary hypertension at rest.[24] In stage B or early C, the pulmonary hypertension is usually present only with exercise. Fairly marked airways obstruction generally accompanies the more advanced case of PMF, even though the patient may have been a lifelong nonsmoker. The obstruction appears to be related to distortion and compensatory overdistension of the remaining lung that is not involved by the large masses. Eventually cor pulmonale may develop. This is usually nonhypoxemic in origin and is due to a reduction of the alveolar-capillary surface rather than hypoxemia.

Radiographic Progression

It is possible to quantitate the risks of occupational dust exposure by relating long-term environmental exposures to appropriate serial medical measurements. In the case of CWP, the latter consists of serial radiographic examinations of the chest. By these means it is possible to calculate an attack rate for CWP and to relate it to a particular cumulative dust exposure. The attack rate is defined as the number of subjects without prior dust exposure who develop pneumoconiosis over a certain working period, eg, 10 years. Alternatively, the rate of progression of established pneumoconiosis over a specified period, eg, 5 years, may be related to dust exposure. In this connection it must be remembered that the rate of progression need not be linear and that the currently available evidence suggests that more dust is required to produce a change from a normal film to category 1 than is required to produce a change from category 1 to category 2. Once the disease is present, progression may occur despite relatively lesser exposure to dust.

Radiographic progression may be measured in two ways—by the independent method and by the side-to-side method.[25] The former method relies on the interpreter classifying a series of paired films presented to him in random order without any knowledge of which film constitutes the pair and in the complete absence of a knowledge of the correct chronological sequence. This method removes the bias introduced by a knowledge of the

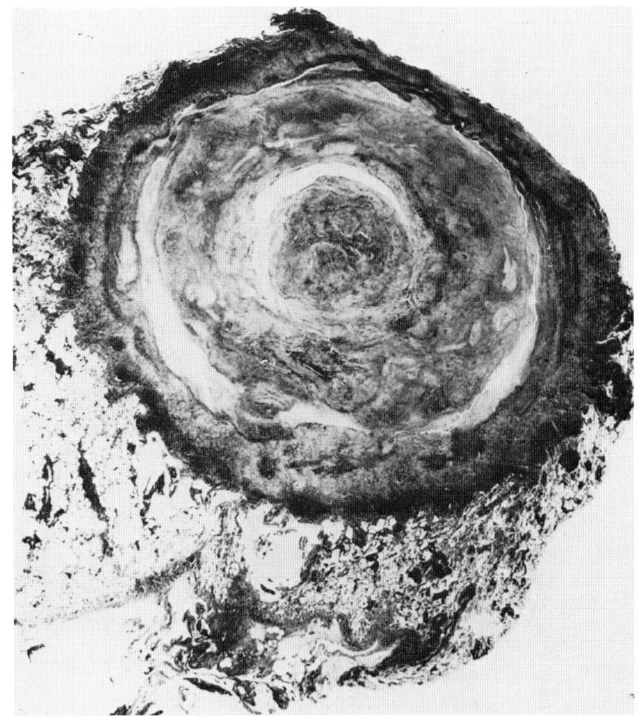

Figure 5.13. Photomicrograph of a Caplan's nodule removed at postmortem. Note the concentric layers of dust and the necrotic center. Although there is a resemblance to the silicotic nodule, the laminated nodule with its dust layers and the obvious coal dust deposition present should easily distinguish it from the true silicotic nodule.

temporal sequence, but does not eliminate bias from other factors, ie, film technique, change in body habitus over the observation period. The side-by-side method places paired films side-by-side with the correct chronological sequence known to the interpreter. As such it introduces bias, since the interpreter knows, or perhaps assumes he knows, that regression never occurs and that only progression is possible.[26] Nevertheless, the side-by-side method provides a means whereby the interpreter can make allowance for changes in technique, ie, overpenetrated or underpenetrated films. The independent method leads to about half as much progression being recorded as does the side-by-side method.[27] It is also more variable and regression is read more commonly.[25] Nonetheless, at the present time the evidence suggests that the side-by-side method, for all its imperfections, is to be preferred.[25,27]

Caplan's Syndrome

Although this radiological curiosity was first described in coal miners, it also occurs in the other pneumoconiosis, in particular, silicosis and asbestosis. In 1952 Anthony Caplan described the syndrome at a meeting of the Thoracic Society of Great Britain.[28] The condition is characterized by certain distinctive radiological abnormalities, in particular, by the presence of a number of rounded, relatively peripherally situated nodules (Fig. 5.12). In many instances it was noted that the opacities had appeared relatively quickly, ie, in the space of 2 to 3 months. Their appearance differed significantly from that seen in typical PMF in that, for the most part, the nodules were multiple, had appeared rapidly, and seldom were more than 2 to 2.5 cm in diameter. Furthermore, they occurred on a background of either minimal pneumoconiosis or, in most instances, on a preivously clear chest radiograph.

Caplan made his observations while interpreting large numbers of routine chest radiographs of working miners and exminers. Stimulated by the unusual radiographic appearances described above, he visited the miners and to his surprise found that more than 50% of them had rheumatoid arthritis. Subsequently, a number of clinical epidemiological studies were carried out and it became obvious that radiographic features often antedated the development of rheumatoid arthritis and that nearly all

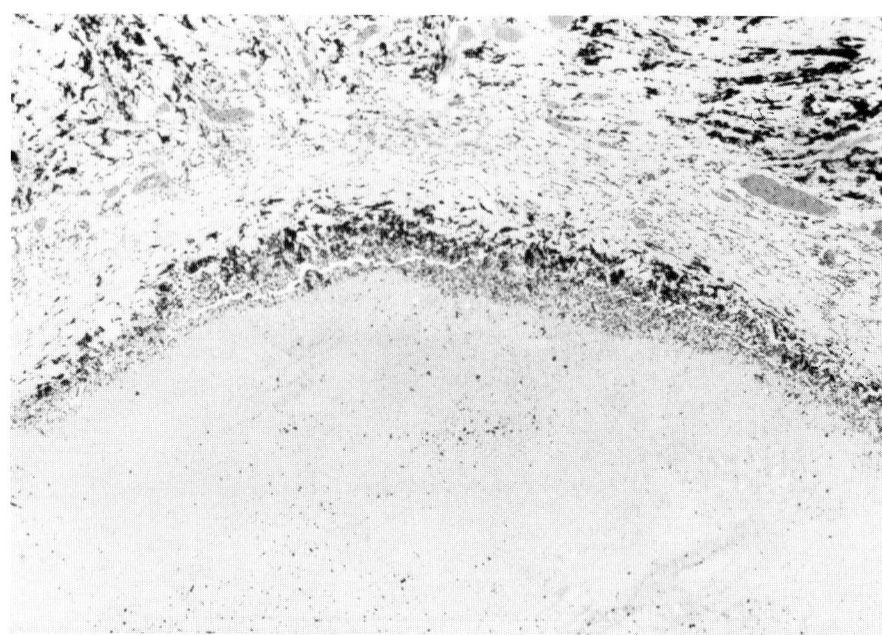

Figure 5.14. Photomicrograph of a Caplan nodule showing the necrotic center and the inflammatory or rheumatoid zone on the periphery. This zone is infiltrated with plasma cells and polymorphs. More peripherally still there is a further zone of dust deposition and some macrophages.

subjects with the characteristic features, even in the absence of overt rheumatoid arthritis, had the rheumatoid diathesis, as manifested by the presence of rheumatoid factor in their serum.[29]

It became evident that occasional crops of nodules would appear in a short time and their their appearance was often indistinguishable from the nodular or r type of opacity that is frequently seen in the radiographs of subjects with silicosis.[30] Occasionally, Caplan nodules would cavitate.

Histologically, there was some resemblance between the Caplan nodule and the typical nodule seen in rheumatoid arthritis, but there were also disparities in that the Caplan nodule was impregnated by dust and possessed some of the features seen in both the coal macule and the silicotic nodule. A characteristic inflammatory zone with plasma cell infiltration was observed in the Caplan nodule, and this was thought to be a reflection of the rheumatoid diathesis (Figs. 5.13 and 5.14).[31] Epidemiological surveys have revealed the presence of Caplan's syndrome in US coal miners; however, it seems to be less prevalent than in Britain.[32] Many miners with Caplan's syndrome also show evidence of antinuclear activity in their serum.

It is suggested that the Caplan nodule develops at a particular site in the lung because of preexisting damage caused by the inhalation of dusts such as coal, silica or asbestos. An analogy is drawn between the development of typical rheumatoid nodules on pressure points such as the tendo achillis or occiput. Whether this is true or not remains debatable. Nevertheless, the Caplan nodule clearly bears a relationship to the rheumatoid nodule, and its appearance portends either the onset or often the exacerbation of preexisting rheumatoid arthritis.

References

1. Morgan WKC, Lapp NL: Respiratory disease in coalminers. Am Rev Respir Dis 1976; 113:531.
2. Morgan WKC: Industrial bronchitis. Br J Ind Med 1978; 35:185.
3. Douglas AM, Lamb D, Ruckley VA: Bronchial gland dimensions in coalminers: Influence of smoking and dust exposure. Thorax. 1982; 37:760.
4. Casswell C, Bergman I, Rossiter CE: The relation of radiological appearance in simple pneumoconiosis

of coal workers to the content and composition of the lung, in Walton WH (ed): Inhaled Particles III, vol 2. London, Unwin Brothers, 1971, p 713.
5. Collins HPR, Dick JA, Bennett JG, et al: Irregularly shaped small shadows on chest radiographs, dust exposure and lung function in coal workers pneumoconiosis. Br J Ind Med 1988; 45:43–55.
6. Liddell FDK, May JD: Assessing the Radiological Progression of Simple Pneumoconiosis. London, National Coal board Medical Service, 1966.
7. Morgan WKC: Coalworkers' Pneumoconiosis: Chapter 14, in Morgan WKC, Seaton A (eds): Occupational Lung Diseases, ed 2. Philadelphia, WB Saunders Co, 1984.
8. Seaton A, Dodgson J, Dick JA, et al: Quartz and pneumoconiosis in coalminers. Lancet 1981;2: 1272.
9. Guidelines for the Use of ILO International Classification of Radiographs of Pneumoconiosis, Occupational Safety and Health Series, No 22, (Revised). Geneva, Switzerland, International Labour Office, 1980.
10. Cockcroft A, Wagner JC, Ryder R, et al: Postmortem study of emphysema in coalworkers and non-coalworkers. Lancet 1982; 2:600.
11. Hankinson JL, Palmes ED, Lapp NL: Pulmonary airspace size in coalminers. Am Rev Respir Dis 1979;119:391.
12. Seaton A, Lapp NL, Morgan WKC: Lung mechanics and frequency dependence of compliance in coal miners. J Clin Invest 1972; 51:1203.
13. Seaton A, Lapp NL, Morgan WKC: The relationship of pulmonary impairment in simple coalworker's pneumonoconiosis to type of radiographic opacity. Br J Ind Med 1972; 29:50.
14. Amandus HE, Lapp NL, Jacobson G, et al: Significance of irregular small opacities in the radiographs of coalminers in the U.S.A. Br J Ind Med 1976; 33:13.
15. Lyons JP, Ryder RC, Campbell H, et al: Significance of irregular opacities in the radiology of coalworker's pneumoconiosis. Br J Ind Med 1974; 31:36.
16. Cockroft A, Lyons JP, Andersson N, et al: Prevalence and relation to underground exposure of radiological irregular opacities and South Wales coal miners with pneumoconiosis. Br J Ind Med 1983; 41:69.
17. Musk AW, Cotes JE, Bevan C, et al: Relationship between type of simple coalworker's pneumoconiosis and lung function: A nine-year follow-up study of subjects with small rounded opacities. Br J Ind Med 1981; 38:313.
18. Cockroft A, Berry G, Cotes JE, et al: Shape of small opacities and lung function in coalworkers. Thorax 1982; 37:765.
19. Carilli AD, Kotzen LM, Fischer ML: The chest roentgenogram in non-smoking females. Am Rev Respir Dis 1974; 29:334.
20. Auerbach O, Stout AP, Hammond EC, et al: Smoking habits and age in relation to pulmonary changes. N Engl J Med 1963; 269:1045.
21. Auerbach O, Garfinkel L, Hammond EC: Relation of smoking and age to findings in the lung parenchyma: A microscopic study. Chest 1974; 65:29.
22. Weiss W: Cigarette smoking, asbestos and pulmonary fibrosis. Am Rev Respir Dis 1971; 104:223.
23. Weill H, Hughes M, Hammad YH, et al: Respiratory health in workers exposed to man-made vitreous fibres. Am Rev Respir Dis 1983; 128:104.
24. Shennan DH, Washington JS, Thomas DJ, et al: Factors predisposing to the development of progressive massive fibroses in coal miners. Br J Ind Med 1981; 38:321.
25. Liddell FDK, Morgan WKC: Methods of assessing serial films of the pneumoconioses: A Review. J Soc Occup Med 1978; 28:6.
26. Reger RB, Butcher DF, Morgan WKC: Assessing change in the pneumoconioses using serial radiographs. Am J Epidemiol 1973; 87:243.
27. Amandus HE, Reger RB, Pendergrass EP, et al: The pneumoconioses: Methods of assessing progression. Chest 1973; 63:736
28. Caplan A: Certain unusual radiological appearances in the chest radiographs of coalminers suffering from rheumatoid arthritis. Thorax 1953; 8:29.
29. Miall WE, Caplan A, Cochrane A, et al: An epidemiological study of rheumatoid arthritis associated with characteristic chest x-ray appearances in coalworkers. Br Med J 1953; 2:1231.
30. Caplan A, Payne RB, Withey JL: A broader concept of Caplan's syndrome related to rheumatoid factors. Thorax 1962; 17:205.
31. Gough J, Rivers D, Seal RME: Pathological studies of modified pneumoconiosis in coal miners with rheumatoid arthritis (Caplan's Syndrome). Thorax 1955; 10:9.
32. Lippman M, Eckert HL, Hahon HN, et al: The prevalence of circulating anti-nuclear and rheumatoid factors in U.S. coal miners. Ann Intern Med 1973; 79:807.

6

Radiological Features of Silicosis

Gerhard K. Sluis-Cremer and Albert Solomon

Introduction

Silicosis is a disease characterized by nodular fibrosis of the lung, caused by the inhalation and deposition in the lung of particles of crystalline quartz (SlO_2) in the respirable size range (generally below 5 μm and certainly below 8 μm in diameter). Naturally occurring quartz is often referred to as alpha quartz.

The word "silica," which describes all physical forms of SlO_2 is used in this chapter to refer to several varieties of crystalline quartz; silica that is not crystalline is referred to as amorphous silica.

The term silicosis has been widely abused in the past, as, for example, its use sometimes for pneumoconioses due to minerals other than silica. The term "silicosis" is still used by some to describe the dust disease coal workers develop, ie, coal worker's pneumoconiosis.[1] The confusion increases when coal workers in the course of coal mining have to mine siliceous rock and develop classic silicosis. The use of correct terms for the different pathological entities is essential.

The toxic qualities of silica are restricted to those varieties possessing a particular crystalline structure (the tetrahedral form). Some varieties of silica, eg, the stishovite polymorph having an octahedral structure, are harmless.[2,3] The physical variations of crystalline polymers of quartz therefore have biological significance.[4] Silica that is not crystalline, ie, amorphous silica, which may be produced in the course of certain industrial processes, such as in the manufacture of ferro alloys, is not thought to cause classic silicosis. Pulmonary injury has been reported in exposed employees, but such disease has neither the radiological nor the histological features of classic silicosis.[5,6]

Source of Human Exposure

Silica is very widespread in nature and is the commonest mineral to cause pulmonary fibrosis. A small amount occurs normally in tissues, including the lungs and especially in the tracheobronchial glands, without apparently inducing fibrosis.[7]

The physician involved in industrial practice should be aware of rock containing free silica that is likely to be released into the atmosphere by the activities of man. Free silica is particularly common in acidic volcanic rocks, such as granites and pegmatites and their detrital derivatives, ie, conglomerates, sandstones, clays, and shales. Many of the veins and lodes containing metal or metal compounds in mining have a high free-silica content. Hence the mining of gold, tin, copper,[8] tungsten, zinc, lead, and other minerals is commonly associated with a silicosis hazard, but iron-ore mining is usually not associated with silicosis because little silica is encountered.

When granites[9–13] and sandstones[14] are quarried, processed, cut, and dressed for building or monuments, respirable free silica in moderate to high concentrations is released. The mining, processing, and use of clay minerals, including bentonite,[15] shales, and slates,[16] are likewise associated with silica exposure. Certain rocks—in general, the ultrabasic rocks and their detrital derivations—do not normally have sufficient free silica to be harmful. Other industrially important rocks with a

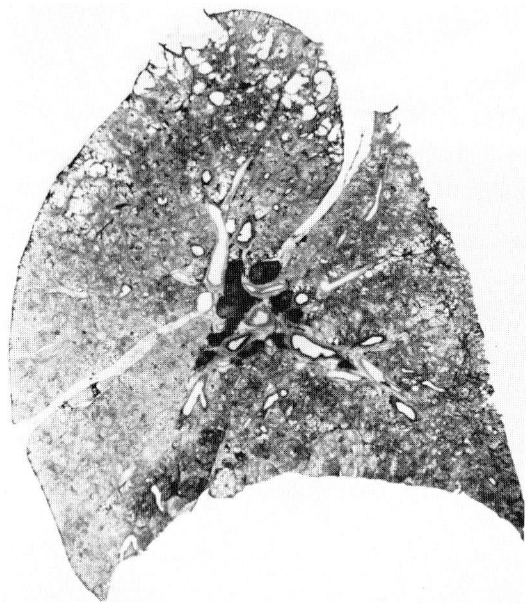

Figure 6.1. A Gough-Wentworth section illustrates modest enlargement of hilar glands in a gold miner with 32 years' service. There is only an occasional silicotic islet in the lung. In silicosis it is very rare for hilar glands to exceed these in size.

very low free-silica content include marble and limestone; therefore, cement has a low free-silica content, although there are exceptions.

In general, the higher the free-silica content of the rock, the higher will be its concentration in the respirable dust and the greater the risk of developing silicosis. When the silica content of a dust is less than 5%, silicosis is most unlikely to occur.

There are also numerous opportunities for exposure to silica in industry, especially in the foundry,[17] ceramic industries (including enameling,[13]) and in the manufacture of refractory bricks.[13] Sand is widely used in foundries to make moulds, and silica parting powders are still used.[17] Fettling and grinding may be associated with a high exposure to silica, even though "sandblasting" is slowly being abandoned, the sand being replaced by safer materials. Quartz itself is mined and milled[18] for use in industry as silica flour (90% pure silica) or for use in preparing scouring powders. The mixture of alkaline soaps and silica appears to be particularly toxic. The ceramic industry uses silica-containing clays and also pure free silica, and silicosis still occurs commonly. Workers in glass factories may also be at risk.[13,19]

Pathogenesis

A detailed discussion of the pathogenesis of silicosis is beyond the scope of this chapter. Free silica particles, particularly those 1 to 3 μm in diameter, induce an inflammatory reaction at their sites of deposition, consisting predominantly of polymorphonuclear leukocytes and macrophages. The role of the former is obscure, although it may be supposed that they release harmful reactive metabolites and enzymes and induce chemotaxis for macrophrages. There seems to be a general consensus that the latter cells play the dominant role in the pathogenesis of silicosis. Silica is believed to first stimulate the macrophages to release a whole series of active chemical mediators that induce further recruitment of macrophages and, by a complicated interaction, induce fibroblast growth and collagen formation. Eventually the macrophages are killed by their ingested silica particles, which are then engulfed by other macrophages, thereby keeping the stimulus to collagen formation going and explaining the progression that so often occurs after cessation of exposure.[20]

There is, however, a lot to learn about the formation of the characteristic "onion-peel" nodule so characteristic of silicosis. Dust reticulation is the first tissue reaction to silica, and this is later replaced by collagen, which becomes remodeled to form the typical silicotic nodule.

The cellular events described are sometimes associated with a rise in angiotensin-converting enzyme[21,22] and lysosomal enzyme[23] in the serum, especially in progressive silicosis. For the same reason there may be increased gallium-67 uptake in active silicosis.[24]

Pathology

The silica particles are transported first to the hilar lymph glands and pleura by macrophages. Silicotic islets form in the hilar lymph glands, which, as a result, become slightly enlarged and give rise to the slight prominence of the hila so commonly seen in x-ray studies of silica-exposed persons (Fig. 6.1).

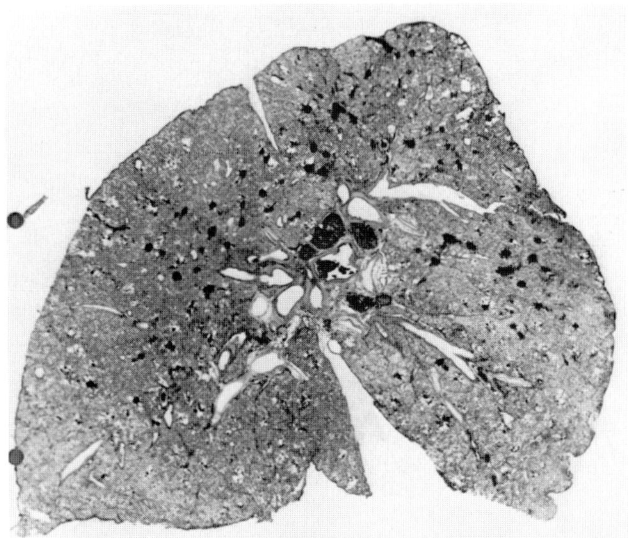

Figure 6.2. Gough-Wentworth section of a gold miner's right lung showing small- and medium-sized nodules predominantly in the upper lobe and in the apex of the lower lobe.

Moderate or marked enlargement of the hilar glands does not usually occur. The hilar glands may, however, become calcified and in some cases give rise to an "eggshell" appearance, the calcification being most marked in the peripheral rim of the glands.

Some thickening of the visceral pleura occurs, but this is commonly slight and seldom demonstrable radiologically. In addition, elongated plaques of 1 or 2 cm in length may occur, nearly always over the upper zones. Histologically they show the features of silicosis. These plaques are on the visceral pleura, unlike the plaques of asbestosis, which are nearly always on the parietal pleura and are uncommonly found in the upper zones. The silicotic pleural plaques may calcify.

There is usually little change in the parietal pleura. There may be small pigmented nodules of lymphoid tissue in the intercostal spaces, and these may contain silicotic islets.

In the lungs the silicotic islets consisting of collagen and hyalin usually appear first in the posterior segment of the upper lobe and the apical segment of the lower lobe (Fig. 6.2). The nodules are situated in the interstititum of the lung in juxtaposition to small arterioles or respiratory bronchioles. Macroscopically they are usually 2 to 6 mm in diameter. They may be grey in color but more commonly are dark or even black, owing to the accumulation of carbon and other pigment. Nodules may be as large as 10 mm. If lesions are larger than this, they are by definition considered as massive fibrosis.

Microscopically the silicotic nodule has a central zone of whorls of hyaline and collagen surrounded by a zone of irregularly distributed collagen fibers (Fig. 6.3). Macrophages and lymphoid cells are present in varying amounts at the periphery; the former frequently contain pigment. On microincineration, free silica can be demonstrated as well as other mineral constituents of the inhaled dust.

The histologically round onion-peel nodules may contain central areas of necrosis. The pathogenesis of the necrosis is uncertain. It was believed in the past that tuberculous infection played a role, and tubercle bacilli were cultured in a few cases. This was in the days when tuberculosis was extremely common in silicotic lungs. There is no available evidence bearing on the relation of tuberculous infection and central necrosis in present times (Fig. 6.4).

The areas of necrosis may calcify in time. Calcified silicosis, which was common in South African gold miners in the earlier decades of this century (Fig. 6.5), is now infrequently seen. The reason for this is not clear. It may well be due to the dramatic fall in silica-dust concentrations in the underground air or to marked reduction in the chance of exposure to tubercle bacilli in the working environment.

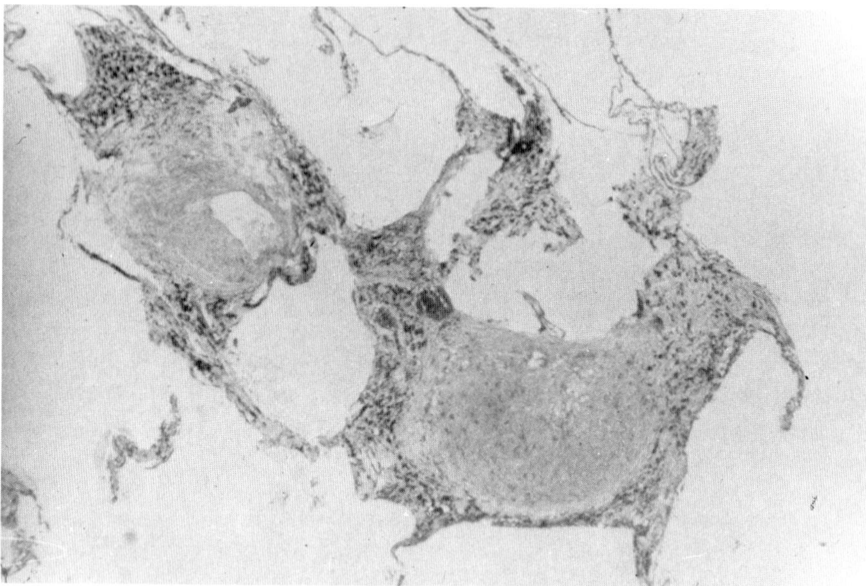

Figure 6.3. Silicotic islet showing central whorls of collagen and at the periphery sparse cellular infiltration.

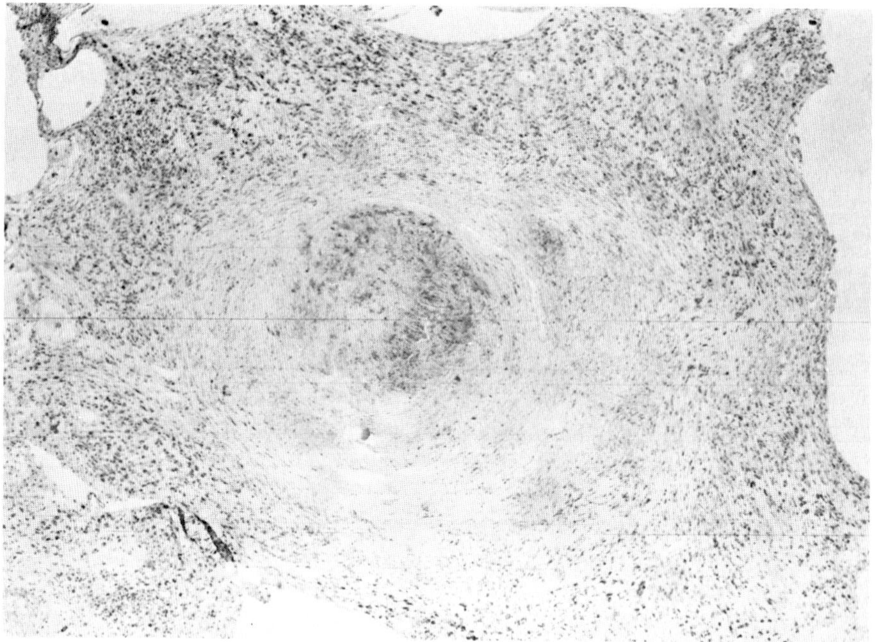

Figure 6.4. Silicotic islet with central necrosis and round-cell infiltration around it. This is not considered evidence of active tuberculosis.

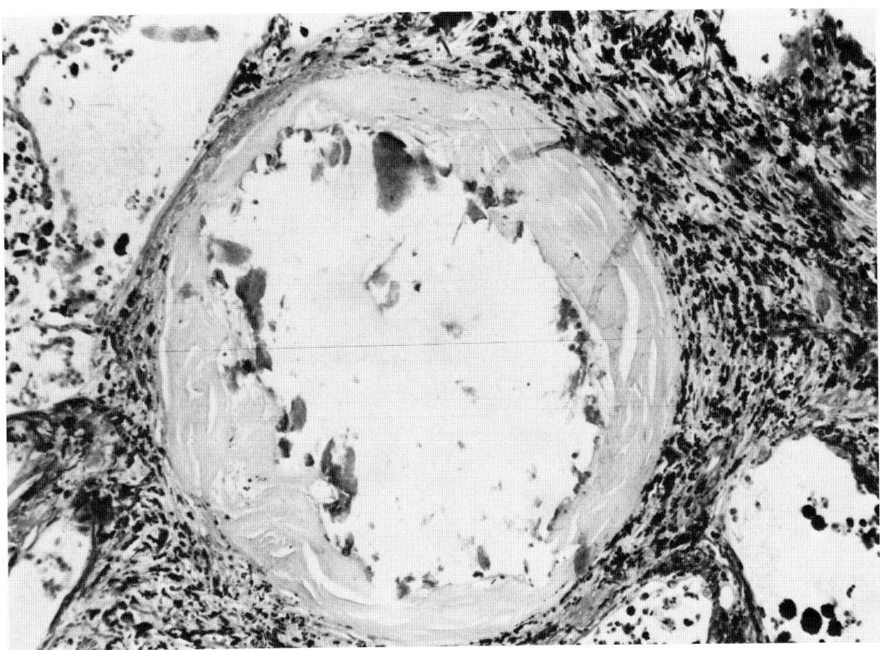

Figure 6.5. Silicotic nodule with remains of the center that was calcified.

In a case-control study on the relationship between silicosis and rheumatoid arthritis, we have also noted that islets with central necrosis occurred twice as frequently in silica-exposed men with rheumatoid arthritis than in equally exposed controls without rheumatoid arthritis among men who came to autopsy. This raises the possibility that immunological factors may be involved in some cases.

Areas of fibrosis more than 1 cm in longest diameter not infrequently associated with some necrosis occur quite commonly and are associated with an aggregation of silicotic nodules. Such areas of fibrosis are by definition called massive fibrosis (Fig. 6.6). We prefer to use the term massive fibrosis instead of progressive massive fibrosis because progression frequently does not occur. These massive areas are probably formed in several ways. Agglomeration of islets with atelectasis of intervening lung tissue has been suggested as one mechanism; in such cases the individual islets can still be recognized in the mass. More commonly, these masses consist of a large homogeneous area of collagen (Fig. 6.7), dust, and pigment, and are thought by many to be due to infection, which is usually or always tuberculous.[25] Histological evidence of tuberculosis is however usually absent. When it occurs it might well be considered a complication rather than a cause. Immunological mechanisms must also be considered as a possible cause. Massive fibrosis, for instance, may develop very rapidly in cases of rheumatoid arthritis associated with silicosis.

Islets may be found to have a round cell infiltrate (lymphocytes and plasma cells) associated with giant cells along the periphery of the islet. This is universally accepted as evidence of a tuberculous infection, although mycobacteria can seldom, if ever, be demonstrated under these circumstances (Fig. 6.8). It has been our experience that the number of areas of massive fibrosis are frequently underestimated on conventional x-ray films taken shortly before autopsy (Fig. 6.9).[120]

Cavitation rarely occurs in areas of silicotic massive fibrosis and is usually tuberculous; unlike the massive fibrosis of coal worker's pneumoconiosis, ischemic necrosis is a very rare cause of cavitation in silicosis.

There is a reasonably good correlation between the size of nodules found at autopsy and the size of the nodules seen on the radiograph. Both at autopsy and on the radiograph, there is usually an

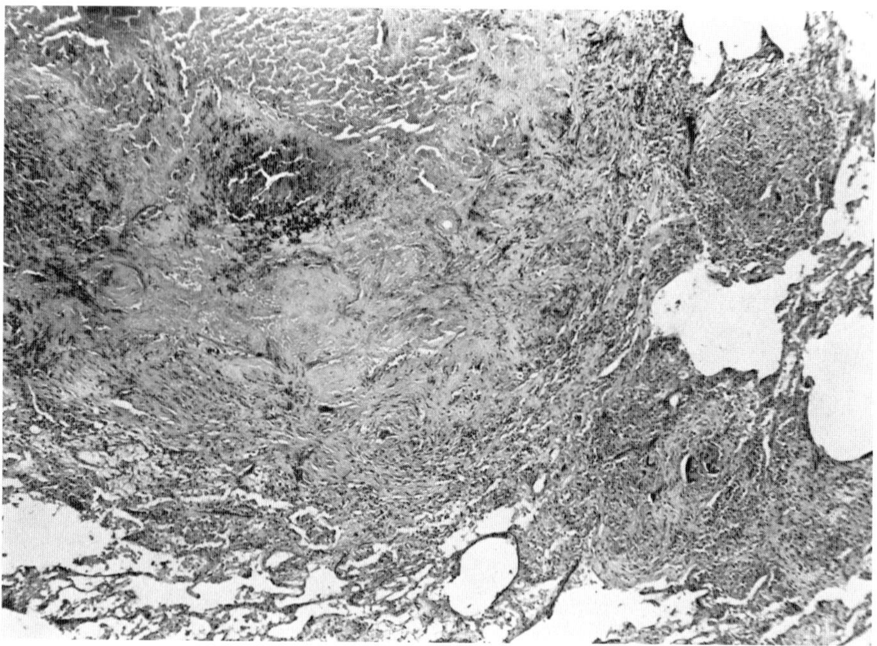

Figure 6.6. Gough-Wentworth section of a lung showing a few pigmented silicotic islets and an area of massive fibrosis.

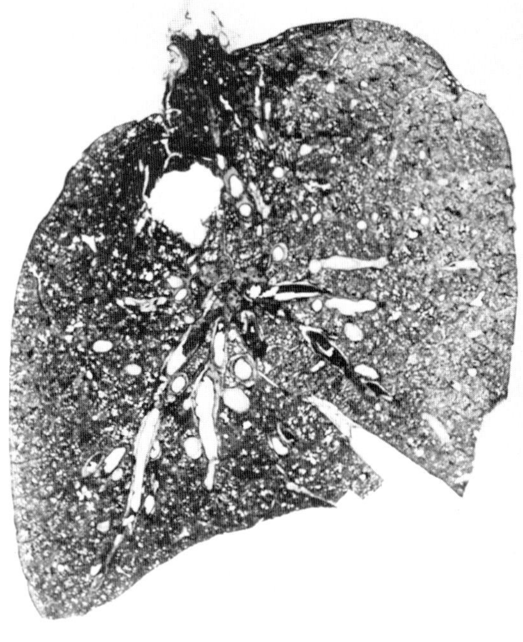

Figure 6.7. Massive fibrosis showing bundles of unorganized collagen and an area of dust deposition. Individual islets cannot be identified in this case, although they can be in Fig. 6.8.

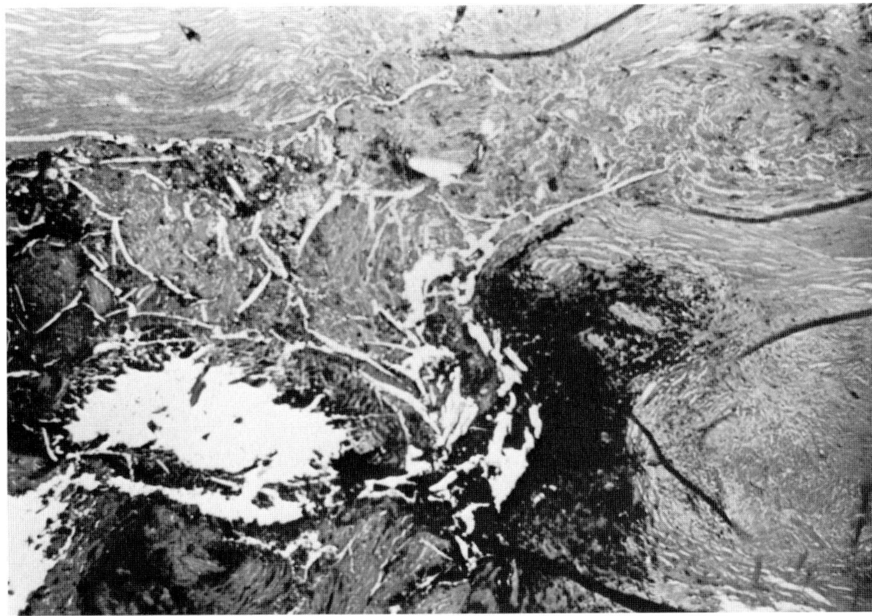

Figure 6.8. Silicotic nodules with necrosis, marked round-cell infiltration, and giant cells in right lower corner. This would be interpreted as silicosis with active tuberculosis. Aggregation of the islets had formed an area of massive fibrosis.

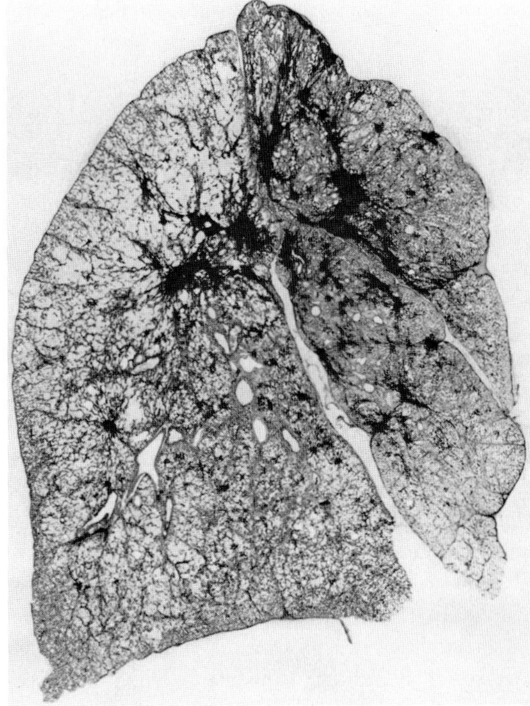

Figure 6.9. Gough-Wentworth section showing multiple areas of massive fibrosis. The number of such areas is often underestimated on the roentgenogram.

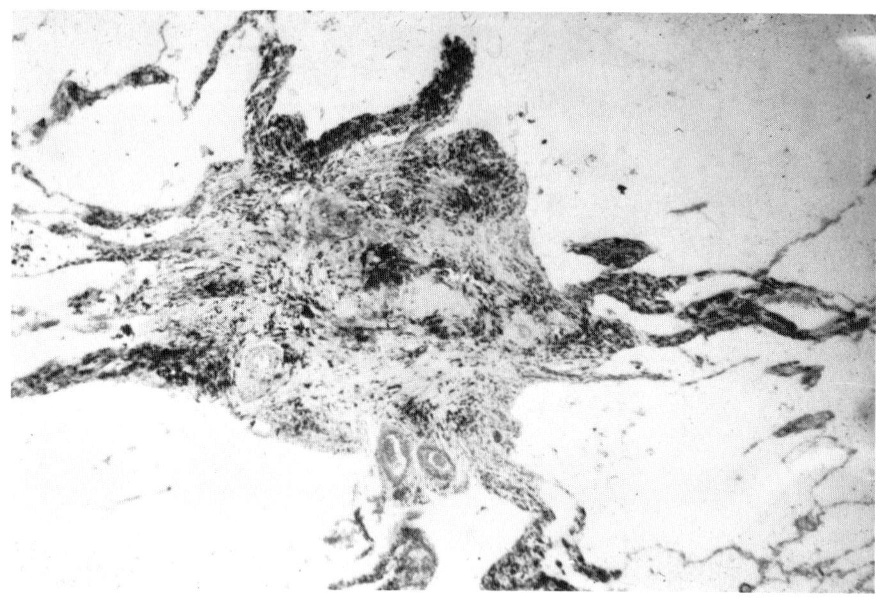

Figure 6.10. Typical stellate nodule seen in mixed dusts pneumoconiosis. The collagen fibers are irregularly distributed in the pigmented dust macule.

admixture of sizes, with one predominating. The radiograph, generally speaking, underestimates the number of nodules found at autopsy. Cases with a small number of nodules commonly have normal radiographs and occasionally a moderate number may be found when a recent radiograph was normal.

The typical silicotic nodules occur particularly when free silica forms a relatively high proportion of the inhaled dust. However, in many mines, and especially in many industries, the silica is admixed with other particulates, ie, silicates, iron, coal, etc. These sometimes modify the tissue reaction in the lungs to produce what are known as mixed dust lesions. These have a stellate rather than a round onion-peel appearance, with irregularly arranged collagen mixed with dust and dust-containing cells. It is not uncommon for these nodules and classical nodules to coexist in the same lungs. There are, to our knowledge, no characteristic radiological features associated with these lesions (Fig. 6.10). Mixed dust lesions are further discussed later in this chapter. The pathological features of acute and subacute silicosis are also reported later in this chapter.

Silicosis and Tuberculosis

Martin Panse described the symptoms and signs of silicosis in Germany in 1614, although respiratory disease in miners had been described before that.[26] Nevertheless, the distinction between silicosis and tuberculosis had not been clarified till early in this century. This was epitomized by the fact that in South Africa the institute set up to examine miners and study the lung diseases from which they suffered in such large numbers was given the official name of "The Miners Phthisis Bureau."

Subsequent studies, among others by Simpson, Strachan, Irwine,[27] and Mavrogordato,[28] in South Africa clarified the pathology of silicosis as a disease separate from tuberculosis. It was then realized that tuberculosis was an important and common complication of silicosis to the extent that in some industries the prevalence of tuberculosis was taken to indicate the extent of the silica hazard.

Tuberculosis complicating silicosis has decreased greatly during this century, where the incidence of tuberculosis in the general population has become low. For instance, in 1916, 75% of white South African gold miners showed evidence of pulmonary tuberculosis at autopsy.[29] When Chatgidakis reported on the same subject in 1963, only 13% of white miners had tuberculosis at autopsy.[30] But among these miners, tuberculosis still occurs in silicotic subjects far more frequently than in silica-exposed men without silicosis. In Sardinia in 1964, morbidity from tuberculosis was 0.12% in the total population, 0.6% among miners, and 5% among men with silicosis.[31] In black South African miners recruited from populations in which the incidence of tuberculosis is still high, the association of the two diseases is common.

In an autopsy study of 3,329 black gold miners regularly screened for pulmonary disease, 4.4% had an occult active tuberculous lesion when silicosis was absent, and 11.1% (N=2,449) when silicosis was present ($P < .001$), a difference not found in asbestos or coal miners and indicating the highly specific nature of the relationship of silica with tuberculosis.[32,99] Paul,[8] studying mostly black copper miners in Zambia, where classic silicosis occurs, found a far higher (30 times) annual incidence of pulmonary tuberculosis in miners with silicosis (3% per annum) than in those without.

Experimentally "healed" tuberculous foci may be reactivated by exposing animals to silica dust[33] probably because macrophages containing silica particles are unable to deal effectively with tubercle bacilli.[34] Animal experimentation has demonstrated the increased incidence and severity of active tuberculosis when challenged with tubercle or attenuated bacilli, such as Gardner's Rl Rv strain or bacillus Calmette-Guérin (BCG) tuberculous vaccine after silica exposure.[36] The usual presentation of pulmonary tuberculosis in persons suffering from silicosis is similar to that in nonminers.

More subtle relationships between silicosis and tuberculosis are, however, postulated by some authorities.[25] Silica dust administered together with BCG (living or dead) or the vole bacillus or even tuberculin[35] increases fibrosis and leads to massive fibrosis in experimental animals. Successfully culturing tubercle bacilli in the sputum of cases of silicotic massive fibrosis in man is, however, most unusual, and histological features of tuberculosis in association with massive fibrosis are uncommon. Moreover, massive shadows seldom persist in silicotics or silica-exposed workers after successful treatment of sputum-positive tuberculosis. In the guinea-pig rendered tuberculin positive by injection of dead BCG, intratracheal silica caused a greater cellular reaction and a faster and more intense fibrosis.[36]

The terms silicotuberculosis and tuberculosilicosis commonly used in the past to describe what were presumed to be different kinds of associations between silicosis and tuberculosis should be abandoned. However, the radiological features of tuberculosis in silicosis surveillance that should arouse suspicion are marked asymmetry of the opacities, involvement of the apices, a "hilar flare" connecting upper lobe silicotic areas to the hilum, greater enlargement of hilar glands than usual in silicosis, and unilateral marked contraction of a lobe apart from obvious diagnostic features such as cavitation.

Tuberculosis in silica-exposed persons with or without radiological silicosis responds well to modern multidrug therapy.[37] Hence, any unusual radiological phenomenon should be viewed with suspicion, and even cases of apparently classic uncomplicated silicosis should have the sputum examined for tubercle bacilli at intervals.

Persons with silicosis, even if occult, may develop tuberculous pleurisy, tuberculous pericarditis, or miliary tuberculosis. This occurs especially in silica-exposed persons who develop immunosuppression, whether from disease or drug induced.

Silicosis and Nontuberculous Mycobacteria

Mycobacterial diseases sometimes occur in persons with silicosis (especially accelerated silicosis).[38] Pneumoconiosis is a disease predisposing to infection with mycobacteria,[39] according to some authors, but their relationship with dust disease is questioned by others.[93] A case-control study in Britain indicated that *Mycobacterium kansasii* infections occurred in excess in persons with current dust exposure, but was not influenced by past dust exposure.[40] In a recent report on 47 cases of pulmonary infection with *Mycobacterium xenopi* from a coal mining area, 75% had preexisting lung disease, but only one had coal worker's pneumoconiosis.[41] The particular organism involved is largely determined by its regional prevalence, eg, in the New Orleans area it is *Mycobacterium kansasii*; in Wisconsin it is *Mycobacterium intracellulare*.[38]

Silicosis and Autoimmune Connective Tissue Disease

Humoral and cell-mediated immunity are disturbed by silica. Autoimmune phenomena occur not infrequently with significant titers of antinuclear antibodies and rheumatoid factor. They are more likely to occur when exposures to silica dust have been extremely high.[42–44]

Scleroderma occurs with increased incidence in silica-exposed persons.[45] Claims have been made in the literature that rheumatoid arthritis occurs with increased frequency in persons with silicosis.[46] There is no published evidence that this is so in silicosis, and there is evidence that it is not so in coal worker's pneumoconiosis.[47] There is also some evidence that diffuse lupus erythematosus may, on occasions, be associated with silica exposure (usually intense exposure).[38,49] The sudden onset and rapid progression of silicotic massive fibrosis has also been reported in association with sarcoidosis in a miner with modest silica exposure.[50]

Prevalence

With adequate dust suppression, the incidence and the severity of silicosis have declined and with it the previous high morbidity and significant mortality. It still remains difficult to estimate the impact of silicosis on health and mortality. The statistics from many countries are impossible to interpret because coal worker's pneumoconiosis is included under the term "silicosis," but not in the United Kingdom, where there were 650 new cases of silicosis in 1977.[55] Statistics are not available for many countries, particularly from some with the highest mortality rate, eg, Indian slate pencil manufacturers.[51]

In South African gold mines, mean lifetime exposure to 0.2 mg/m^3 is still associated with an appreciable incidence of silicosis, although deaths directly due to silicosis are very rare. Thus in a cohort of white miners who worked from January 1, 1934 to December 31, 1938, 48% of those working in the most dusty occupations – ie, miners at the face, had developed radiological silicosis by 1968.[52]

Nevertheless, in a cohort of 3,970 white gold miners in these mines born between January 1, 1916, and December 31, 1930, there were no deaths due to silicosis or tuberculosis to the end of 1978, when they were 48 to 62 years old.[53] Deaths due to silicosis, especially when tuberculosis is a complication, may not be recognized in black miners as the follow-up on migrant workers retiring to their own countries of origin is lacking.

Prevalence rates also vary from country to country and industry to industry. The most important factors causing such variations are undoubtedly the intensity and duration of exposure. Other factors – ie, genetic variation in susceptibility as suggested by familial aggregation of cases[54] and a relationship to ABO blood groups[55] – do not appear to be important. However, identical twins are more frequently concordant for silicosis than nonidentical twins, according to one report.[13]

There is no evidence of any racial susceptibility. Women may, however, be more susceptible than men.[117] Concurrent inhalation of other mineral dusts (some of which may promote silicosis and others retard its development[56,57]) are of little importance.

In 1900 Betts described an epidemic of silicosis with many deaths in a quartz mill.[58] Outbreaks of silicosis have occurred among tombstone sandblasters[49] and shipping sandblasters,[38] and at a brick company handling silica, all associated with a high mortality.

Sometimes an industry associated with a low silicosis risk suddenly produces a high incidence of the disease owing to a change in processing the siliceous rock: eg, a change in the crushers in a granite quarry in Austria brought about a great increase of production of crushed stone, but also a large increase in dust.[59]

Radiological Features

The radiological features of silicosis are described under the following headings, according to the structures involved: pleura, hilar lymph nodes,

Figure 6.11. Nodular opacities 1/2 profusion r/r. *Visceral* (lesser fissure) thickening. Mid-zonal nodulation considered atypical for silicosis, however, culture for *M tuberculosis* negative. Exposure to siliceous dust, 18 years. Posterior junction line markedly thickened and irregular (probable plaques).

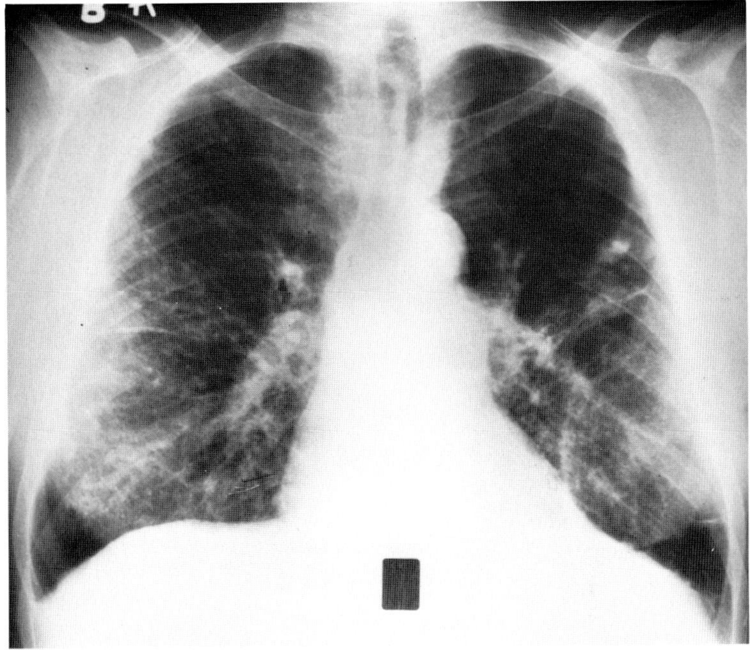

lymph nodes in the parenchyma, and lung parenchyma.

Pleura

Slight general thickening of the visceral pleura is common but infrequently demonstrated radiologically (Fig. 6.11).

Hyaline localized pleural plaques which sometimes calcify and appear as flat elliptical symmetrical plaques over both upper zones in apical views (Figs. 6.12 and 6.13). These features are reasonably characteristic. Although uncalcified and calcified plaques also occur after exposure to asbestos, they are rare at this site, ie, the upper zones, and have not been symmetrical, as occurs with silicotic plaques.

The Hilar Lymph Nodes

Hilar lymph nodes are commonly *slightly* enlarged, with "fuzzy" margins. However, the radiological appearance of marked hilar gland enlargement with a clear margin is not, as a rule, due to silicosis.

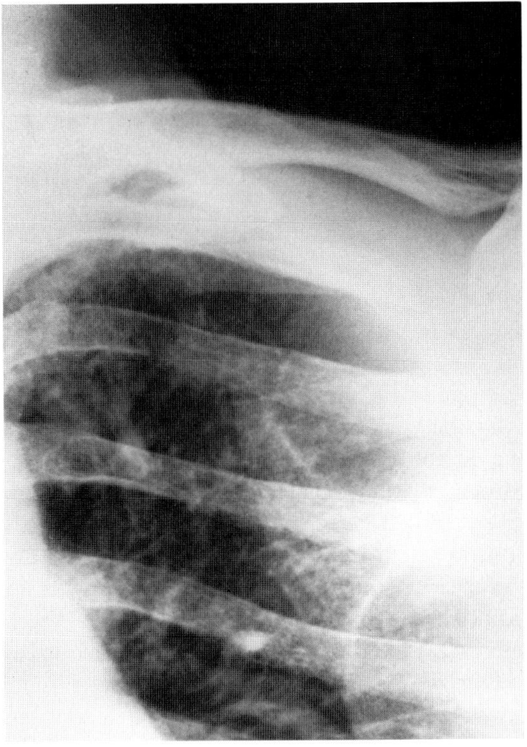

Figure 6.12. Opacities profusion 1/1 q/r. Uncalcified hyaline plaque, left upper zone (magnified view).

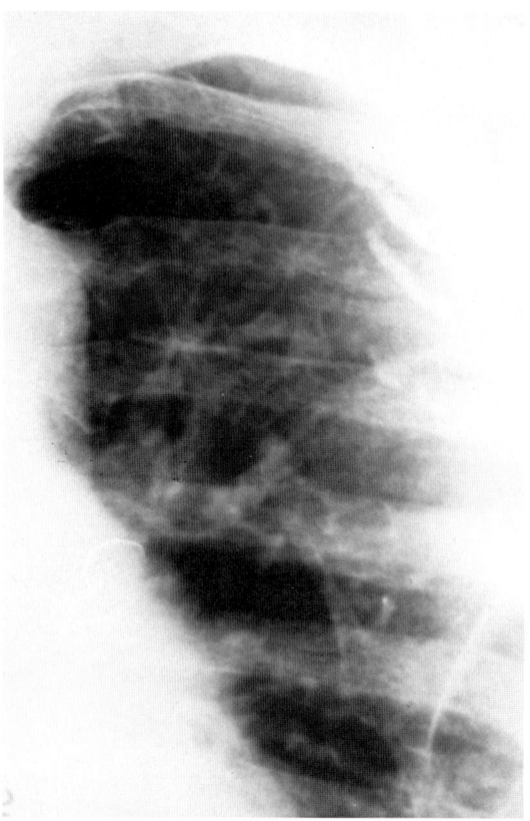

Figure 6.13. Magnified left upper lung field. Symmetrical flat calcified elliptical plaques, both upper lung zones. Plaques appeared after 42 years of exposure to silica dust and were unassociated with any other features of silicosis.

Diffuse symmetrical hilar node calcification may occur, but eggshell hilar gland calcification is the more common and sometimes the only manifestation of silicosis.

Eggshell nodes are not pathognomonic of silica exposure, but occur in a number of other diseases, particularly tuberculosis and sarcoidosis. More rarely they occur in amyloidosis, scleroderma, postirradiated Hodgkin's disease, blastomycosis and histoplasmosis.[69] The eggshell appearance is, however, sufficiently characteristic of silica exposure to warrant taking a careful history of industrial exposure. Our autopsy evidence indicates that eggshell nodes are not due to associated tuberculous infection.[60] Diffuse calcification of the lymph glands is more indicative of tuberculous infection.

Calcified nodes are usually free of complications, but may compress bronchi (especially the right middle lobe bronchus), producing a middle lobe syndrome, which may also be produced by active tuberculous infection of these lymph glands in subjects with silicosis.[61] A calcified node may also erode into bronchi, cause obstruction, or be expectorated. Dangerous hemoptysis may occur (Fig. 6.14). Rarely other structures may be affected, for example, esophageal compression.[62] Bronchoesophageal fistula,[63] tracheobronchial stenosis,[64] bronchoarterial fistula,[65] and compression of the superior vena cava have all been reported.[66]

Parenchymal Lymph Nodes

Bronchial lymph nodes occur far out in the lungs. Silicotic islets may occur in these lymph nodes, which may then become enlarged[67] and calcify and may appear typically "eggshell," even at the lung periphery (Figs. 6.15 and 6.16).

Parenchymal Lung Change

There are two kinds of parenchymal lesions in silicosis: small opacities and massive shadows. The small opacities are nearly always rounded, though often with fuzzy borders and may be p, q, or r initially (see Chapter 2) (Figs. 6.17 and 6.18). They appear in the upper lung zones at first, often more profuse on the right, but later the distribution of the opacities tends to become characteristically symmetrical.[13] The extreme apices are usually spared and changes there should arouse the suspicion of possible associated tuberculosis. With progression, the round opacities—being far the commonest—spread into the midzones and uncommonly into the lower zones. Rarely, one side is spared, particularly with reduced ventilation to one lung, as in Macleod's syndrome.

The profusion of nodulation does not correlate with lung function tests as is the case in coal workers' pneumoconiosis. In coal workers' pneumoconiosis, associated usually with emphysema, impaired carbon-monoxide diffusion has been reported when there are p nodules.[68,69] The various sizes are not fixed, small ones may, with time, become larger (Fig. 6.18), and there

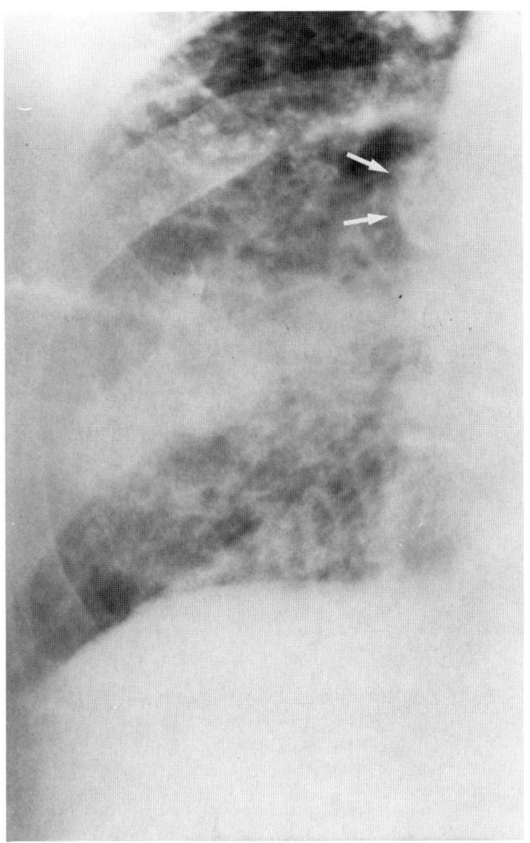

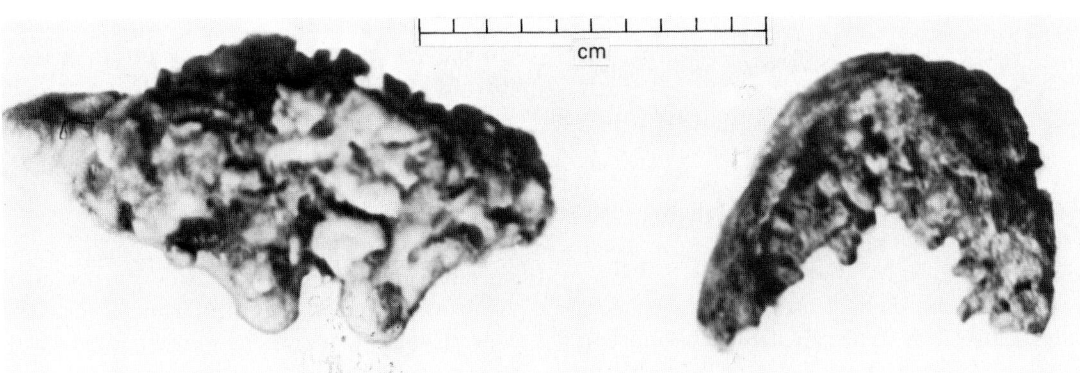

Figure 6.14. A. Calcified pleural plaques: sparse lung nodulation (1/1 q/q) and eggshell hilar glands on the right (*arrow*). Collapse and fibrosis of the right middle lobe. Coughed-up calcified hilar gland with hemoptysis. Expectorated gland shown in **B**.

are exceptions to the rule that the opacities occur most profusely in the upper zones. Sometimes the atypical distribution in the midzones persists through life.

Although silicosis classically presents first in the right upper zone and sometimes remains more prominent in that region, this is by no means invariable. The radiological onset of silicosis is usually insidious, and difficulty may be experienced in determining the exact year of onset. The x-ray appearance of silicosis may be sudden, especially when associated with immunological disease. Cases are seen, however, where no definite explanation is found for the sudden onset.

While the rounded opacities of silicosis often have fuzzy and indistinct borders, true irregular opacities are also seen as in coal workers' pneumoconiosis.[70] The small round opacities of silicosis

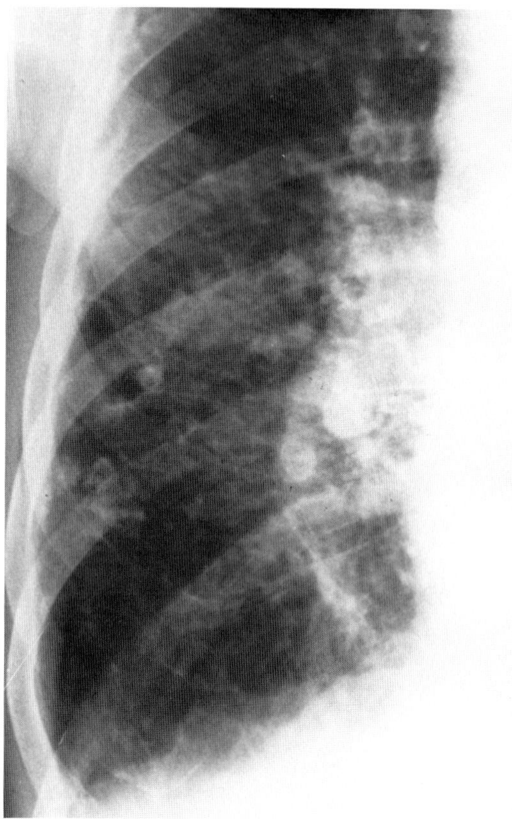

Figure 6.15. Silica dust exposure, 35 years. Radiograph shows early silicosis (1/1 r/r) and eggshell calcification in the pulmonary parenchyma (magnified right lung).

may calcify because of necrosis in the silicotic islet, a phenomenon that was commonly seen in the past in gold miners, but has now become infrequent.

In 1930 Simpson et al. isolated *Mycobacterium tuberculosis* from some silicotic islets with central necrosis.[27] However, this central necrosis may have been due to the far higher dust exposures in those days and not to the associated tuberculosis. Calcification of silicotic nodules may become very widespread and produce a "snow storm" effect on x-ray study (Fig. 6.20).

Radiological opacities greater than 1 cm are termed "large opacities" and massive fibrosis and progressive massive fibrosis are often used as synonyms (Fig. 6.21). Although the condition is often progressive,[71] it may remain static for years and even decades. Typically large opacities appear after silicosis has been seen on the radiograph for many years, and as they increase in size, the background of small opacities get sparser, being incorporated into the massive opacity, with an apparent diminution of profusion. Bullous emphysema, which often accompanies the large opacities, also results in the small opacities becoming difficult to see. With the passage of time it is usual for large opacities to involve both lungs, almost invariably in the upper zones, but not the apices (Figs. 6.22 and 6.23). On the rare occasions when they are unilateral, and especially when a background of small opacities is not visible, they may pose extremely difficult problems in differential diagnosis.

Silicotic massive shadows eventually tend to migrate to the hilum or to the mediastinum (Fig. 6.26). Unlike massive opacities in coal workers' pneumoconiosis, cavitation in silicotic massive fibrosis is rare, and when seen in silicosis, it is due to tuberculosis. Cavitation in coal workers' pneumoconiosis is due to ischemic necrosis in the masses,[72] but is extremely rare in silicosis and this could be explained by the findings on arteriography of a rich vascular supply to the massive silicotic lesions.[73]

In general, large opacities occur more frequently as the profusion of the small opacities increases. Age may be an independent factor, as in coal worker's pneumoconiosis,[74] possibly because of changes that occur in the immune system with age.

Progression of Silicosis

The factors determining the rate of progression of nodulation and massive fibrosis are not well understood. Unquestionably, small opacities may progress in profusion and size after cessation of exposure, and nodulation and even large opacities may appear radiographically for the first time many years after exposure has ceased. A unilateral large opacity can result in unnecessary resections in cases of progressive massive fibrosis.[77] This is avoidable if a thorough occupational history is obtained and fine-needle aspiration cytology or biopsy performed.

Normally, silicosis progresses slowly, but may remain static for many years. It is not even known

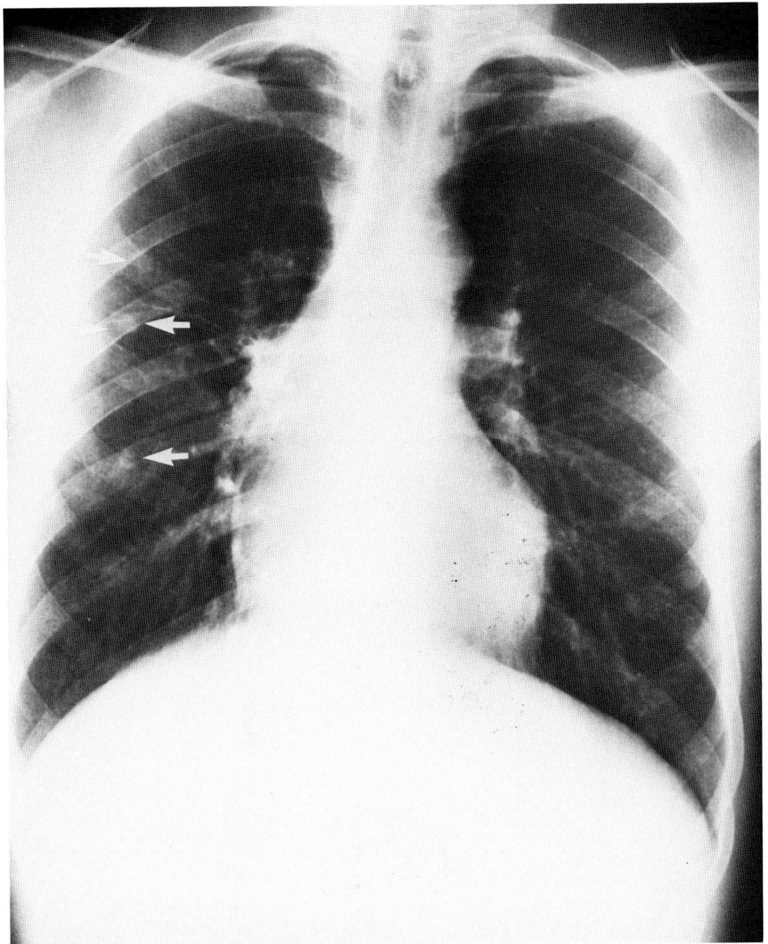

Figure 6.16. Subject had only 2 years' exposure to high siliceous dust. Several nodules 1 cm in diameter noted on the radiograph (*arrows*). No clinical clue to their etiology; erythrocyte sedimentation rate (ESR) was normal. Thoracotomy performed and nodules went to histology, which showed they were parenchymal lymph nodes infiltrated with silicotic islets.

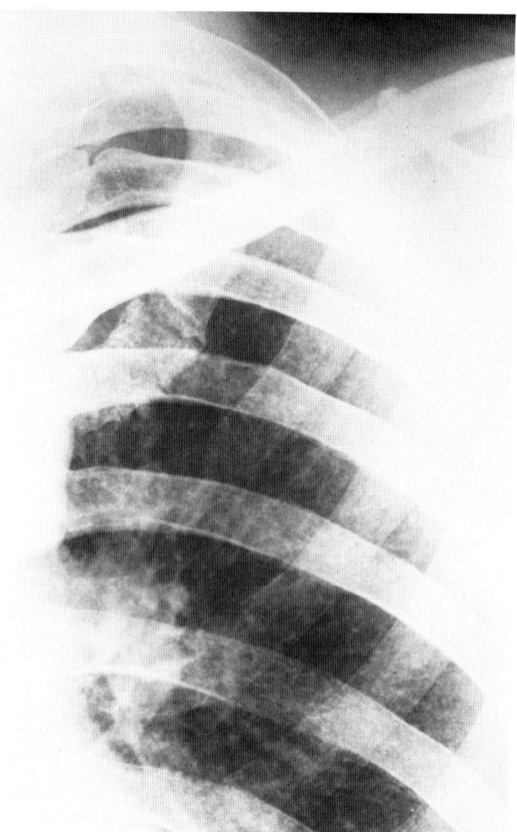

Figure 6.17. Silicosis with profusion 1/1 and p/p nodulation after 28 years' exposure to silica dust. Lung function tests: normal.

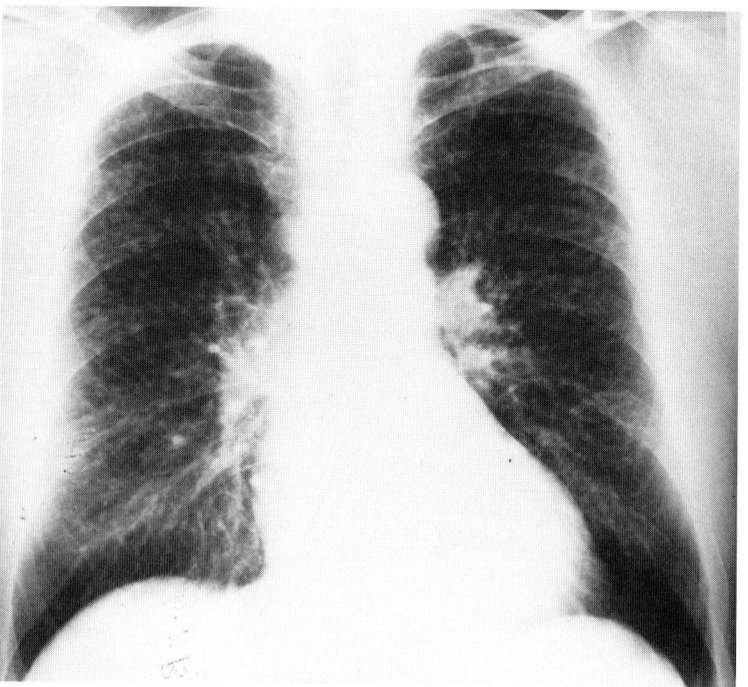

Figure 6.18. Lung nodules profusion 2/3 r/r upper zones. There is relative sparing of the apices and bases on chest radiograph. Exposure to moderately high-intensity silica dust over 33 years with rather sudden onset of silicosis. Lung function tests: normal.

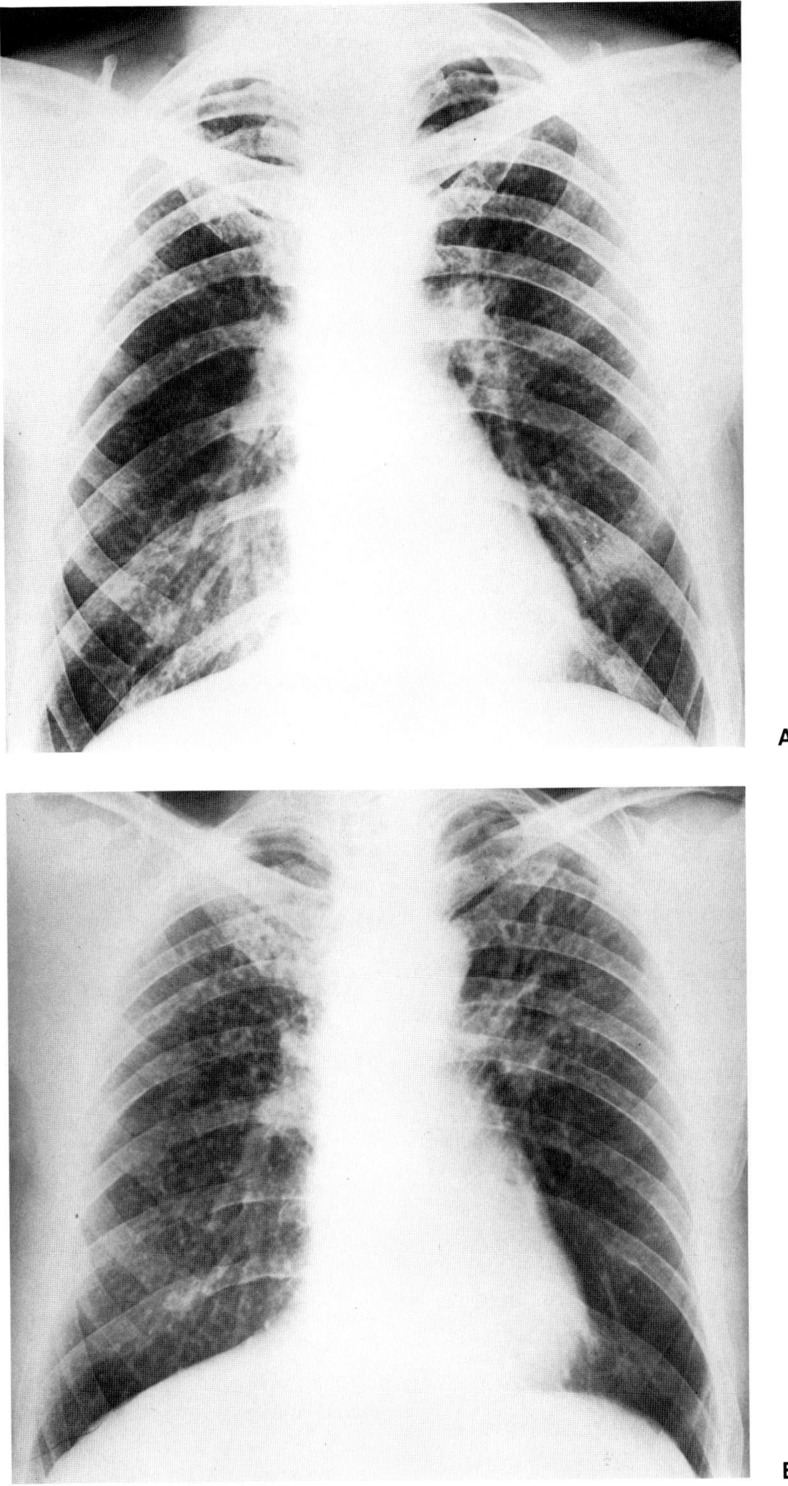

Figure 6.19. **A.** q/q nodules have enlarged to r/r. Patient had 36 years' exposure to highly siliceous dust. **B**. The change in size took place over 4 years, but patient remained clinically well. Twelve sputum cultures for *M tuberculosis* were negative.

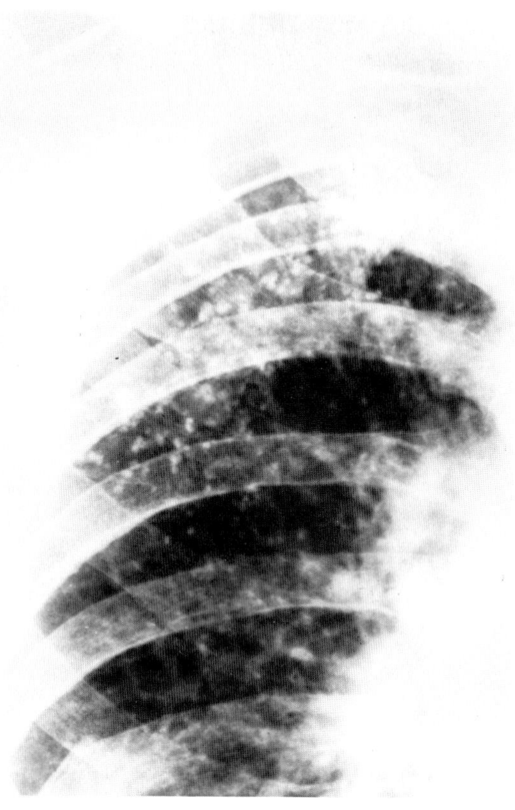

Figure 6.20. Nodules (profusion 2/2 type q/r) with calcification. Eleven years after initial development of silicosis, nodules became calcified. Sputum cultures for tuberculosis were negative.

with certainty whether progression is more likely to occur in those who continue with moderate silica exposure after onset, compared with those who terminate exposure,[75] though the available evidence favors the latter group.[76] It is probable that the most important factor determining progression is the cumulative silica dust exposure. However, the physicochemical state of the silica crystals[4] and host factors, including blood groups, may play a role,[54] as may the presence of other mineral dust in the lung.[56,57,68,78]

Acute and Subacute (Accelerated) Silicosis

Acute silicosis is a rare disease provoked by an exposure to very high silica doses. It develops the radiological and histological features of alveolar proteinosis (silico-proteinosis), possibly associated with ill-defined atypical silicotic nodules.[80] The radiological features are those of alveolar infiltration and obliteration with possible air bronchograms.[81] The lung opacities have poorly defined margins and are not homogeneous, often resembling alveolar pulmonary edema. Nodulation and evidence of fibrosis may be associated with the above changes.[82,83] This condition has been seen in sandblasters, ceramic workers, and open-cast coal miners working in siliceous rock.[89] It has also been produced in animal models by inhalation of high doses of silica.[84]

Subacute (accelerated) silicosis refers to a characteristic histological appearance, usually associated with unusual radiological features[85] (Figs. 6.24 and 6.25). Such cases may follow very high silica exposures, but they also occur in persons exposed to doses to which fellow workers either get no radiological silicosis or the classic relatively benign disease. In 1933 Gardner described similar cases following exposure to high silica dust inhalation as "acute silicosis"[86] prior to recognition of alveolar proteinosis.[13]

Silicosis, Emphysema, and Chronic Airway Disease

Perifocal emphysema as seen in coal worker's pneumoconiosis does not occur with silicosis, but bullous emphysema quite commonly occurs near areas of massive fibrosis.

Silica-exposed workers smoke as frequently and as much as the general male population and develop chronic obstructive airways disease with or without emphysema. There is, in addition however, a large body of evidence—both epidemiological and pathological—showing that exposure to many dusts, including silica-containing dust,[87] is a significant risk factor for the development of air-flow limitation. South African gold miners, for instance, develop dust-related airway obstruction whether they have radiological silicosis or not when total dust exposure has been standardized for.[88]

All lung function tests, including spirometry and flow-volume studies, in silicotics are, however,

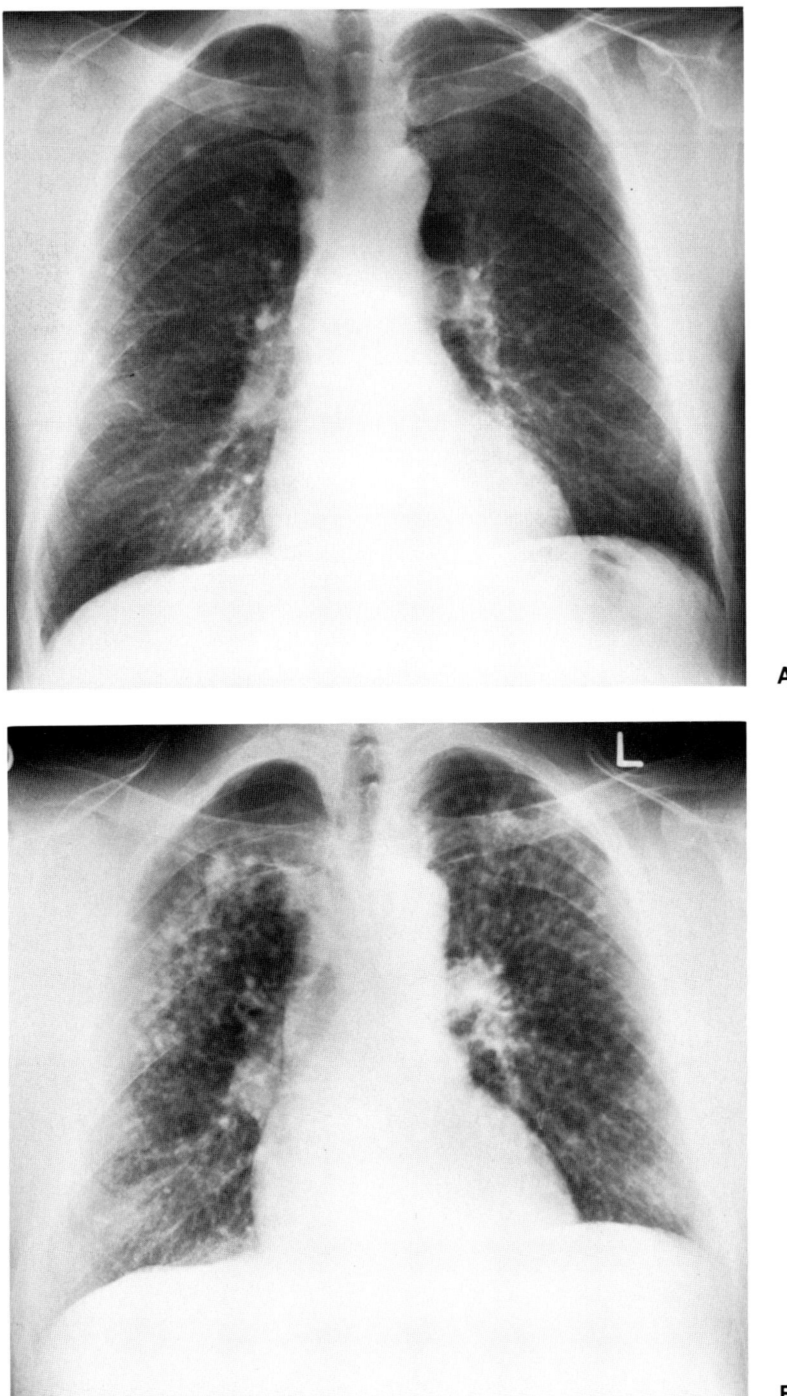

Figure 6.21. A. q/r nodules in the midlung zone. Initial presentation after 15 years of silica exposure. **B**. A shadow of massive fibrosis appeared 14 years after previous radiograph. The ESR was 23 mm/1 h, but repeated cultures for tubercle bacilli were negative.

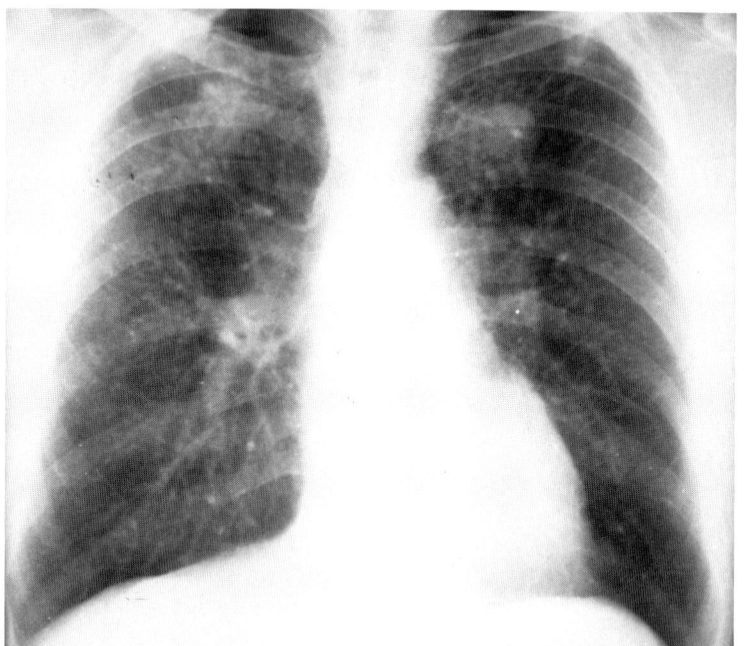

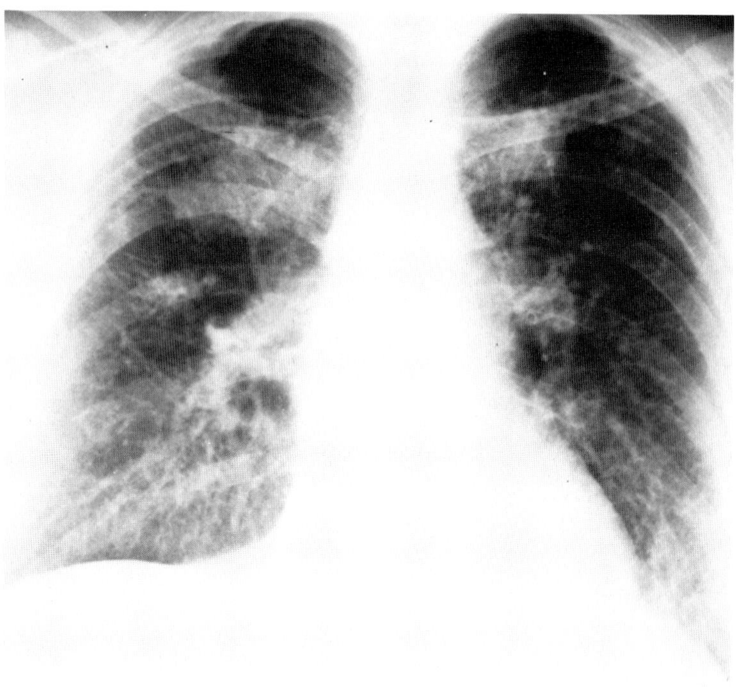

Figure 6.22. A. Rounded opacities 1/1 q/q, right upper zone and left upper zone massive opacities. Subject had 34 years' exposure to siliceous dust. **B**. Development of third massive opacity in the right hilum. Laboratory findings: Mantoux text, positive (1.5 cm); ESR, 26 mm/1 h; rheumatoid tests, negative; cultures for tuberculosis, negative; scalene node biopsy negative for sarcoid, tuberculosis, and malignancy. Case shows diagnostic difficulties in cases of massive fibrosis as hilar mass was thought to be malignant or tuberculous.

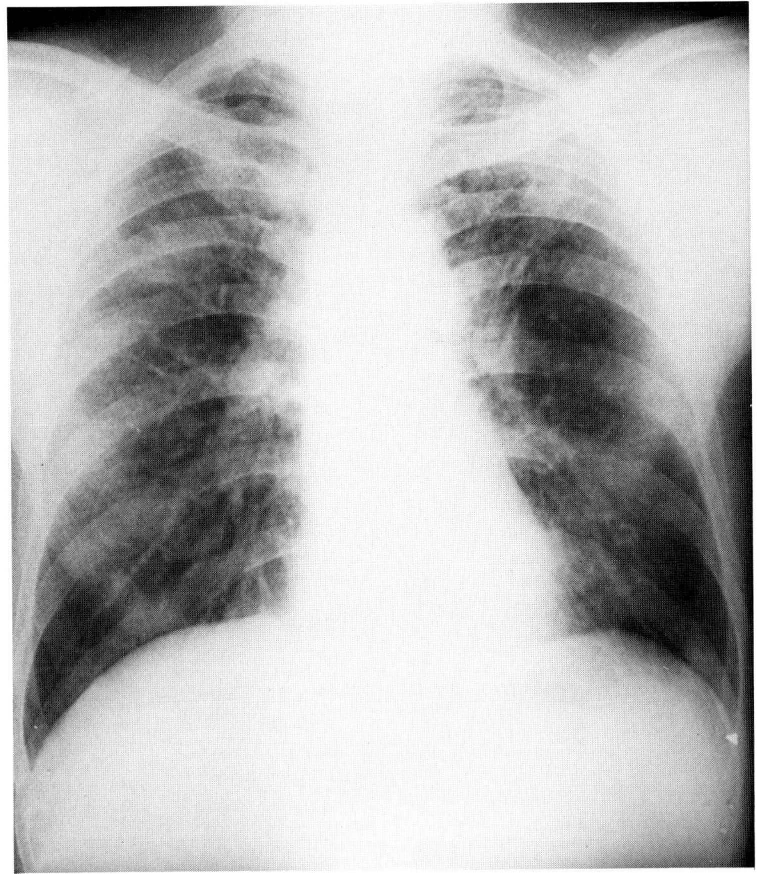

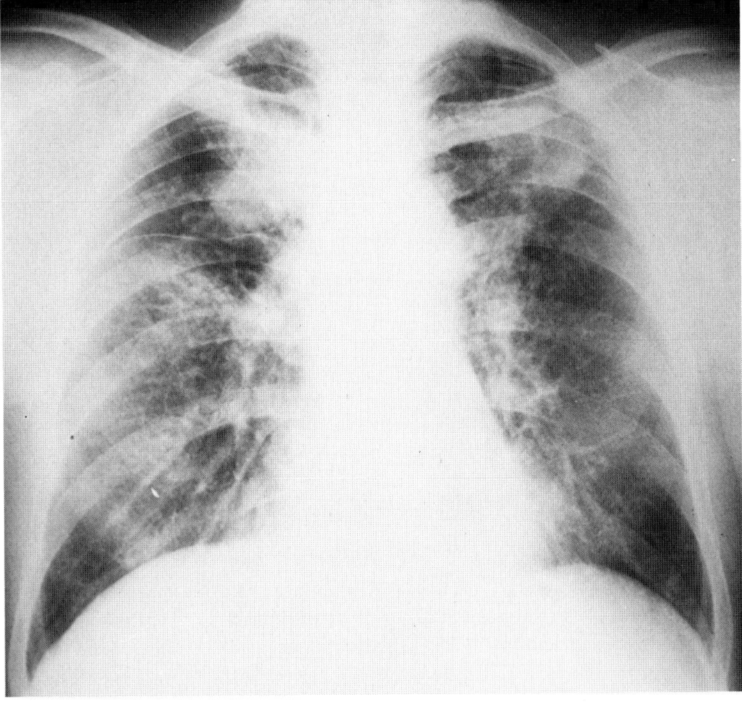

Figure 6.23. A. Radiograph 1/1 q/q with massive fibrosis (MF), type A. Exposed to high silica dust for 21 years. **B**. Radiograph profusion 3/4 type r/r nodules with early MF (type A), rapidly progressed to MF, type C. Changes occurred 2 years after above radiograph. Laboratory findings: Mantoux test, positive; ESR normal; eight sputum cultures for mycobacteria, negative. Early subclavicular opacity might have been tuberculosis that reactivated.

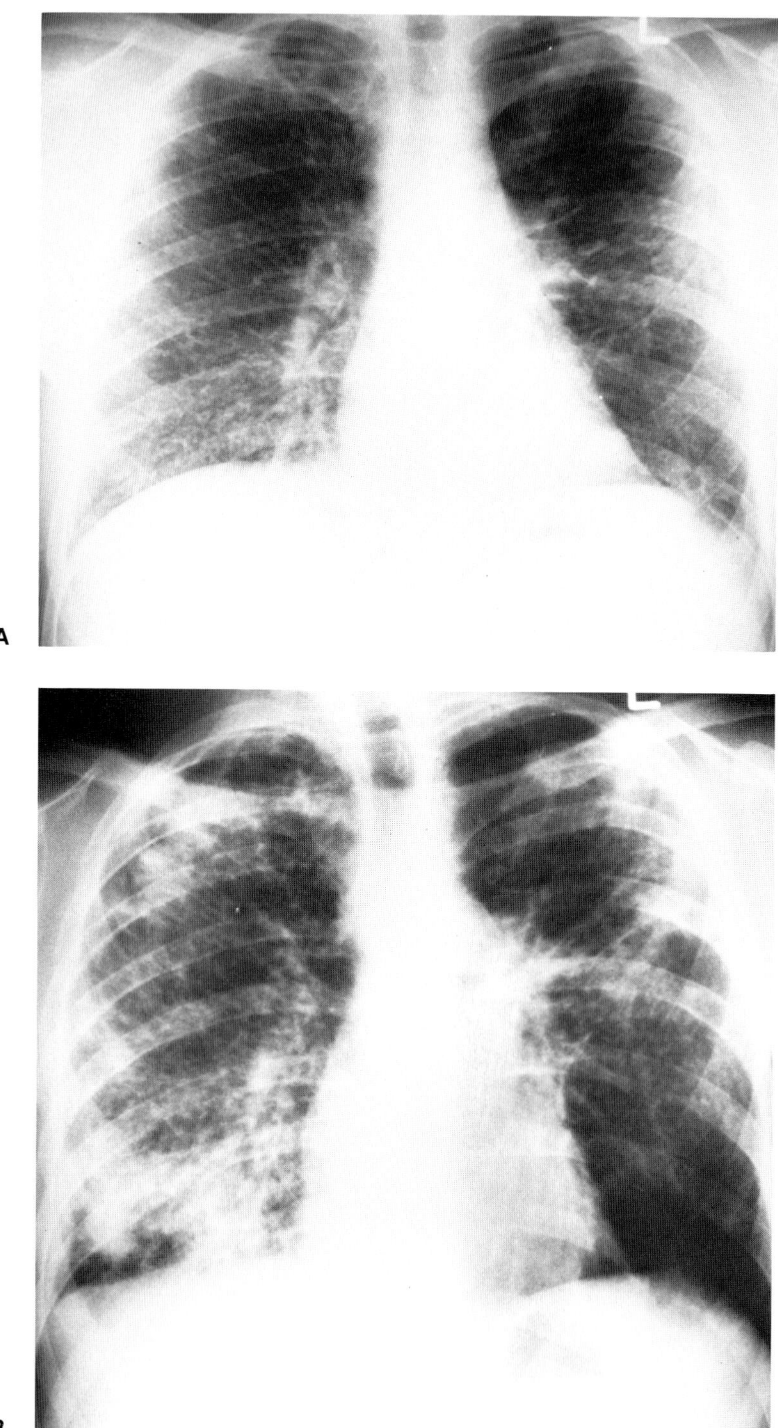

Figure 6.24. A. q/r nodules profusion 1/2. Left midzonal vascular distortion (parenchymal scarring). The subject had an 11-year history of exposure to silica dust. Lung biopsy: islets and plaques of silicotic collagenization, with perivascular and interstitial histiocytes and lymphocytes, and reticulin and collagen deposition. Birefringent particles present. The features are those of subacute silicosis. **B**. Three years later shows rapid progression and profusion of opacities. Cultures for *M tuberculosis* were negative on eight occasions; ESR, 43 mm/1 h (Westergren).

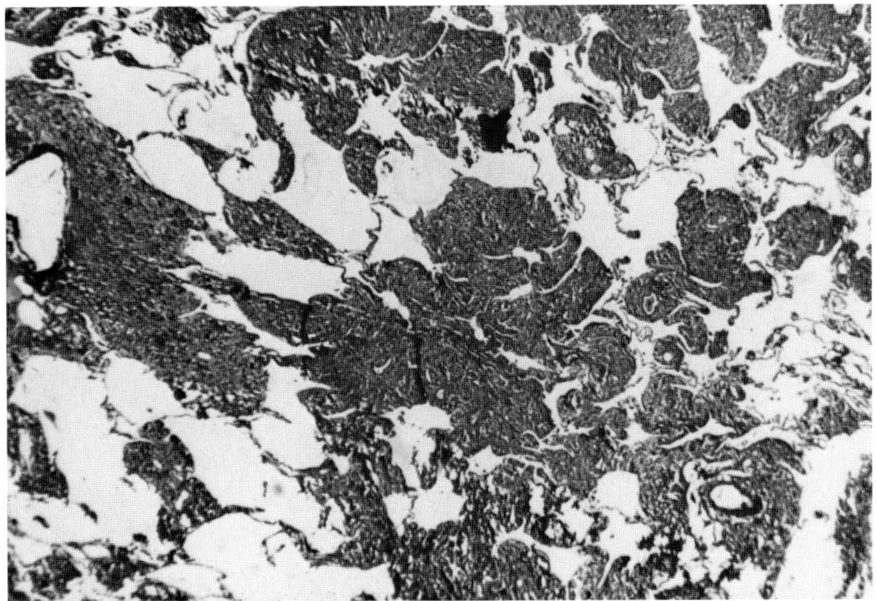

Figure 6.25. Subacute silicosis. There are immature islets and perivascular interstitial cell infiltration with collagen deposition.

quite often within normal limits or nearly so, especially in nonsmokers. Lung function tests in silicotics when abnormal, far more commonly show obstructive features and hyperinflation than restrictive features in the absence of massive fibrosis. Massive fibrosis itself may be associated with a restrictive pattern, but even in this case an obstructive pattern is not rare, especially when only A shadows are present. A mixed pattern in advanced silicosis is not unusual.[89] The increase in residual volume, which becomes more marked with profusion of small opacities in coal miners who show no evidence of obstruction,[89] has not been shown to occur in silicosis.[90] Air-flow limitation at low lung volumes may be the only parameter that is abnormal–possibly due to small airway lesions due to local dust deposition.[91] It is therefore not rare for silicosis to be associated with radiographic features of hyperinflation (Fig. 6.27).

Spontaneous pneumothorax is excessively rare as a complication of silicosis with or without evidence of emphysema and signs of cor pulmonale are only seen with advanced massive fibrosis, or when the silicosis is associated with marked emphysema or advanced tuberculosis.

Silicosis and Tuberculosis

Tuberculosis in silicosis may present in several ways,[93] including the development of cavitation in areas of massive fibrosis, with sputum-positive *M tuberculosis*, but may occasionally be positive when no cavitation is demonstrable. Active tuberculous lesions are occasionally found at autopsy in silicotic subjects who have shown no radiographic suggestion of tuberculosis in life . A sparse growth of tubercle bacilli, eg, one to five colonies, raises a very difficult therapeutic dilemma in silicosis, as it may be due to contamination, especially if further sputum examinations are repeatedly negative.

Tuberculous infiltration is similar to that in a nonsilica-exposed person, both in site and appearance (Fig. 6.29). Tuberculosis should also be suspected if unusual radiological features occur during the progress of silicosis. Even in the presence of p-sized nodulation, monitoring for *M tuberculosis* should be carried out.

A high degree of suspicion should also be exercised when a silicotic subject develops a disease or is subjected to treatment that may be associated with immunosuppression (Fig. 6.28).

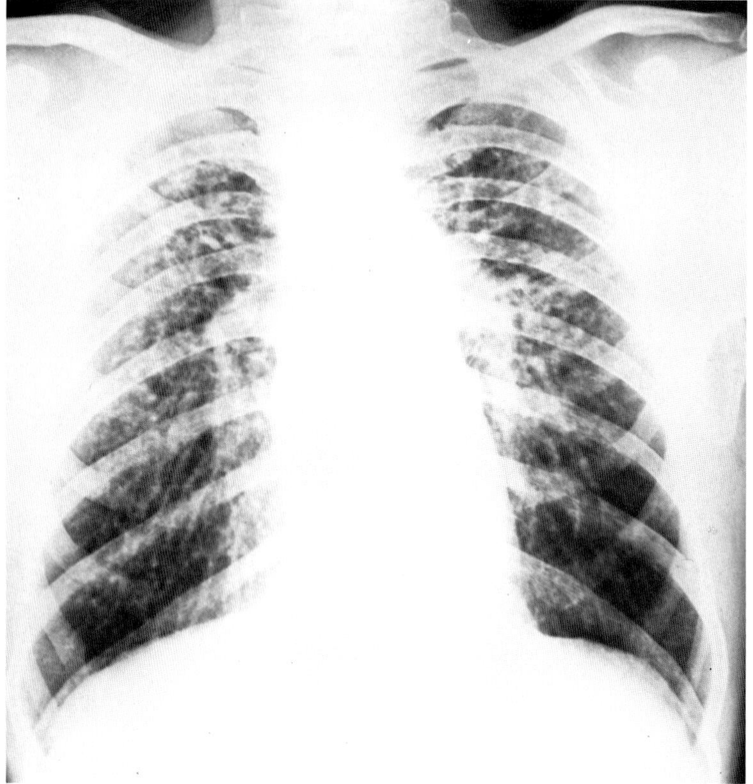
A

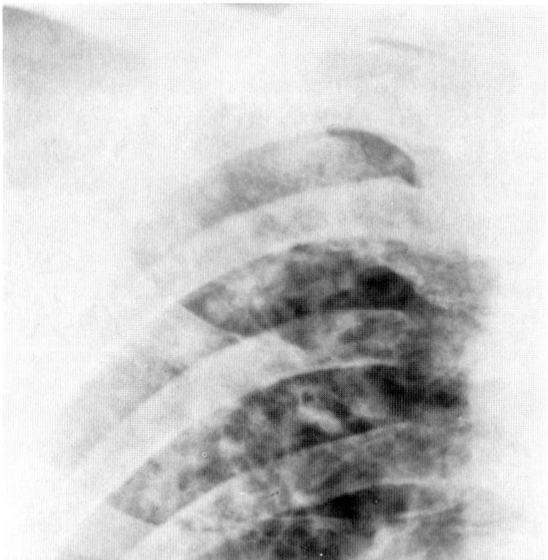
B

Figure 6.26. A. Round opacities (3/3 r/q). Large subclavicular opacities. **B**. Early massive opacity on right. **C**. Right opacity now embedded in mediastinum; hila are markedly elevated. Associated emphysema with tenting of diaphragms probably due to upper zone volume loss and pleuritic traction in the overinflated lower lobes.

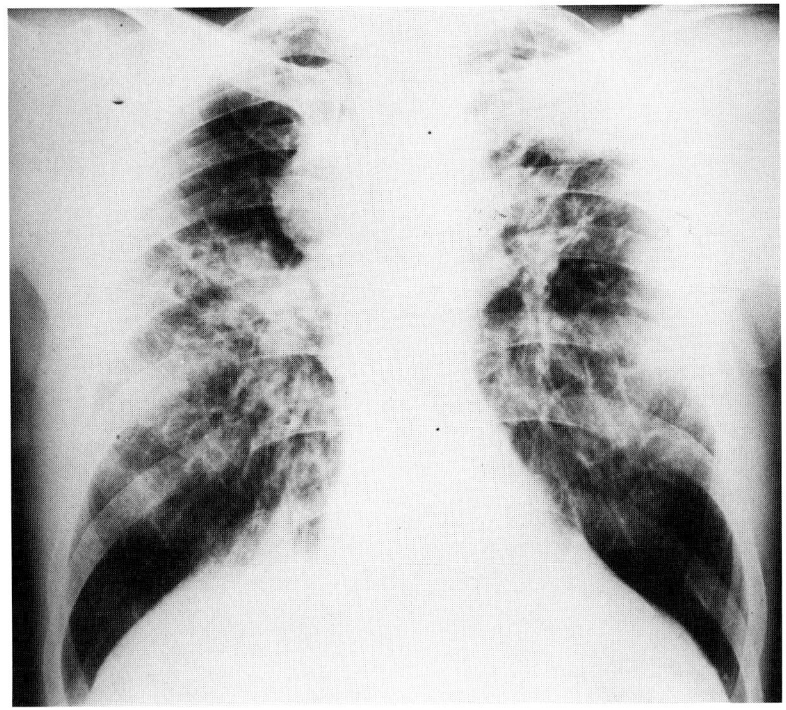

Figure 6.26

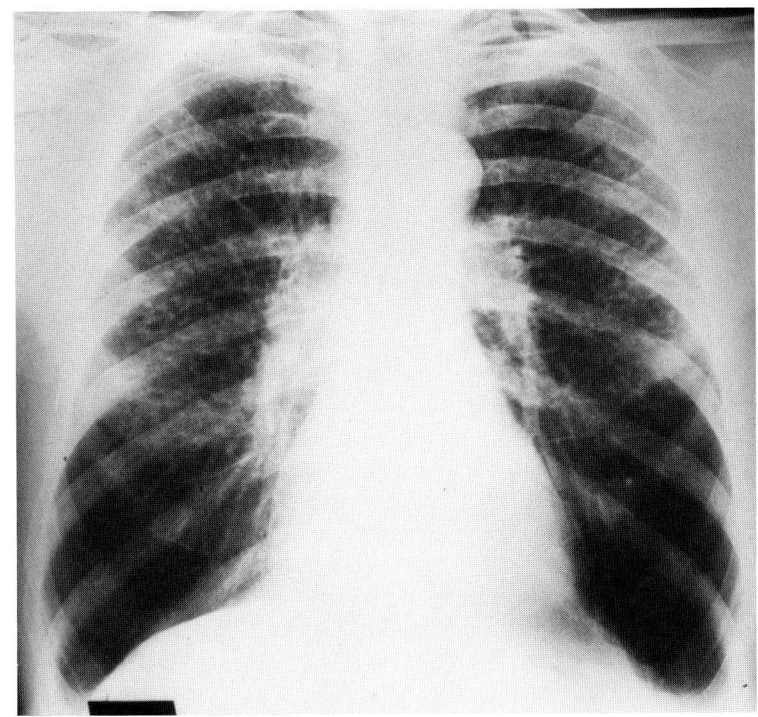

Figure 6.27. Round opacities 3/2 profusion: size q/q. Exposure, 40 years. Associated hyperinflation of lungs: flattened diaphragms and hypertransradiancy with subcardiac air trapping at bases. History of cigarette smoking as a youth, followed by pipe smoking for last 20 years. Lung function test: marked airways obstruction.

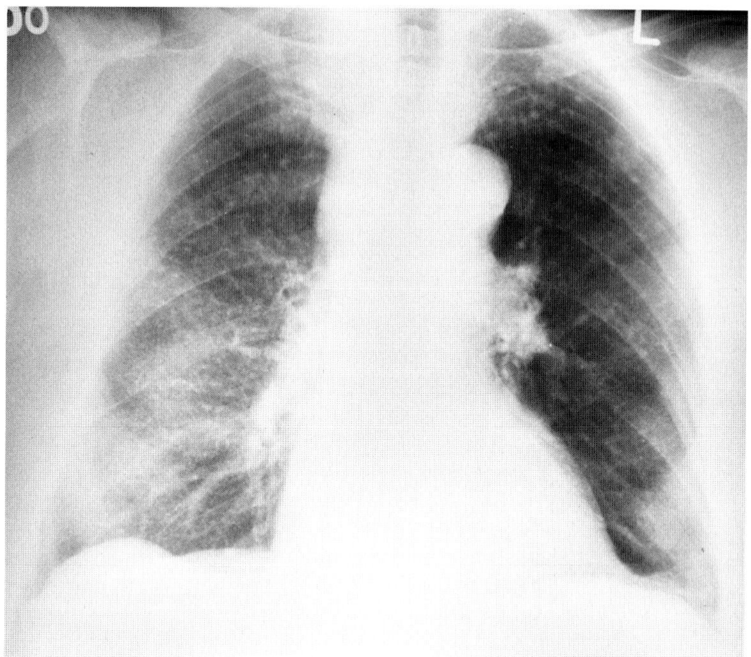

Figure 6.28. Calcified silicotic nodules and an enlarged right paramediastinal mass of lymph glands. Exposure to siliceous dust, 31 years. Developed lymphoma with features of chronic lymphatic leukemia; treated with immunosuppressants. Developed tuberculous pericardial effusion; organisms isolated from pericardial fluid. Responded to appropriate antituberculosis therapy. Autopsy findings: marked silicosis, non-Hodgkins lymphoma. No signs of tuberculosis.

Occasionally, tuberculosis in silicotic lungs may result in the appearance of large opacities after successful treatment (Fig. 6.30).

Silicosis and Bronchial Carcinoma

Goldsmith et al. made a case for an association between silicosis and lung cancer.[92] A recent case-control study, which included smoking habits of South African gold miners exposed to a mean of 0.2 mgm/m³ of free silica, showed no association between lung cancer and silicosis or lifetime silica dust exposure.[79] Hepplestone also concluded that no casual relationship exists between bronchial cancer and silica dust exposure.[104] However, there are recent reports that maintain that there is an excess of bronchial cancer in sufferers from silicosis, particularly in the mining, tunneling, and quarrying operations.[94–96] In hard rock mining (iron, tin, and gold) low but significant exposure to radon occurs, producing an extra confounding factor.[97–99] In such circumstances it is not surprising that elevated standardized mortality ratios for bronchial carcinoma occur in such exposed populations, with a not uncommon coexistence of silicosis and bronchogenic carcinoma, where both are common diseases. Other carcinogens are present in many other industries where exposure to silica occurs, eg, polycyclic hydrocarbons in foundries. However, sharply lowering dust levels reduced an excess of bronchial cancers in Vermont granite workers.[121]

Carcinoma can arise in an area of silicotic fibrosis, so-called scar carcinoma, as described by Boyd et al. in Cumberland hematite mines.[100] Boehm et al. reported 41 cases of scar cancer found at autopsy and provided criteria for the diagnosis. However, their cases probably had "anthracosilicosis."[101] Scar carcinoma in silicotics is, in our experience, extremely rare. In the last 30 years, about 3,000 pairs of lungs per year have been examined at autopsy, and there have only been two cases of scar carcinomas associated with an area of silicotic fibrosis[102] (Figs. 6.31 and 6.32).

Scars associated with a carcinoma often do not have the characteristic features of silicosis, and in fact may be a response to the carcinoma.[103] It is also possible that the host cellular response to the carcinoma may preferentially cause dust accumulation at that site with resultant silicotic nodules or silicosis and bronchial cancer may coexist.

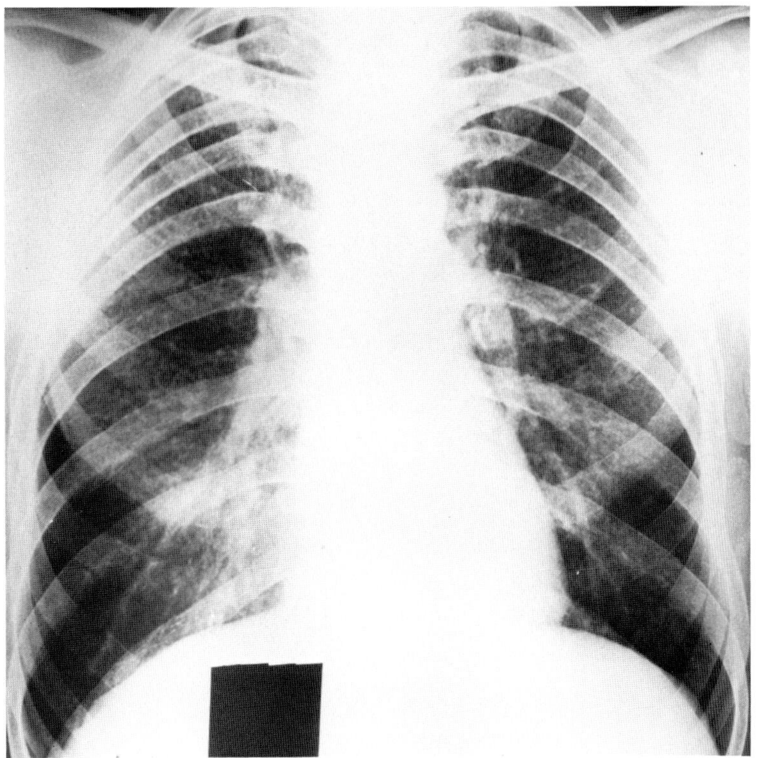

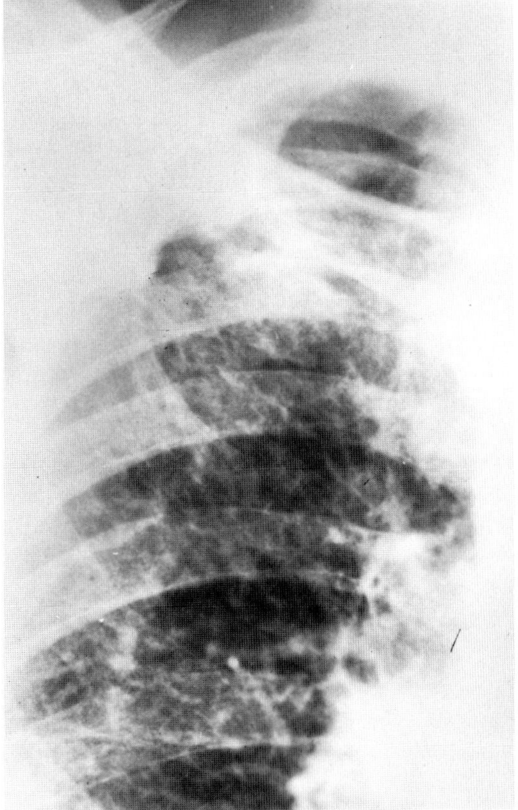

Figure 6.29. A. X-ray nodulation profusion 3/3 q/q. High siliceous dust exposure, 20 years. **B**. After 40 years the subject developed agglomeration of nodules to form A-sized large opacity right subclavicular region. Sputum culture highly positive for *M tuberculosis*.

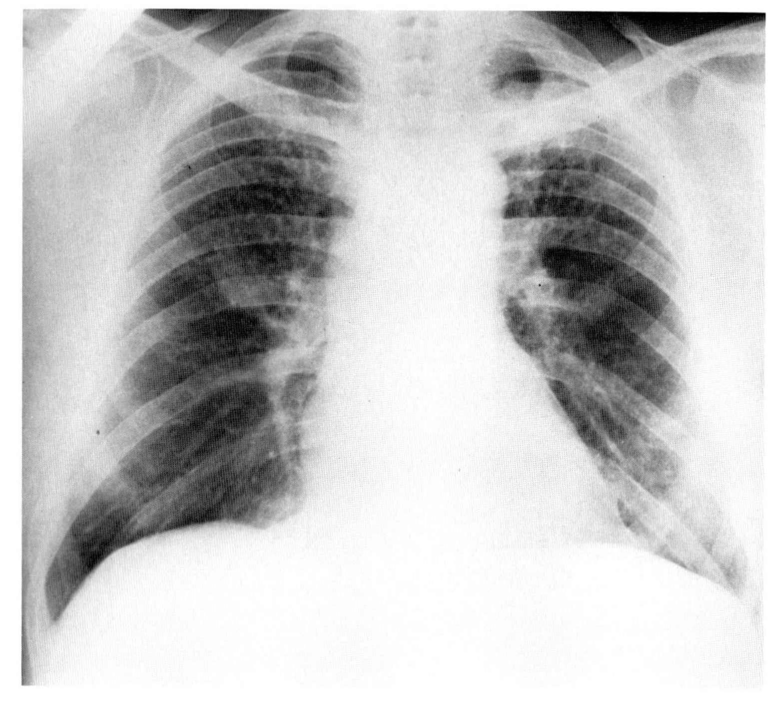

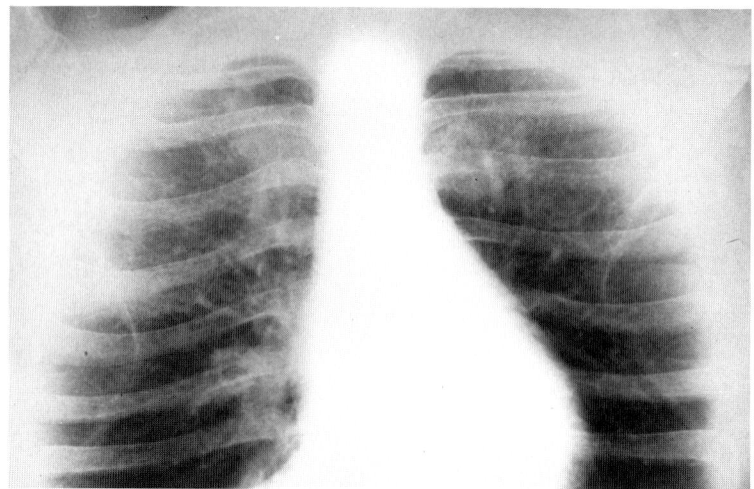

Figure 6.30. A. X-ray study with small nodules profusion 1/1 type p/p. Exposure to siliceous dust, 31 years. **B**. Developed apical opacities. Sputum positive for *M tuberculosis*: treated. Bilateral apical opacities persisted despite antituberculous treatment. Extremely rare event.

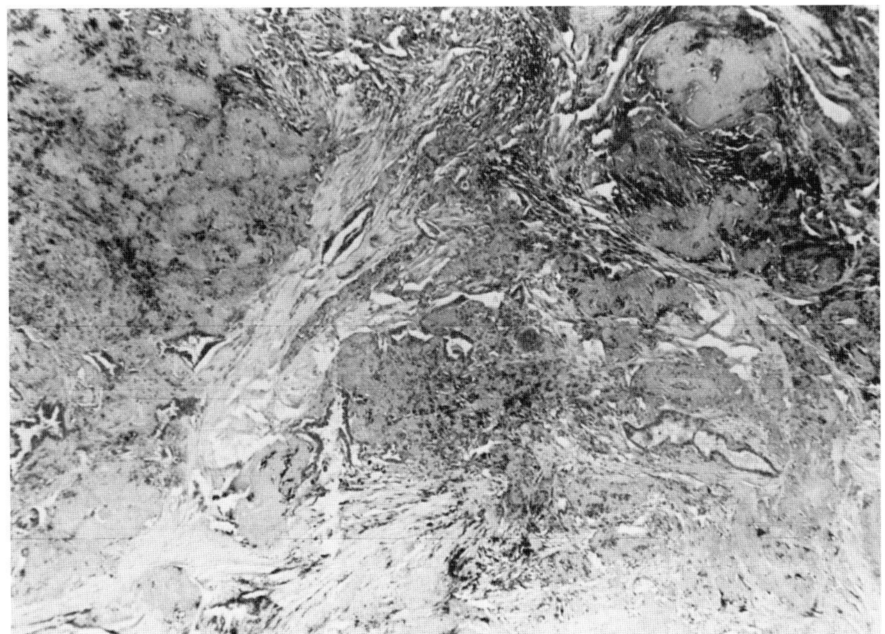

Figure 6.31. Adenocarcinoma in a scar associated with silicotic islets.

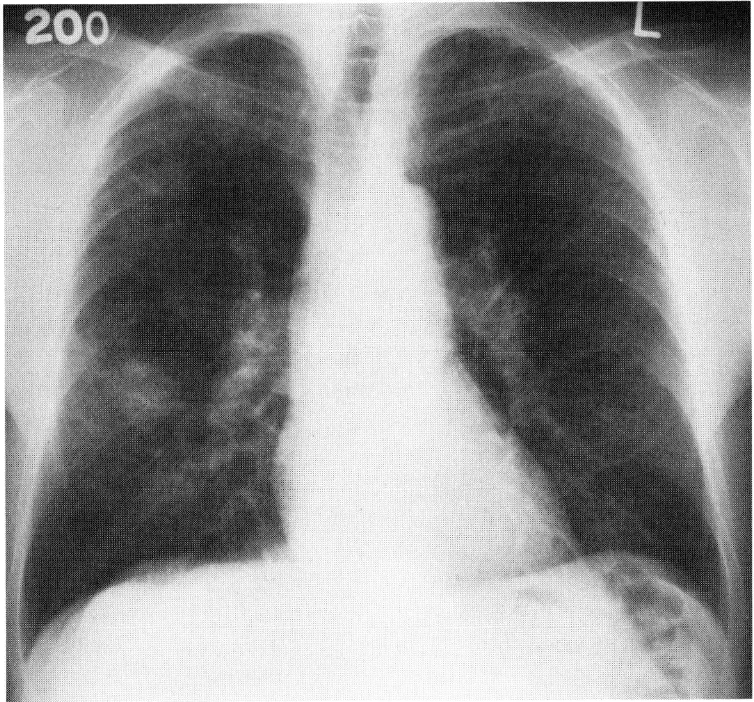

Figure 6.32. Silicotic nodules and right lower zone massive opacity that developed 6 years after the nodules. Subject was heavy smoker with 32 years exposure to siliceous dust. Autopsy performed within days of death due to multiple injuries. Right lower lobe: Massive silicotic opacity (1.0 × 1.5 cm) with neoplastic cells, consistent with scar carcinoma. Extremely rare in our experience.

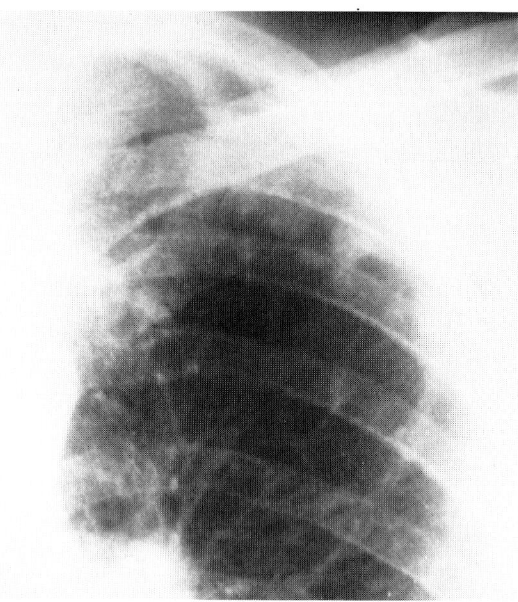

Figure 6.33. Magnified left upper field: Evidence of bilateral peripheral nodules in upper lung fields (0.5 × 1.0 cm). Siliceous dust exposure, 30 years. Developed rheumatoid arthritis. At that time chest findings were normal. Ten years later lung changes appeared.

Silicosis and Rheumatoid Arthritis

Rheumatoid arthritis does not in our experience (others[122] disagree) occur more commonly in silica-exposed workers, but silicosis has unusual features or progresses in an unusual manner in rheumatoid sufferers.[105]

Large peripheral upper zonal nodules develop,[106,107] usually bilateral (Fig. 6.33). Silicotic nodules of Caplan's syndrome may remain static for many years, may calcify, cavitate, or even disappear. Successive crops of large nodules may appear. Characteristically, on histology there are necrotic centers and concentric zones of macrophage infiltration, fibroblasts, and collagen.[105] The fibroblasts may show palisading. Unusually, Caplan's nodules may be unilateral (Fig. 6.34). The syndrome may take on a more serious form with a rapid increase of nodules and rapid progression of the joint disease. The radiographic changes may present diagnostic difficulties. Differentiating large opacities from pulmonary neoplasms or large cavitary neoplasms from rheumatoid necrobiotic opacities, or *M tuberculosis* cavities may require intensive clinical investigation (Fig. 6.35). Nodules associated with rheumatoid arthritis are more likely to progress to large opacities. These can appear suddenly and progression is more rapid than usual, taking into account cumulative silica dust exposure.[108] At autopsy, such cases often show pathological features of silicosis and not of Caplan's syndrome which is illustrated in Fig. 6.36.

Silicosis and Scleroderma

There are a number of reports on the coexistence of silicosis and scleroderma.[109] Erasmus reported a high incidence of scleroderma in gold miners, with 6 of his 17 cases showing radiological features of silicosis.[115]

In some reports there is uncertainty as to whether the association is with silicosis or coal worker's pneumoconiosis, hence the title of Rodnan et al.'s report, "The Association of Progressive Systemic Sclerosis (Scleroderma) with Coal Workers' Pneumoconiosis and Other Forms of Silicosis."[110] In their experience with 60 men with progressive systemic sclerosis, 26 had worked as coal miners or in "other occupations marked by prolonged and heavy exposure to silica dust." In fact, 16 of the 26 men were coal miners. Coal workers can under unusual mining conditions develop silicosis, ie, in those mining areas where drills used by the miners enter strata of silica bearing rock, above or below the coal seam.

A more recent case-control study on 79 cases of progressive systemic sclerosis occurring in gold miners failed to show an association between radiographic silicosis and progressive systemic sclerosis. There was, however, a significant association between cumulative silica dust exposure and progressive systemic sclerosis, and an even stronger positive association with the intensity of silica exposure.[45] Intense exposure may be associated with silicotic lesions in extrathoracic immunologically active organs—ie, liver, spleen, bone marrow—and so be involved in the pathogenesis of scleroderma.[118,119]

Unusual clinical and radiological features may occur in silica-exposed persons. Radiographs may show markedly unusual manifestations (Figs. 6.37 to 6.39).

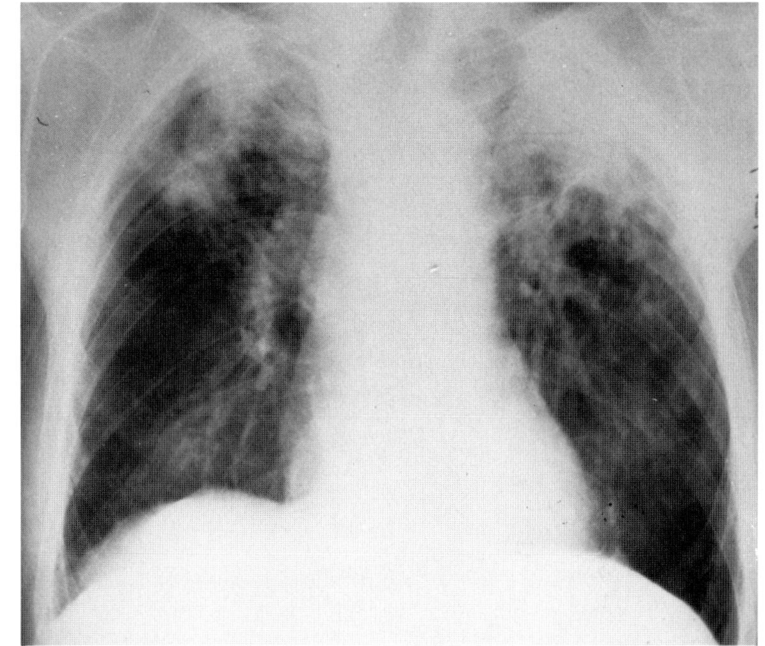

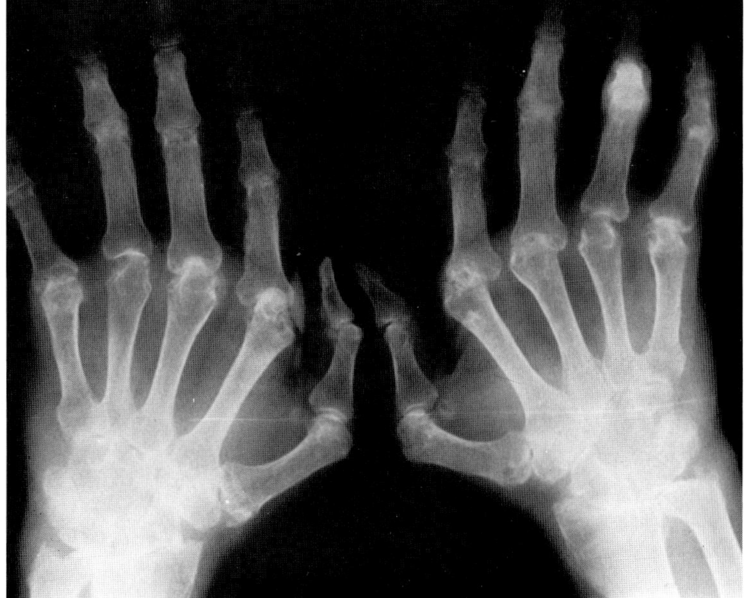

Figure 6.34. A. Early x-ray change nodules 1/1 q/q. The subject subsequently developed a right-sided pleural effusion and the abrupt appearance of large nodules and massive opacities. Exposed to siliceous dust for 30 years. **B**. Radiograph of hand with characteristic rheumatoid erosions.

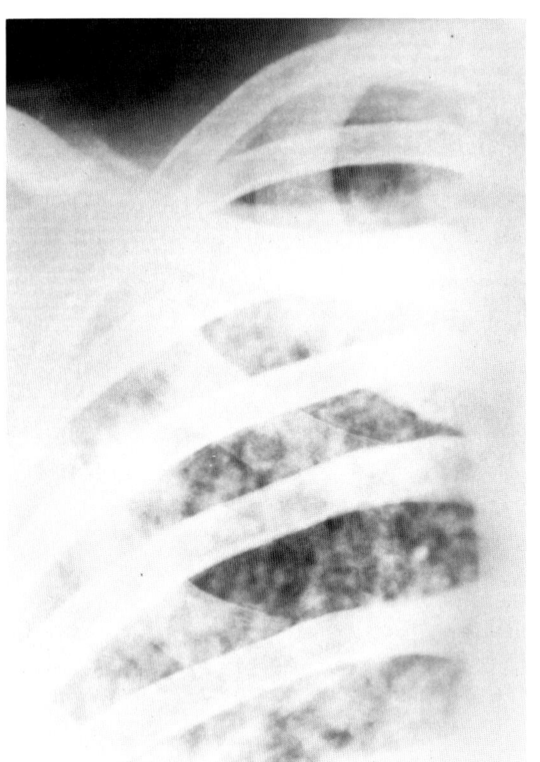

A

Figure 6.35. Successive radiographs of a man exposed to siliceous dust over 43 years. Developed rheumatoid arthritis 33 years after initial silica dust exposure. Small upper zonal nodular opacities (early). **A**. Four years later. Nodules 1/1 q/r . Massive opacity. All tests for tuberculosis were negative. **B**. Three years later. Profuse opacities 2/2 r/r C. **C**. X-ray hands – rheumatoid changes. Patient died following a myocardial infarction. Postmortem examination: Silicotic islets present and large areas of massive fibrosis in both upper zones. Size: Right side 3 × 2 cm; left side 5 × 4 cm. Right upper zone massive fibrosis revealed a 2.0-cm cavity. Histology confirmed the silicosis, but the diffuse fibrosis and areas of necrosis had the features of fibrocaseous tuberculosis with infiltration by epitheliod cells and Langhans' giant cells. The cavity was also tuberculous. This illustrates the difficulties in differential diagnosis in this situation.

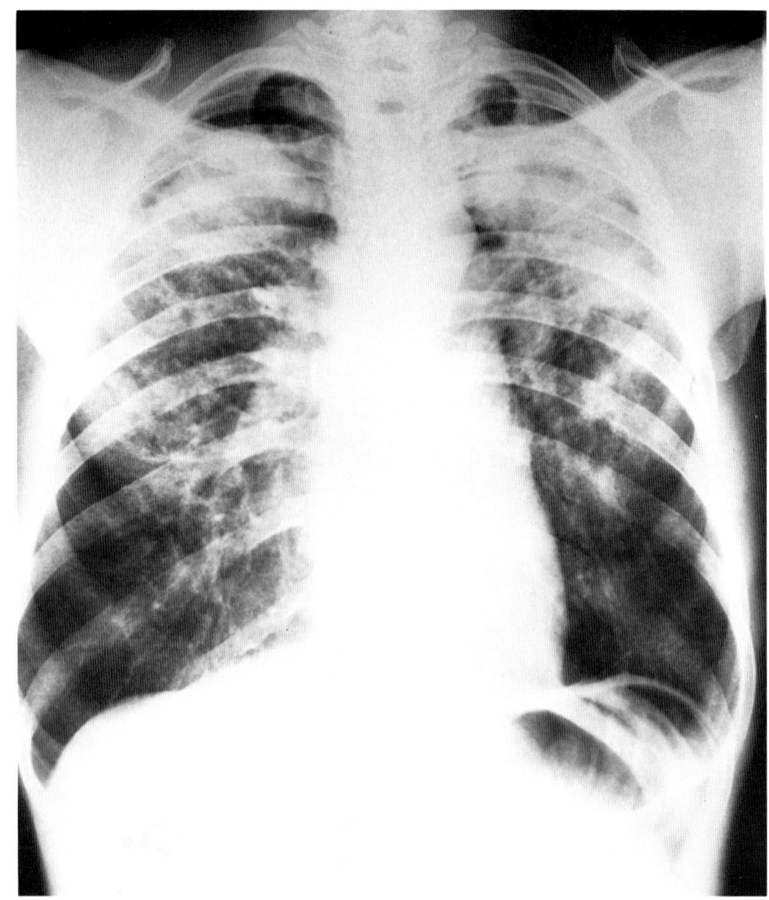

B

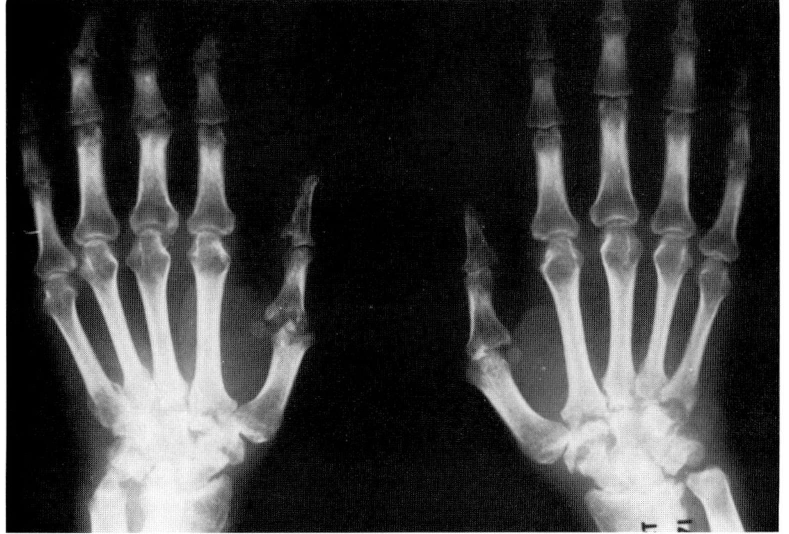

Figure 6.35

Figure 6.36. Photomicrograph of a section through a rheumatoid silicotic nodule. A large nodule with central necrosis, concentric pigmented zones with macrophage infiltration. On the periphery, deposition of collagen with some palisading by fibroblasts on the right edge of the nodule.

Mixed Dust Pneumoconiosis

McLaughlin described a specific histological appearance of pneumoconiotic nodules differing from both silicosis and coal worker's pneumoconiosis.[111] The fibers of reticulin and collagen are arranged in a linear and radial manner, forming a stellate and irregular nodule. "Mixed dust pneumoconiosis," therefore, described a particular histological feature and not a disease entity and should not be used for radiographic abnormalities consistent with pneumoconiosis because the patient has been exposed to a mixture of potentially harmful dusts, either concurrently or sequentially.

McLaughlin's cases were foundry workers exposed to low levels of silica, together with carbon and iron, whose lesions appeared to occur only when the silica content of the dust was less than 10%. But similar lesions have been detected in a number of gold, coal, and asbestos miners, sometimes alone, and sometimes associated with classic silicotic lesions. In gold miners it is unlikely that the silica content in the dust was less than 10%.[112,113] "Mixed dust pneumoconiosis" was also reported from an iron mine in Labrador, where the dust contained up to 8% of silica, iron oxide and some amphibole asbestos.[114]

The fibrogenic effect of crystalline silica may possibly be modified by other dusts inhaled simultaneously; the protective effect of iron, as originally described by Kettle, has been repeatedly confirmed.[56,78] Aluminium silicates may have a similar effect.

In our experience the radiological appearances of mixed-dust pneumoconiosis are similar to silicosis and coal worker's pneumoconiosis, and one cannot predict the histology from the radiological appearances. Massive shadows occur sometimes, rather irregular in outline, but commonly indistinguishable from those of silicosis (Fig. 6.40).

Differential Diagnosis

Many lung diseases may mimic the small rounded opacities of silicosis. The most important, and the one causing the most difficulties, is tuberculosis. Sarcoidosis and histoplasmosis may also occur in the lungs of persons with a silica exposure and produce appearances consistent with silicosis, but there are usually some features that would be unusual in silicosis, such as sudden manifestation of nodules on the radiograph or enlarged hilar lymph nodes, or specific biological or biochemical tests suggesting other pathology. A lung biopsy may infrequently be needed to make a definitive diagnosis.

Infections, carcinomatosis, and autoimmune diseases are usually associated with specific clinical features to indicate a diagnosis other than silicosis.

Bilateral massive opacities are sufficiently characteristic of dust inhalation. Other diseases causing massive opacities in the lung, such as Wegener's granulomatosis or sarcoidosis, have other clinical and laboratory signs. Silicosis cannot be diagnosed without an occupational history.

A bronchogenic carcinoma cannot be excluded by radiographic signs when there is a large unilateral opacity, but can be suspected if serial films show rapid enlargement. Percutaneous aspiration cytology with a fine needle usually provides the required information.

Bizarre radiographic appearances associated with rheumatoid arthritis and scleroderma may pose difficulties, but are usually resolved by follow-up films.

Most errors can be avoided through a thorough occupational history,[116,117] though occasionally the exposure is unusual and not readily obtained. An example is "Transkei lung," where silicosis occurred in black women from grinding maize in traditional hollowed-out stone boulders with a high silica content,[116] indicating that silicosis is a very ancient disease. Rarely a hobby, such as polishing semiprecious gems, leads to siliceous dust inhalation.

Computed tomography (CT) scans of the chest in the assessment of silicosis have not as yet yielded better scores for the detection of nodules, nor has CT as yet identified more "silicotic patients" with minimal parenchymal disease. But significantly more coalescence and large opacities have been identified in patients with simple silicosis.[120]

Acknowledgments. Many of the x-ray photographs were derived from the Medical Bureau for Occupational Diseases Museum. Others were material borrowed from the National Centre for

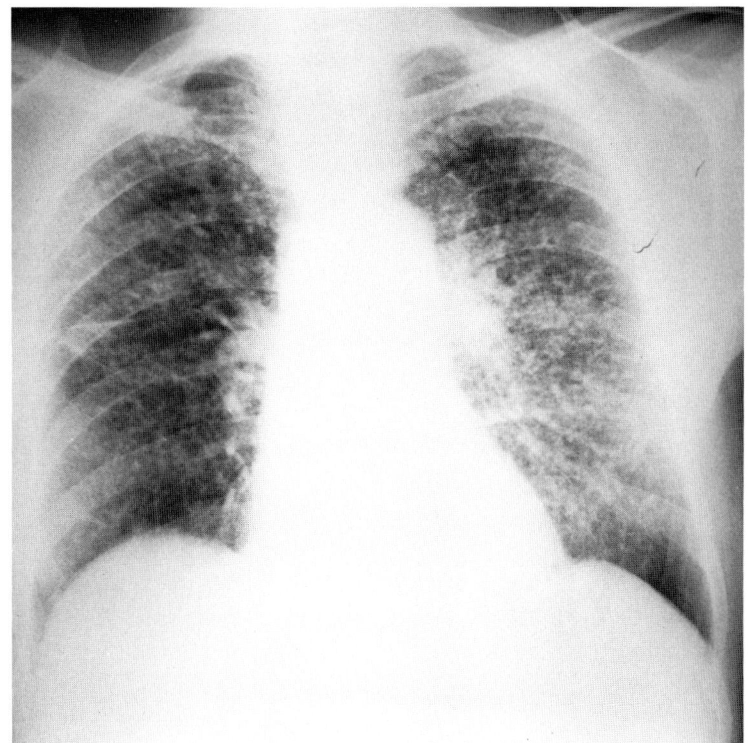

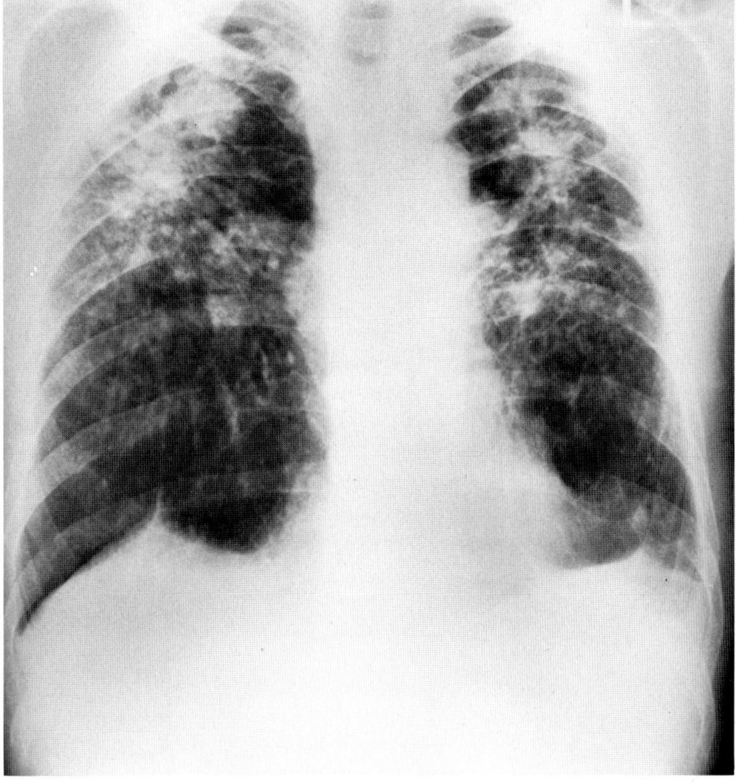

Figure 6.37. Silicosis and scleroderma. Exposure: low siliceous dust for 27 years. Scleroderma developed 8 years before radiographic changes in lung. *Clinically*: Early rheumatoid-like symptoms in hands. Latex test positive 1 year later. Four years later: scleroderma of hands and forearms, chest and perioral region. Esophagogram: loss of tone in esophagus. *Radiographs*: Early normal. **A**. One year later: Rounded opacities 3/3 q/r. **B**. Three years later: Gross massive opacities. *Autopsy*: Numerous silicotic nodules and gross bilateral massive opacities.

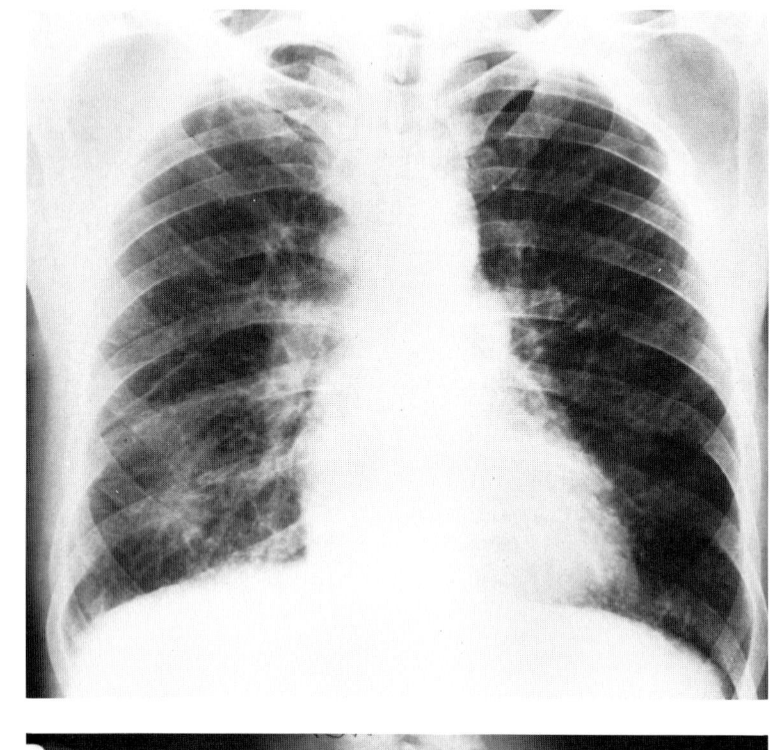
A

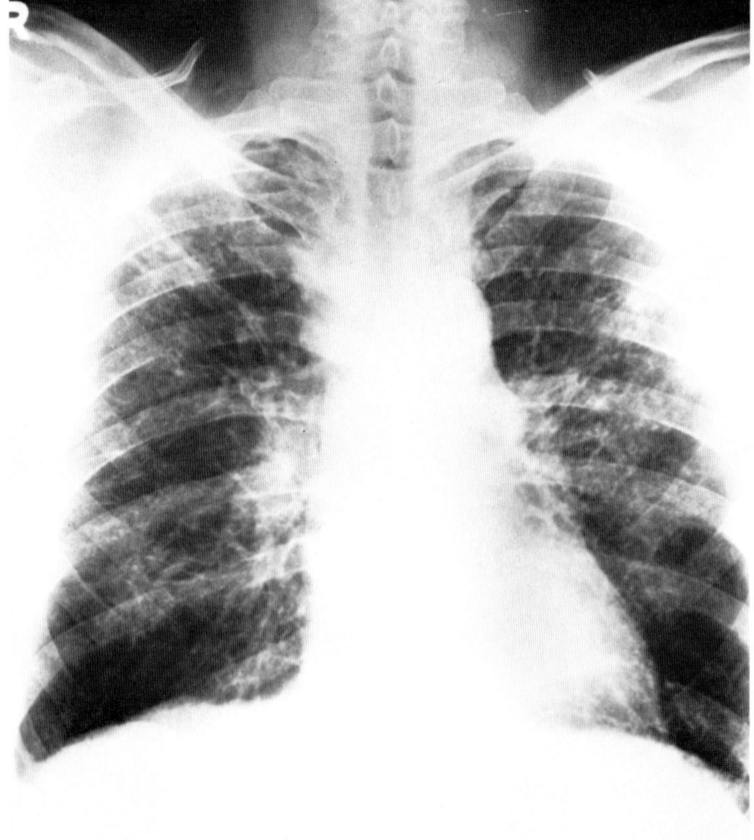
B

Figure 6.38

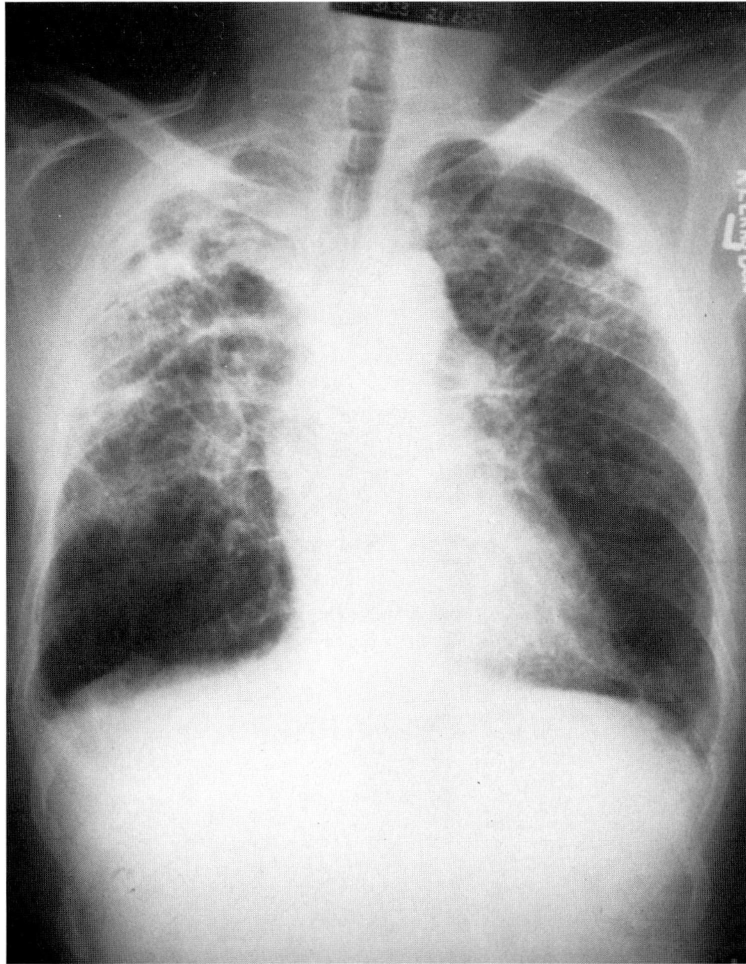

C

Figure 6.38. Silicosis in a man with scleroderma. **A**. X-ray study, 1975. Basal irregular opacities and an ill-defined massive opacity. **B**. Appearance of sparse upper zonal rounded opacities (q/q 1/1), ie, indicative of silicosis. **C**. X-ray study, 1983. Massive upper zonal opacities. Exposure history to silica: 1944–1975. *Clinically* 1974: Raynaud's phenomenon; sclerodactyly; whole-body pigmentation. Restricted movement of small joints of hand. Esophagogram, loss of tone in lower esophagus. Antinuclear antibody present. Skin biopsy consistent with scleroderma. Lung function test: Restrictive pattern normal diffusion. Lung biopsy: Internal and medial thickening of small arteries, which may be a feature of scleroderma.

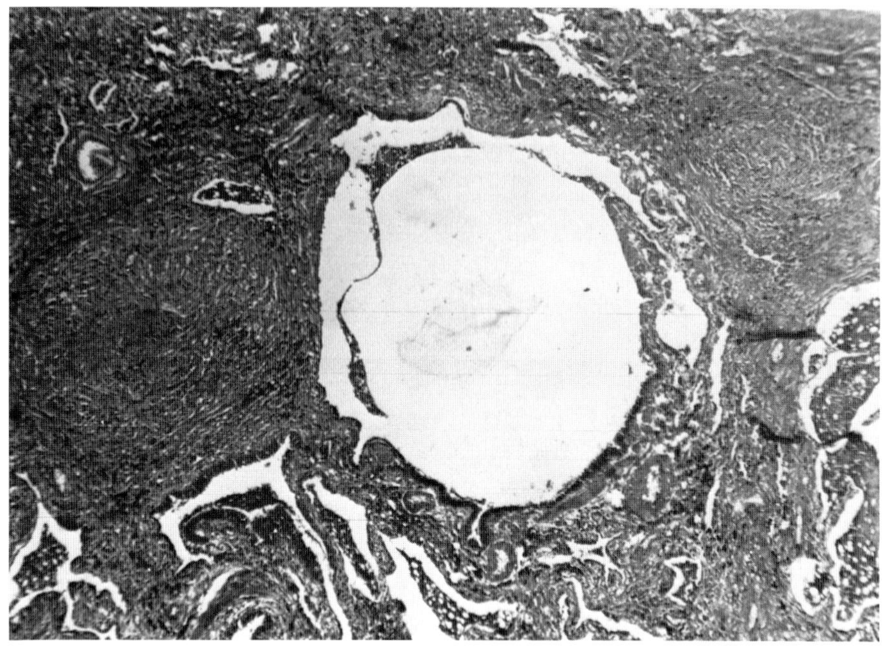

Figure 6.39. Lung section from a man with progressive systemic sclerosis demonstrating honeycombing, gross interstitial fibrosis and a silicotic islet in the right upper corner.

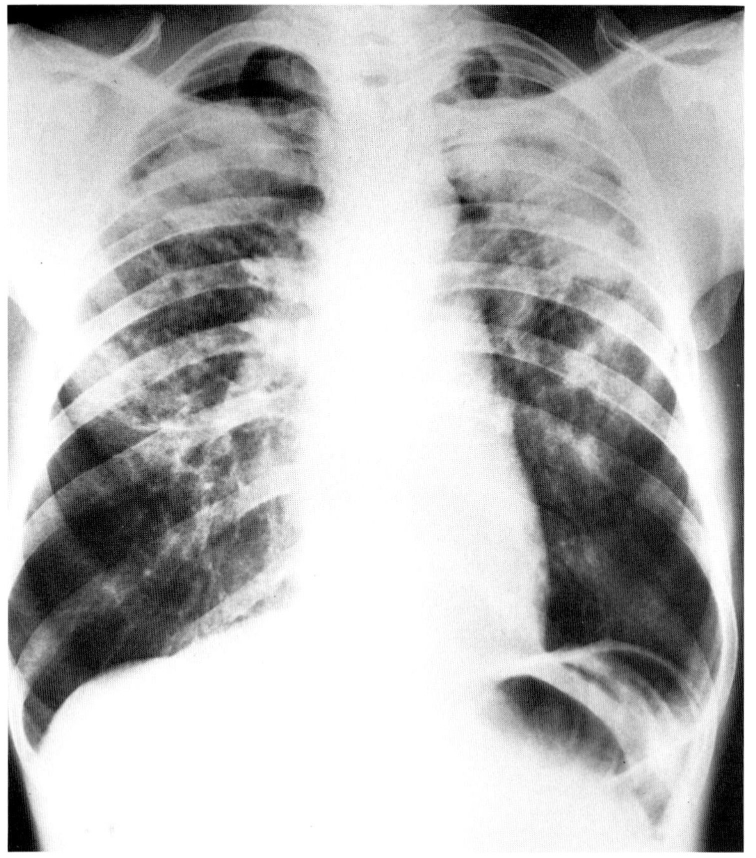

Figure 6.40. Bilateral symmetrical large opacities and some irregular midzonal massive opacities. Foundry worker: grindstone manufacturing, 18 years. Lung function tests: moderate airway obstruction. Histology: Silica particles in large numbers; interstitial linear collagenization; foci of nodular fibrosis associated with marked hemosiderin and carbon-dust deposition. Diagnosis: Mixed-dust pneumoconiosis.

Occupational Health, factories, and mines. To all concerned we proffer our thanks.

We would also like to thank Dr. F.J. Wiles and Professor M.R. Becklake for reading the manuscript and making very valuable comments.

Neither the persons mentioned above nor the medical institutions with which we are or have been associated, necessarily subscribe to the viewpoints put forward in this chapter.

References

1. Ulmer WT: Die silikose (coal worker's pneumoconiosis): Entwicklung einer Krankheit, in: VI International Pneumoconiosis Conference, 1983, vol 1. Bochum, Bergbau-berufsgenossenschaft, 1984, pp. 75–81.
2. Bateman ED, Emerson RJ, Cole P, et al: The mechanisms of fibrogenesis in occupational lung diseases. Research approaches and methods. New York, Marcel Dekker, 1981, p. 237.
3. Stober W, Breiger H: On the theory of silicosis. Arch Environ Health 1968; 16:706–708.
4. Langer AM: Crystal faces and cleavage planes in quartz as templates in biological processes. Q Rev Biophys 1978; 11:543–575.
5. Swensson A, Kvarnströmk BT, Edling NPG, et al: Pneumoconiosis in ferrosilicon workers. A follow up study. J Occup Med 1971; 13:427–432.
6. Princi F, Miller L, Davis A, et al: Pulmonary disease of ferroalloy workers. J Occup Med 1962;4: 301–310.
7. Belt TH, Irwin D, King EJ: Silicon and dust deposits in the tissues of persons without occupational exposure to siliceous dusts. Can Med Assoc J 1936; 34:125–133.
8. Paul R: Silicosis on Northern Rhodesia Copper Mines. Arch Environ Health 1961; 2:10–23.
9. Ahlmark A, Bruce T, Nyström A: Silicosis from quarrying and working of granite. Br J Ind Med 1965; 22:285–290.
10. Ashe HB: Silicosis and dust control. Public Health Rep 1955; 70:10.
11. Lloyd Davies TA, Doig AT, Fox AJ, et al: A radiographic survey of monumental masonry workers in Aberdeen. Br J Ind Med 1973; 30:227–231.
12. Yee HT, Bourne HG: Survey of monument industry in Ohio. Am Ind Hyg Assoc J 1970; 31:501–505.
13. Worth G, Schiller E: Die Pneumokoniosen. Köln, Staufen Verlag, 1954.
14. Gupta SP, Beja A, Jain AL, et al: Clinical and radiological studies in silicosis based on a study of the disease among stone-cutters. Indian J Med Res 1972; 60:1309–1315.
15. Phibbs BP, Sundin RE, Mitchell RS: Silicosis in Wyoming bentonite workers. Am Rev Respir Dis 1971; 103:1–17.
16. Glyn Thomas J, Emlyn Owen T, Corrado HA: Respiratory tuberculosis and pneumoconiosis in slate workers. Br J Dis Chest 1967; 61:138–143.
17. Clarke NE: Silicosis and diseases of retired iron foundry workers. Ind Med 1972; 41:6:22–25.
18. Banks DF, Morring KL, Boehlecke BA, et al: Silicosis in silica flour workers. Am Rev Respir Dis 1981; 124:445–450.
19. Wani KM, Niyogi AK: Environment and silicosis in glass factories. Indian J Public Health 1968; 3:131–139.
20. Vigliani EC: La patogenesi della silicosis. Schweiz Med Wochenschr 1983; 113(suppl 15):43–46.
21. Nordman H, Koskinen H, Fröseth B: Increased activity of serum angiotensin enzyme in progressive silicosis. Chest 1984; 86:203–207.
22. Bucca C, Veglio F, Rolla G, et al: Serum angiotensin converting enzyme (ACE) in silicosis. Eur J Respir Dis 1984; 65:477–480.
23. Koskinen H, Nordman H, Fröseth B: Serum lysozyme concentration in silicosis patients and workers exposed to silica dust. Eur J Respir Dis 1984; 65:481–485.
24. Siemsen JK, Sargent EN, Grebe SF, et al: Pulmonary concentrations of Ga^{67} in pneumoconiosis. AJR 1974; 120:815–820.
25. Attygale D, Harrison CV, King EJ, et al: Infective pneumoconiosis. Br J Ind Med 1954; 11:245–259.
26. Engel H: Occupational medicine in Germany. J Soc Occup Med 1985; 35:14–16.
27. Simpson FW, Strachan AS, Irwine LG: Proc Transvaal Mine Medical Officers Assoc (Suppl) 1931; 10:118.
28. Mavrogordato A: Contributions to the study of miners' phthisis. Publ S Afr Inst Med Res 1926; 3:1–84.
29. Watkins-Pitchford W, Moir J: On the nature of the doubly refracting particles seen in microscopic sections of silicotic lungs and an improved method for disclosing siliceous particles in such sections. Publ S Afr Inst Med Res 1916; 1:207–230.
30. Chatgidakis CB: Silicosis in South African white gold miners. Med Proc 1963; 9:383–392.
31. Monaco A: Antituberculosis chemo-prophylaxis in silicotics. Bull Int Union Tuberc 1964;35:51–56.
32. Sluis-Cremer GK: Active pulmonary tuberculosis discovered at post-mortem examination in the lungs of black miners. Br J Dis Chest 1980;74:374–378.
33. Gardner LU: Will the inhalation siliceous dusts activate a partially healed focus of tuberculous infection? An experimental study. Public Health Rep Wash 1930; 45:282–288.

34. Allison AC, D'Arcy Hart P: Potentiation by silica of the growth of mycobacterium tuberculosis in macrophage cultures. Br J Exp Pathol 1968; 49: 465.
35. Gross P, Westrick ML, McVerney JM: Experimental tuberculo-silicosis. Am Rev Respir Des 1961; 83:510–527.
36. Schepers GWH: Silicosis and tuberculosis. Ind Med Surg 1964; 33:381–399.
37. Howlett KS, Warring FC: Response to treatment in silico-tuberculosis. Arch Environ Health 1964; 9:343–354.
38. Barley WC, Brown M, Buechner HA, et al: Silicomycobacterial disease in sandblasters. Am Rev Respir Dis 1974; 110:115–125.
39. Wolinsky E: Non tuberculous mycobacteria and associated diseases. Am Rev Respir Dis 1979; 119:107–159.
40. Kaniat SR, Rossiter CE, Gilson JC: A retrospective clinical study of pulmonary disease due to anonymous mycobacteria in Wales. Thorax 1961; 16: 297–308.
41. Banks J, Hunter AM, Campbell IA, et al: Pulmonary infection with mycobacterium xenopi. Thorax 1984; 39:376–382.
42. De Shazo RD: Current concepts about the pathogenesis of silicosis and asbestosis. J Allergy Clin Immunol 1982; 70:41–49.
43. Doll NJ, Stankus RP, Hughes J, et al: Immune complexes and auto-antibodies in silicosis. J Allergy Clin Immunol 1981; 68:281–285.
44. Turner-Warwick M: Immune reactions in pulmonary fibrosis. Schweiz Med Wochenschr 1977; 6:171–175.
45. Sluis-Cremer GK, Hessel PA, Hnizdo E, et al: Silica, silicosis and progressive systemic sclerosis. Br J Ind Med 1985; 42:838–843.
46. Dickie HA: Asbestos and silica. Their multiple effect on the lung. DM 1982; 28:37–45.
47. Miall WE: Rheumatoid arthritis in miners. Ann Rheum Dis 1955; 14:150.
48. Ziskind M, Jones RN, Weill H: Silicosis. Am Rev Respir Dis 1976; 113:643–665.
49. Suratt PM, Winn WC, Brody AR, et al: Acute silicosis in tombstone sandblasters. Am Rev Respir Dis 1977; 115:521–529.
50. Roegel E, Paul G, Dechoux J, et al: Silicose d'evolution rapide et pseudotumoralegreffe sur une sarcoidose pulmonaire evolutive. Poumon Coeur 1981; 37:195–202.
51. Saiyed HN, Chatterjee BB: Rapid progression of silicosis in slate pencil workers. Am J Ind Med 1985; 8:135–142.
52. Beadle DG, Harris E, Sluis-Cremer GK: The relationship between the amount of dust breathed and the incidence of silicosis, in Shapiro HA (ed): Pneumoconiosis. Proceedings of the International Conference, Johannesburg, 1969. Cape Town, Oxford University Press, 1970, pp. 473–477.
53. Wyndham CH, Bezuidenhout BN, Greenacre MJ, et al: Mortality 1970–1978 among middle aged white South African goldminers. Br J Ind Med 1986; 43:677–684.
54. Noweir MH, Moselhi M, Amine EK: Role of family susceptibility, occupational and family histories and individuals' blood groups in the development of silicosis. Br J Ind Med 1980; 37:399–404.
55. Sherson D: Silicosis. Br J Ind Med 1981; 38:397.
56. Parkes WR: Occupational Lung Disorders. ed 2. London, Butterworths, 1982, p 159.
57. Martin JC, Daniel-Moussard H, Le Bouffant L, et al: The role of quartz in the development of coalworkers pneumoconiosis. Ann NY Acad Sci 1972; 200:127–141.
58. Bettts WW: Chalicosis pulmonum or chronic interstitial pneumonia induced by stone dust. JAMA 1900; 34:70–74.
59. Gründorfer W, Raber A: Progressive silicosis in granite workers. Br J Ind Med 1970; 27:110–120.
60. Rubilina EE: Progression of silicosis and risk of silicotuberculosis in mine workers in Kazakhstan. Gig Trud 1977; 4:36–39.
61. Ellis RH: Disease of the right middle lobe in pneumoconiosis. Br J Dis Chest 1964; 58:169–172.
62. Longley EO: Oesophageal compression due to silicotic mediastinal lymph nodes. Trans Soc Occup Med 1970; 20:69.
63. Cavasso B, Couropmitree C, Heredia R: Egg-shell silicotic calcification causing bronchoesophageal fistula. Am Rev Respir Dis 1973; 108:1384–1387.
64. Olivieri PG, Ortone PG, Cielo R: Alcuni aspetti clinico-radiologici di stenosi tracheo-bronchiale nella silicotica. Med Lav 1971; 62:323–335.
65. Loehr J: Ungewoehnliche toedliche broncho-arterielle fistel bei hilus silikose. Med Welt 1972; 49:1854–1855.
66. Picart N, Lanoy N, Courtoy P: Une cause inhabituelle de compression de la veine cave superieur. Acta Cardiol 1972; 27:648–653.
67. Kradin RL, Spirn PW, Mark EJ: Intrapulmonary lymph nodes. Clinical, radiologic and pathologic features. Chest 1985; 87:662–667.
68. Ruckley VA, Fernie JM, Chapman JS, et al: Comparison of radiographic appearances with associated pathology and lung dust content in a group of coalworkers. Br J Ind Med 1984; 41:459–467.
69. Gross BH, Schneider HJ, Proto HV: Egg-shell calcification of lymph nodes. An update. AJR 1980; 135:265–268.
70. Lyons JP, Ryder RC, Campbell H, et al: Signifi-

cance of irregular opacities in the radiology of coalworkers pneumoconiosis. Br J Ind Med 1974; 31: 36–44.
71. Solomon A: Massive fibrosis in goldminers: A radiological evaluation. Environ Res 1977; 13:47–55.
72. Parkes WR: Occupational Lung Disorders. ed 2. London, Butterworths, 1982, p 185.
73. Tada, S, Yasukochi H, Shida H: Bronchial artery in silicosis. AJR 1974; 120:810–814.
74. Sheunar DH, Washington JS, Thomas DJ, et al: Factors predisposing to the development of progressive massive fibrosis in coalminers. Br J Ind Med 1981; 38:321–326.
75. Ahlmark A: Silicosis, dust conditions and dust control in Sweden. Staub-Reinhalt Luft 1969; 29: 1–6.
76. Hessel PA, Sluis-Cremer GK, Hnizdo E, et al: Progression of silicosis in relation to silica dust exposure. Presented at Inhaled Particles VI Cambridge 1985 (in press). Dodson J: Pergamon Press, Oxford.
77. Capezzuto A: Considerazioni su un caso di silicosi pseudotumorale isolata. Med Lav 1970; 63:587–593.
78. Kettle EH: The interstitial reactions caused by various dusts and their influence on tuberculous infections. J Pathol Bacteriol 1932; 35:395–405.
79. Hessel PA, Sluis-Cremer GK: Case-control study of silicosis, silica exposure and lung cancer in South African gold miners, in Goldsmith DF, Winn DM, Shy CM (eds): Silica, Silicosis and Cancer: Controversy in Occupational Medicine. (Cancer Research Monographs) vol 2, Praeger Scientific (1986). pp 351–355.
80. Buechner HA, Ansari A: Acute silico-proteinosis. A new pathologic variant of acute silicosis in sandblasters. Dis Chest 1969; 55:274–284.
81. Rubin E, Weisbrod GL, Sanders DE: Pulmonary alveolar proteinosis. Relationship to silicosis and pulmonary infection. Radiology 1980; 135:35–41.
82. Xipell JM, Ham KN, Price CG, et al: Acute silicolipoproteinosis. Thorax 1977; 32:104–111.
83. Dee P, Suratt P, Winn W: The radiographic findings in acute silicosis. Radiology 1978; 126:359–363.
84. Heppleston AG: Animal model: Silica induced pulmonary alveolar lipoproteinosis. Am J Pathol 1975; 78:171–174.
85. Michel RD, Morris JF: Acute silicosis. Arch Intern Med 1964; 113:850–855.
86. Gardner LU: Pathology of so-called acute silicosis. Am J Public Health 1933; 23:1240–1249.
87. Wiles FJ, Faure MH: Chronic obstructive lung disease in gold miners, in Walton WH (ed): Inhaled particles IV. Proceedings of an International Symposium organised by the British Occupational Hygiene Society, Edinburgh 1975. Oxford, Pergamon Press, 1977, pp 727–734.
88. Irwig LM, Rocks P: Lung function and respiratory symptoms in silicotic and non silicotic gold miners. Am Rev Respir Dis 1978; 117:429–435.
89. Morgan WKL, Seaton A: Occupational Lung Diseases, ed 2. Philadelphia, WB Saunders Co, 1984, pp 404–406.
90. Theriault GP, Peters JM: Pulmonary function and roentgenographic changes in granite dust exposure. Arch Environ Health 1974; 28:23–27.
91. Churg A, Wright JL: Small airway lesions in patients exposed to non-asbestos mineral dusts. Hum Pathol 1983; 14:688–693.
92. Goldsmith DF, Guidotti TL, Johnston DR: Does occupational exposure to silica cause lung cancer? Am J Ind Med 1982; 3:423–440.
93. Morgan WKC: The relationship between tuberculosis and silicosis. Am Rev Respir Dis 1979; 119: 319–320.
94. Finkelstein M, Kusiak R, Surany LG: Mortality among miners receiving compensation for silicosis in Ontario 1940–1975. J Occup Med 1982; 24: 663–667.
95. Westerholm P: Silicosis. Observations on a case register. Scand J Work Environ Health 1980; 6(Suppl 2):1–86.
96. Westerholm P, Ahlmark A, Maasing R, et al: Silicosis and lung cancer—a cohort study, in: VIth International Pneumoconiosis Conference 1983. vol 1. Bochum: Bergbau-Berufsgenossenschaft, 1984, pp 217–227.
97. Axelson D, Sundell L: Mining, lung cancer and smoking. Scand J Work Environ Health 1978; 4:46–52.
98. Edling C: Lung cancer and smoking in a group of iron ore miners. Am J Ind Med 1982; 3:191–199.
99. Fox AJ, Goldblatt P, Kinlen LJ: A study of the mortality of Cornish tin miners. Br J Ind Med 1981; 38:378–380.
100. Boyd JT, Doll R, Faulds JS, et al: Cancer of the lung in iron ore (haematite) miners. Br J Ind Med 1970; 27:97–105.
101. Böhm E, Rutemeyer E, Könn G, et al: Das silikotischen narbencarcinom, in: VIth International Pneumoconiosis Conference 1983, vol I. Bochum: Bergbau-Berufsgenossenschaft, 1984, pp 237–249.
102. Goldstein B: Personal communication.
103. Madri JA, Carter D: Scar cancers of the lung. Human Pathol 1984; 125:625–631.

104. Heppleston AG: Silica, pneumoconiosis of the lung. Am J Ind Med 1985; 7:285–294.
105. Chatgidakis CF, Theron CP: Rheumatoid pneumoconiosis (Caplan's syndrome). Arch Environ Health 1961; 2:397–408.
106. Caplan A: Certain unusual radiological appearances in the chest of coal miners suffering from rheumatoid arthritis. Thorax 1953; 8:29–37.
107. Gough J, Rivers D, Seal RMF: Pathological studies of modified pneumoconiosis in coal miners with rheumatoid arthritis (Caplan's syndrome). Thorax 1955; 10:9–18.
108. Sluis-Cremer GK, Hessel PA, Hnizdo E, et al: The relationship between silicosis and rheumatoid arthritis. Thorax 1986; 41:596–601.
109. Devulder B, Plouvier B, Martin JCL, et al: The association of scleroderma-silicosis or Erasmus' syndrome. Nouv Presse Med 1977; 6:2877–2879.
110. Rodnan GP, Benedek TG, Medsger TA, et al: The association of progressive systemic sclerosis (scleroderma) with coal workers pneumoconiosis and other forms of silicosis. Ann Intern Med 1967; 66:323–334.
111. McLaughlin AIG: Pneumoconiosis in foundry workers. Br J Tuberc 1957; 51:297–309.
112. Goldstein B, Rendall REG: The relative toxicities of the main classes of minerals, in Shapiro HA (ed): Pneumoconiosis. Proceedings of the International Conference, Johannesburg, 1969. Cape Town, Oxford University Press, 1970, pp 429–434.
113. Goldstein B, Webster I: Mixed dust fibrosis in mineworkers, in Walton WH (ed): Inhaled Particles III, vol 2. Old Woking, Unwin, 1971, pp 705–711.
114. Edstrom HW, Rice DMD: "Labrador lung" an unusual mixed dust pneumoconiosis. Can Med Assoc J 1982; 126:27–30.
115. Erasmus LD: Scleroderma in gold miners on the Witwatersrand with particular reference to pulmonary manifestations. S Afr J Lab Clin Med 1957; 3:209–231.
116. Palmer PES: Transkei silicosis. S Afr Med J 1967; 41:1182–1188.
117. Gerhardson L, Ahlmark H: Silicosis in women. J Occup Med 1985; 27:347–350.
118. Slavin RE, Swedo JL, Brandes D, et al: Extrapulmonary silicosis. Human Pathol 1985; 16:393–412.
119. Cisno F, Azzalini M, Camagna MT: Considerazioni su 16 casi di silicosi del fegato e della milza. Med Lav 1971; 8-9:378–385.
120. Begin R, Bergerson D, Samson L, et al: CT assessment of silicosis in exposed workers. AJR 1987; 148:509–514.
121. Costello J, Graham WGB: Vermont granite workers mortality study. Am J Ind Med 1988; 13:483–497.
122. Klockars M, Koskela RS, Jarrinen E, et al: Silica exposure and rheumatoid arthritis. Brit Med J 1987; 294:997–999.

7

Nonmining Inhalation of Silica and the Silicates

David S. Feigin*

Introduction

There are a multiplicity of silicas and silicates that cause pulmonary disease by inhalation during occupational exposure or, occasionally, by accidental or environmental dust inhalation. Asbestos, a form of combined silica, is an unsuspected hazard in many circumstances. Mining silicosis has been extensively discussed in the preceding chapter. This chapter is concerned with nonmining exposure to silica and with any inhalation of the many silicates in addition to asbestos.

There are many different classifications of silicates, usually based on the nature of the inhaled particle or on the pathology of resulting disease. A common classification into "fibrous" or "nonfibrous" forms is based on particle shape. "Fibrous silicates," either mineral or man-made materials, are inhaled as a "fiber," ie, its length is at least three times its width.[1] The overall diameter of the fiber is usually less than 3 μm, so passage through the tracheobronchial tree is common. Fiber size and shape are probably important determinants of the prevalence and nature of the disease produced by the inhaled substance.

Substances not qualifying as "fibrous" are often considered less likely to cause disease than fibrous substances, but many important nonfibrous silicates, such as talc and kaolin, are also known disease producers.[2] Radiologic abnormalities associated with inhalation of fibers typically have an interstitial pattern. When visible, these abnormalities are usually associated with obvious symptoms, including dyspnea and chronic cough. Inhalation of nonfibrous material characteristically manifests as pulmonary nodules and are often found in asymptomatic patients.

The distinction between fibrous and nonfibrous silicates is not entirely clear.[3] Talc, for example, is usually considered nonfibrous, but may appear in some circumstances as a fibrous form. There are also several man-made substances obtained by melting rock into vitreous fibers, including fiberglass and rock wool.[4] The radiographic manifestations of man-made fibers resemble those of naturally occurring nonfibrous minerals–ie, as small, well-defined nodules without lymph node enlargement or linear, reticular densities in the lung. Natural fibrous minerals, in contrast, more often produce reticulations, large irregular masses and lymph node enlargement.

Another system of classification for silicates and similar minerals is based upon the production of significant inflammation and fibrosis ("fibrogenesis") in the lung.[3] Unfortunately, fibrogenesis is highly variable and inconsistent and many substances are partially or mildly fibrogenic; examples include fiberglass and many forms of coal. Further, different types of pulmonary inflammation and fibrosis occur, resulting in marked differences in the clinical, pathologic, and radiologic manifestations; an example of a distinct type of reaction is the granuloma formation of beryllium. Airway disease may be an important source of symptoms and disability[4a] and is usually considered independent of fibrogenesis. Airway irritation alone can produce significant symptoms

---

* The opinions and assertions contained herein are solely those of the author and in no way represent those of the Department of the Army or Defense, or the Veterans Administration.

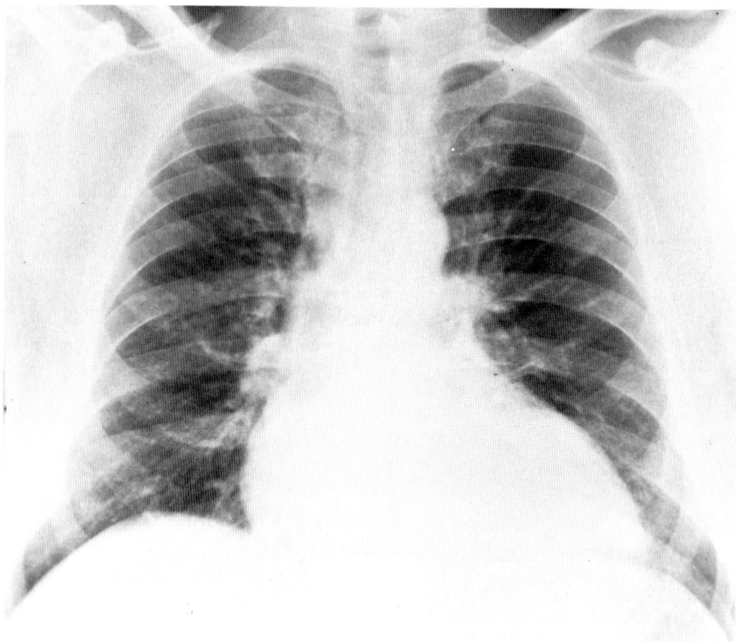

Figure 7.1. Simple silicosis in a rubber factory worker. A diffuse, fine, nodular infiltrate is present throughout the lungs. There is no significant lymphadenopathy present, and there are no nodules larger than 1 cm in diameter. (AFIP Negative No. 80-5976.)

without any radiologic changes at all, further complicating the correlation of clinical and radiographic evidence.[5] Finally, fibrogenic and nonfibrogenic dusts are commonly inhaled together, precluding separation of the effects specifically related to each dust and adding yet another complication.

Because of these problems with classification, this chapter first considers the nonmining exposure to silica, including the acute form "silicoproteinosis," a distinct type of silicosis generally associated with nonmining exposure. The silicates are then discussed in order of their relative importance, with special emphasis on talc. Particle description, ie, nonfibrous or relative fibrogenicity, is mentioned but not emphasized because it does not contribute to an understanding of the diseases or their roentgenographic manifestations.

Nonmining Silicosis

Nonmining exposure to significant inhalation of free silica (silicon dioxide) is now at least as common as mining exposure in recent years.[1,6] The most important nonmining source is foundry work involving abrading and polishing surfaces of metal castings and replacing silica brick linings of furnaces.[2] Ziskind et al[7] include eight circumstances where exposure to free silica occurs, including mining; quarrying and tunneling; stonecutting and polishing (especially monumental masonry); manufacture of metal castings with adherent sand from molds; manufacture of glass; foundry work using sand molds and abrasive blasting; manufacture of pottery, porcelain, and firebricks; boiler scaling with pneumatic impact tools; and vitreous enameling involving use of high temperature and air jets. "Sandblasting" is abrasive cleaning of metals including molds where a stream of sand is projected by compressed air against a metal surface producing dust clouds with almost all the particles respirable.[8] Sandblasting is thus involved in several of the forms of exposure.[2]

Nonoccupational exposure to silica has been reported only rarely. Intentional or unintentional use or abuse of abrasives, such as household cleansers, may cause disease identical with occupational exposure.[9]

Foundry work, especially the operation called "fettling," in which sand is removed from metal castings, is nearly as common as mining as a source

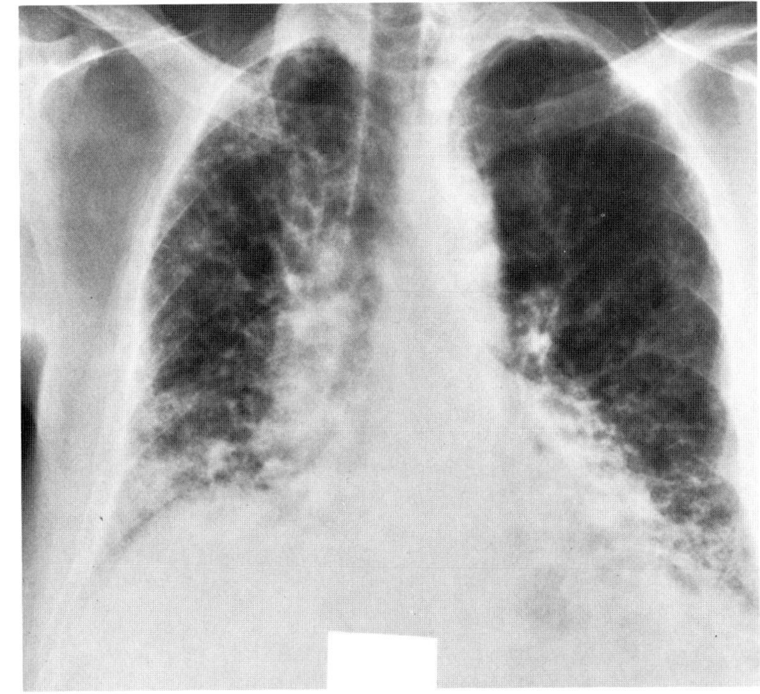

A

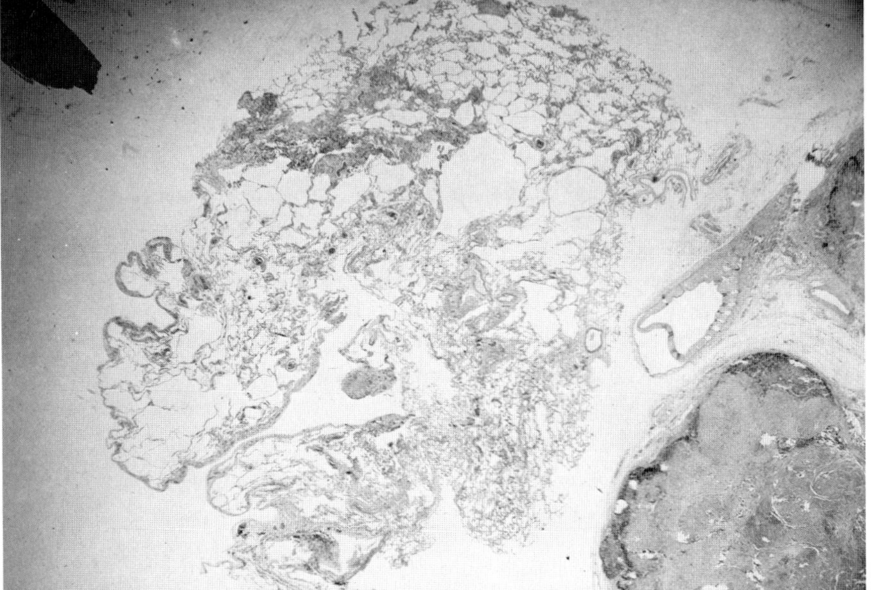

B

Figure 7.2. Severe simple silicosis in a foundry worker. **A**. Frontal radiograph with chronic interstitial infiltration accompanied by scattered nodules of varying sizes and shapes. Hilar enlargement is present bilaterally, especially on the right. Some nodules may exceed 1 cm in diameter. Appearances indicate marked pulmonary destruction, called "honeycomb" or "end-stage" lung. (AFIP Negative No. 79-5653.) **B**. Histologic slide of an area with no significant destruction showing patchy, irregular interstitial thickening, especially in the upper portion of the specimen. Portions of enlarged lymph nodes containing silica are seen on the right. (AFIP Negative No. 76-7471.)

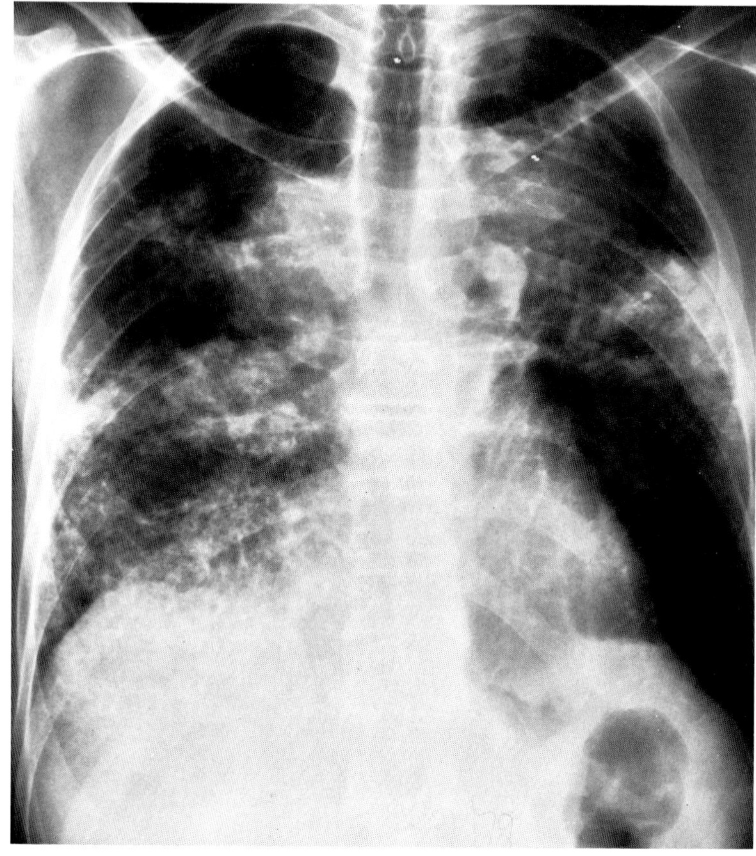

Figure 7.3. Complicated silicosis in an aluminum and iron foundry worker. **A**. Large, ill-defined masses are present in both lungs. These are scattered calcifications within a diffuse interstitial infiltrate. Peripheral emphysema, typical of complicated silicosis, is also obvious and the hila are both enlarged and distorted bilaterally. (AFIP Negative No. 82-1470.) **B**. Low-power histology (50 ×) from right lower lobe shows diffuse interstitial thickening that correlates with the reticular pattern seen roentgenographically. (AFIP Negative No. 76-7488.) **C**. High-power (200 ×) histology shows typical granulomas with clefts containing particles of silica as well as giant cells. Between the granulomas diffuse interstitial thickening caused by inflammation and fibrosis is visible. (AFIP Negative No. 76-7439.)

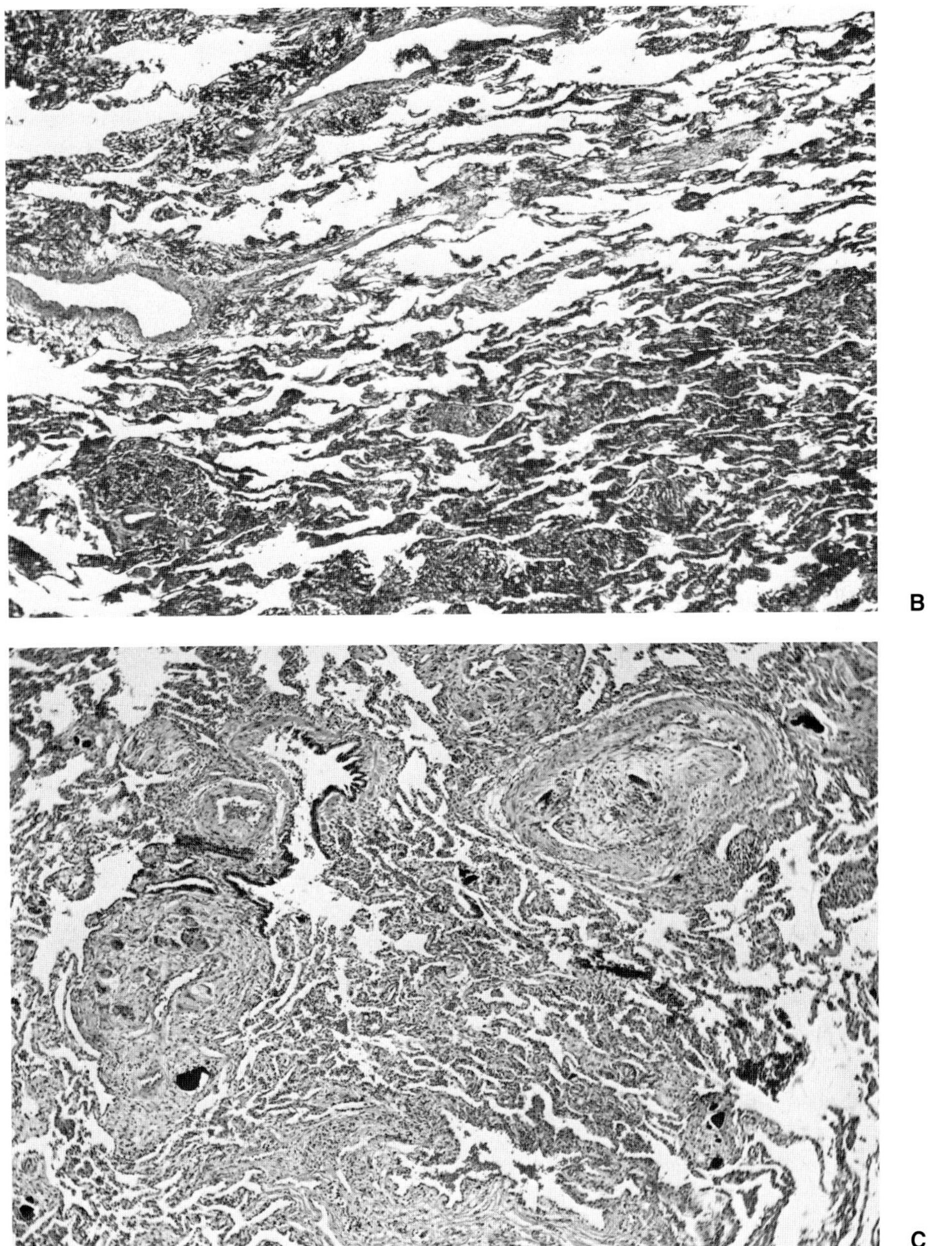

Figure 7.3

of exposure to free silica.[10] Many far less common occupational exposures have also been recently described, including the manufacture in Japan of a material called "tonoko," which is used as a wood filler containing nearly 80% free silica.[11] Slate pencil workers in India are exposed to material containing almost 70% free silica.[12] "Silica flour" used for abrasives is crushed quartz rock and consists of nearly 100% free silica in extremely small, easily respirable particles.[13] Ceramic manufacture principally involves the use of kaolin, very low in free silica, but exposure to silica may be high over the years particularly where basic principles of prevention to dust exposure have not prevailed, as documented in Israel.[14]

The pathogenesis of disease is similar in both mining and nonmining exposure to free silica.[8] Whenever particles of silica are smaller than 5 μm in diameter, they easily pass through the tracheobronchial tree into the lungs, and significant symptoms result. Chronic nonmining exposure produces clinical, radiologic, and pathologic pulmonary disease identical to chronic mining exposure (Figs. 7.1 to 7.3).

Acute and accelerated disease is more common in nonmining than mining exposure because of the greater opportunities for a worker to be exposed to high concentrations of finely divided silica. "Accelerated silicosis" is a rapidly progressive form of silicosis in which symptoms and findings are the same as in chronic silicosis, but clinical and radiographic progression is far more rapid[1] and occurs most commonly with sandblasting. Accelerated silicosis has also been associated with exposure to silica flour or abrasive soap powders. High exposure results in marked chronic silicosis becoming manifest within a few years instead of requiring a decade or more.

Acute silicosis, or "silicoproteinosis," can result from overwhelming exposure; symptoms and findings manifest themselves in as brief a period as a few weeks. First described from exposure to abrasive soap powders[15] in 1929, cases of acute silicosis have been documented in sandblasters and many other occupations. Sudden, dramatic onset of dyspnea, fever, cough, and weight loss may result in death even after the administration of steroids, bronchial lavage, and other treatment. Use of high-dose steroids has been effective in some cases.

Acute silicosis appears to represent a disease distinct from other forms of silica inhalation and may involve an immune mechanism not affected in either accelerated or chronic silicosis.[16]

Radiologic changes (Fig. 7.4) in both chronic and accelerated silicosis are indistinguishable for mining and nonmining exposure, both producing simple and complicated forms. A period of two or more decades is usually required to produce nodules larger than 1 cm, described as complicated silicosis. Radiologic manifestations appear to be most common with increased duration and concentration of silica exposure and are especially common with the initial abnormal film obtained at a relatively young age.[16] Roentgenographic abnormalities correlate best with forced vital capacity and forced expiratory volume and fail to correlate with other measures of pulmonary function. A few reports describe less radiologic abnormalities in nonmining exposures,[17] but most studies show no such difference.

Radiographic signs in acute silicosis (Fig. 7.5) differ significantly from those in accelerated or chronic forms. There is usually consolidation, especially in the lower zones, sometimes accompanied by pleural effusions. Lymph-node enlargement is not present in most early cases, but may be seen because of preceding chronic changes. The findings resemble alveolar proteinosis, including the possibility of an interstitial pattern of reticulations occurring as the dominant abnormality in a minority of patients. The more typical alveolar pattern, the principal manifestation of this disease, results from proteinaceous exudate filling alveoli, but interstitial inflammation may be marked and may produce an interstitial pattern, especially at the periphery of lung most involved by the alveolar pattern.

Diatomaceous Earth

Diatomaceous earth is amorphous free silica that can be heated to the point at which it crystallizes; is often called cristobalite.[18] Cristobalite, also known as kieselguhr in Sweden, is approximately 65% to 90% free silica in fibrous form, being thus greatly fibrogenic and causing pulmonary disease in every way identical with other forms of silicosis. Diatomaceous earth originates from the remains of

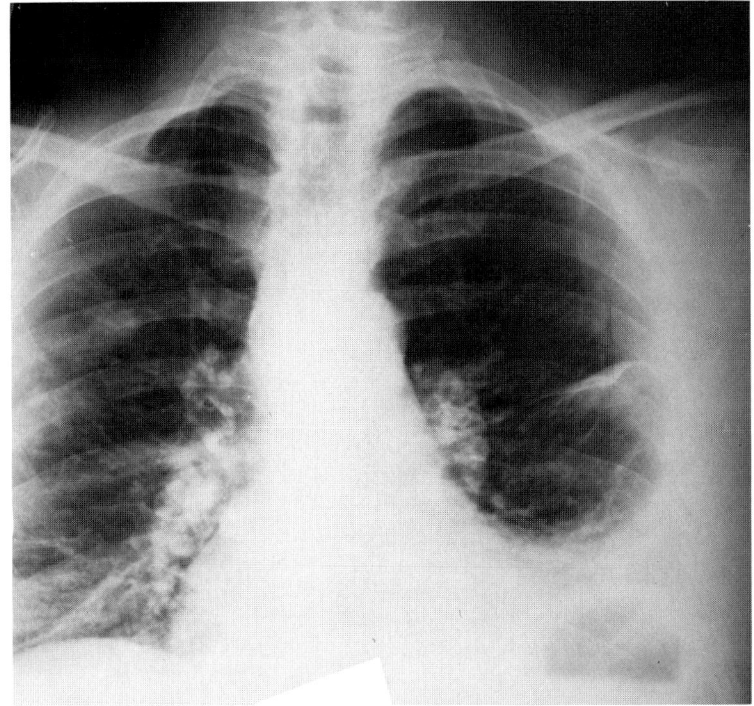

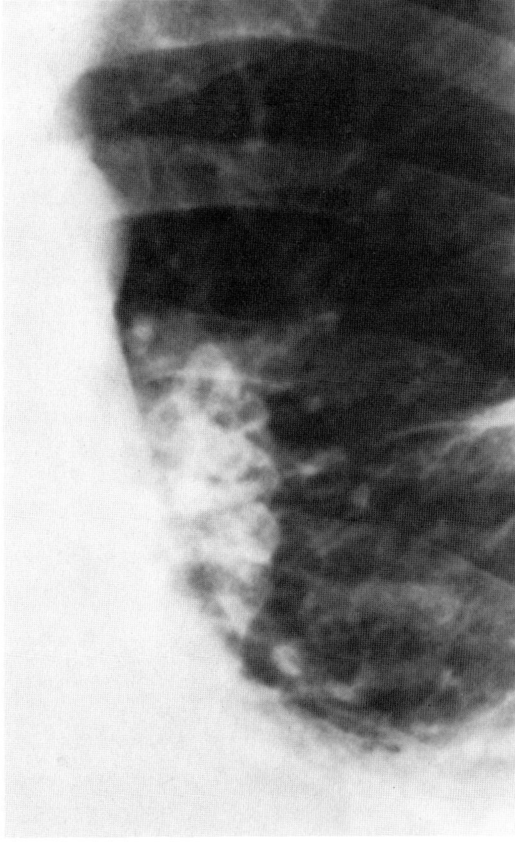

Figure 7.4. Chronic, complicated silicosis in a mill worker with prominent eggshell calcified lymph nodes. **A**. Frontal view. (AFIP Negative No. 78-5311.) **B**. Close-up of left hilum with numerous eggshell calcifications in lymph nodes. Scattered nodules of varying sizes are present, especially in the right lung. Marked scarring of the left lower zone and pleura is also evident, probably the result of old inflammatory disease rather than the silica exposure. (AFIP Negative No. 78-5311.)

A

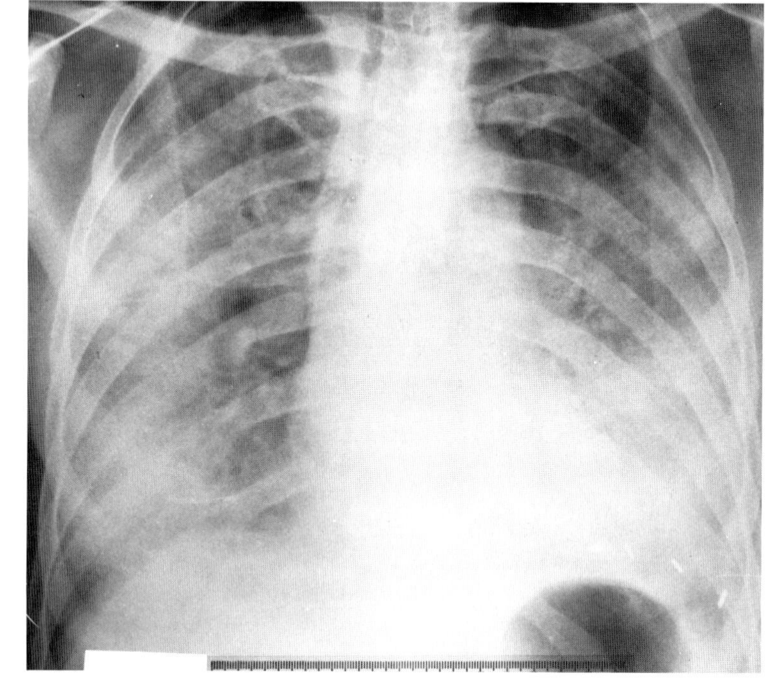

B

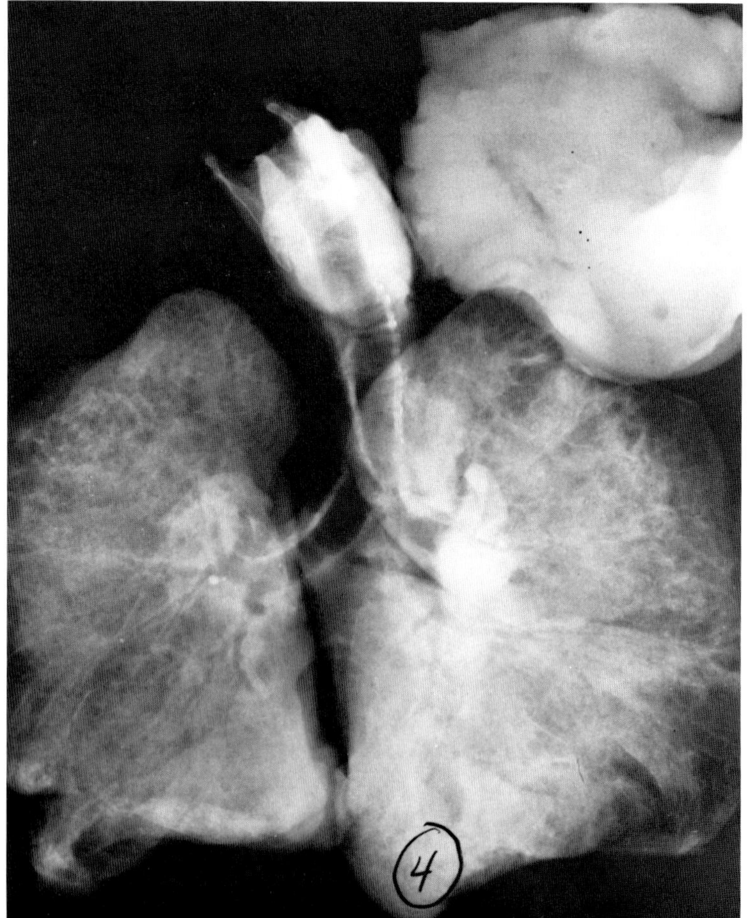

Figure 7.5

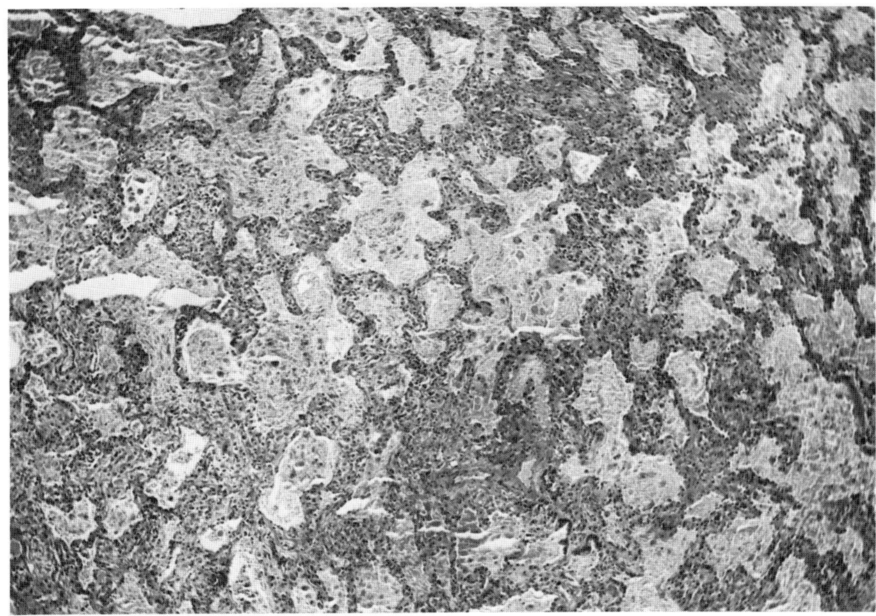

Figure 7.5. Acute silicosis (silicoproteinosis). **A**. Frontal chest film shows bilateral consolidations, especially in the lower and midzones. (AFIP Negative No. 64-2762.) **B**. Autopsy specimen of lungs with diffuse bilateral consolidation caused by filling of alveoli with proteinacious exudate, causing the consolidative pattern. (AFIP Negative No. 64-2762.) **C**. Medium-power view of histology (70 ×) shows exudate filling alveoli and inflammation of interstitium. (AFIP Negative No. 76-7497.)

aquatic plants, principally unicellular algae, called diatoms.[19,20] Diatomaceous earth is used in filters, abrasives, insulation materials, lubricants, and absorbants, and is obtained by strip mining, usually in the western portion of the United States.

Clinical disease appears identical with other forms of silicosis, although long-term, continued exposure is apparently necessary for significant disease to be manifest.[18] Radiographic findings are usually those of simple silicosis (Fig. 7.1), although masses of complicated silicosis also occur after very prolonged exposures. Lesions were found only in mill workers with 27 to 46 years of exposure, according to Cooper.[18] There has been a marked decrease in the occurrence in recent years.

Other Forms of Silica

Nepheline

This is a complex silicate mined in Canada as a hard rock and milled into a powder for use in glazing pottery.[21] Nepheline may contain a high proportion of free silica and can be a cause of silicosis in both simple and complicated forms.[1] Alunite is another complex silicate, composed primarily of aluminum silicate and used as cat litter in Australia.[22] It also may contain free silica, consequently producing silicosis.

Talc

The term "talc" is applied to both a pure silicate of magnesium and to a mixture of minerals containing the pure substance and many other constituents, with mineral talc as only a minor component.[23] In its pure mineral form, talc occurs as microscopic plates or sheets; the shape is responsible for its lubricant quality.[1] It is thus not a fibrous silicate, but individual particles may appear as a fibrous form in some instances; this has led to the confusion in classifying talc as both fibrous and nonfibrous silicate.

Four distinct forms of pulmonary disease, with clearly different radiographic appearances, may be defined. Confusion among the distinct forms has led to considerable misunderstanding of clinical,

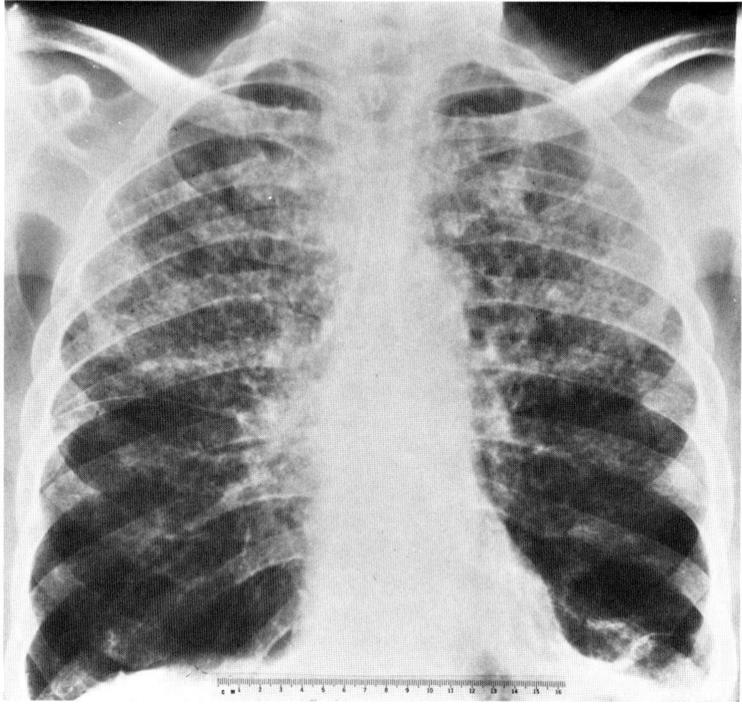

Figure 7.6. Talcosilicosis. Frontal chest film of a Californian talc miner shows numerous small nodules in both upper lung fields, accompanied by hilar lymphadenopathy, resembling simple silicosis. (AFIP Negative No. 81-604.) From D.S. Feigin: TALC: Understanding its manifestations in the chest. AJR, 146: 295–301 February 1986, © by ARRS.

pathologic, and radiologic manifestations of talc in the lungs. The four forms of talc disease are talcosilicosis, talcoasbestosis, pure talcosis, and intravenous administration of talc.

Talcosilicosis (Fig. 7.6). Produced by exposure to talc associated with free silica and other nonasbestiform minerals.[24] The clinical and radiologic manifestations resemble those of silicosis, probably because of the high free silica content of the inspired air, which in Italian mining operations is as high as 18%.[24] The only documented difference between silicosis and talcosilicosis is the histological presence of talc.[25] Radiologic changes are indistinguishable from those of silicosis and may appear as both simple and complicated forms. Thus, the contribution of the talc to the production of disease in these patients is questionable whenever the silica content of the inhaled dust exceeds the levels that generally produce silicosis.

Talcoasbestosis (Fig. 7.7). Produced by the inhalation of talc with asbestiform fibers. Some of the best documented cases are from the Gouveneur region in upper New York State where talc is mined with tremolite and anthophyllite.[23] The clinical, radiologic, and pathologic manifestations of asbestos in exposed workers have been documented, however, only after a decade following initial exposure, as cough and dyspnea become manifest. The radiographic signs are those typical of interstitial lung disease, with linear and reticular densities and septal lines typically predominate in the lower zones especially adjacent to the heart, as in pure asbestosis. Bilateral pleural thickening, mainly involving the lower portion of the lateral lung fields on frontal views, is also common and identical with asbestos pleural thickening[26]; the apical pleura and costophrenic angles are relatively spared. Calcifications occur on the diaphragm as well as in lateral pleural plaques. In fact, diaphragmatic calcification in talc exposure is only seen in talcoasbestosis and not in any of the other three forms of talc disease. Talcoasbestosis is also associated with malignancies, including bronchogenic carcinoma and malignant mesothelioma,[24] but not in as high an incidence as in asbestos exposure. The incidence may well vary with the type of asbestos inhaled with the talc.[27]

Pure talcosis. Well documented in both occupational and nonoccupational exposure to talc free of silica and asbestiform minerals. Pure talc is mined

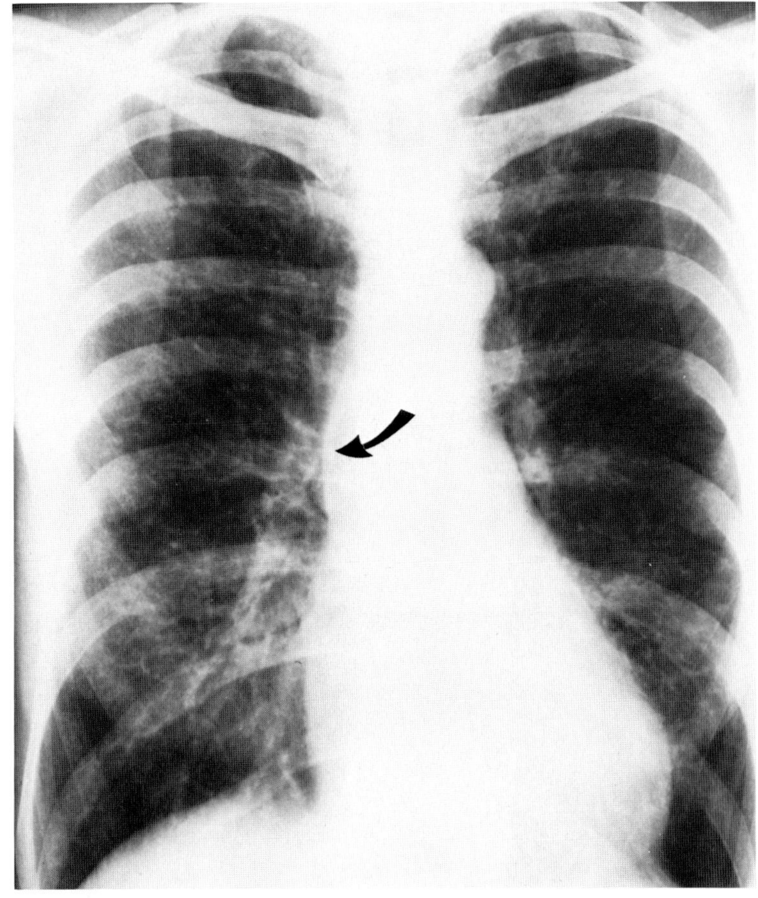

Figure 7.7. Talcoasbestosis in a long-term talc worker, using talc from upper New York. Frontal film shows diffuse reticulations throughout both lungs and a pleural plaque, especially obvious on the medial aspect of hilum (*arrow*). (AFIP Negative No. 60-5439.) From D.S. Feigin: TALC: Understanding its manifestations in the chest. AJR, 146: 295–301 February 1986 © by ARRS.

in Vermont, Montana, portions of California, and other areas.[23] In addition, pure talcosis may result from exposure to talc mixed with other minerals, such as carbon in Texas, in which the impurities do not themselves commonly produce disease. Pure talc is mostly used in cosmetics and skin powders and has not proved harmful. It is considered fibrogenic by some.[28] Other reports do not agree, despite symptoms and findings of pulmonary function tests that are consistent with restrictive pulmonary disease and that are well documented in pure talc exposure. Airway obstruction may also occur.[29] Miners, associated workers, and those exposed in processing pure talc are most likely to be affected, but the disease has also been documented from the cosmetic industry, but only when exposure has been very heavy and prolonged.[25,30]

Pure talc inhalation can also cause acute pulmonary symptoms when large quantities are aspirated, accidental exposure occurring more frequently in infants.[24,31] Pleural installation of pure talc may result in pleural thickening and fibrosis[24,32] and may cause significant pulmonary disease if the talc enters the lung. Radiographic abnormalities associated with pure talc inhalation consist of small nodules, usually seen in the lower zones. Reticulations may also occur but appear less commonly[33] (Fig. 7.8). Pleural thickening secondary to pure talc has been described but its incidence is very uncertain[23,29,33]; however, calcifications have not been reported and lymphadenopathy rarely, if ever, occurs. Pathologic changes of pure talc include granuloma formation[25] as well as interstitial inflammation; the granulomas are probably responsible for the radiographic nodularity.

Intravenous administration of talc, the fourth form of pulmonary disease, is commonly a result of self-administered intravenous injections of tablets diluted with talc and meant for oral medication.[34]

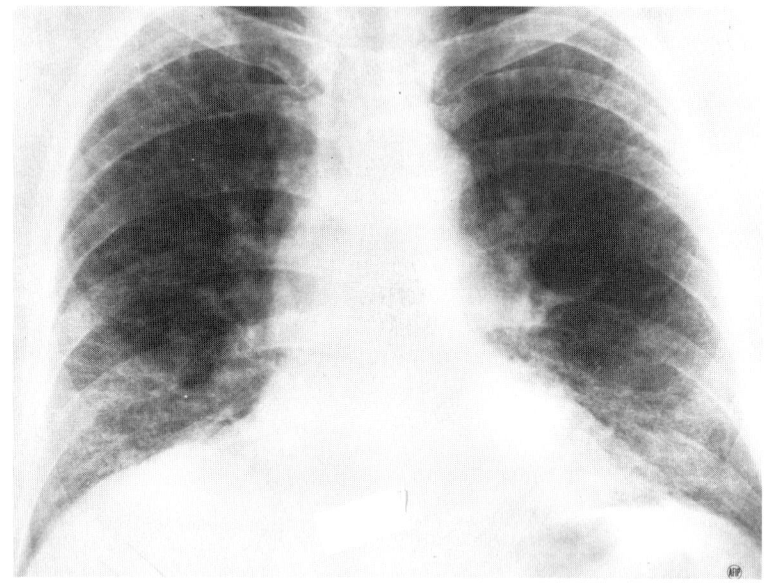

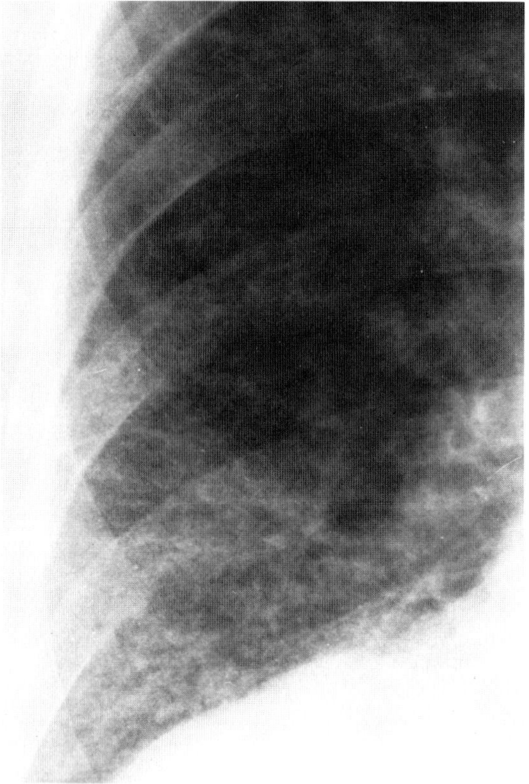

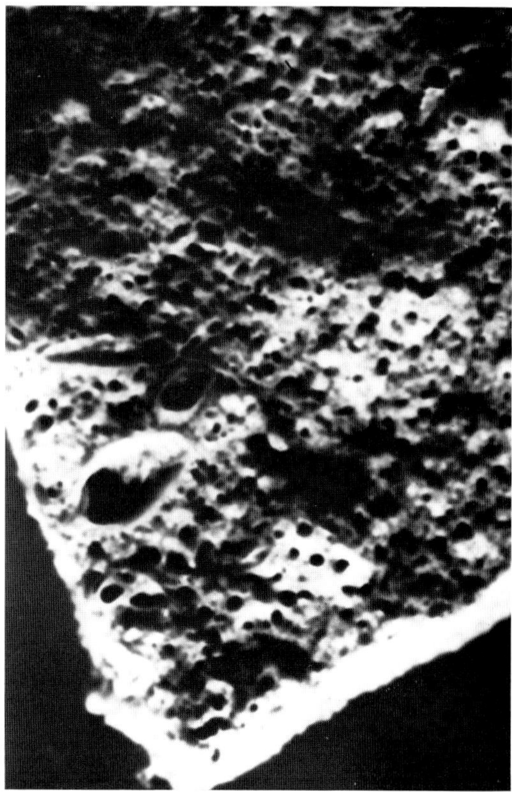

Figure 7.8. Pure talcosis in a soapstone worker from California. **A**. Frontal chest film shows diffuse reticular densities, most marked in the lower zones at the periphery of the lung. (AFIP Negative No. 69-2216.) **B**. Close-up of right lower lung shows the reticular pattern and tiny nodules. (AFIP Negative No. 69-2216.) **C**. Gross specimen of lung demonstrates diffuse thickening of pulmonary interstitium by deposition of talc. Histology also showed diffuse inflammation. (AFIP Negative No. 69-2216.) From D.S. Feigin: TALC: Understanding its manifestations in the chest. AJR, 146: 295–301 February 1986, © by ARRS.

Such abused medications include pentazocine and methadone. Severe dyspnea and other manifestations similar to those of pulmonary emboli occur because of the formation of vascular and perivascular granulomas in the lung as well as pulmonary abscesses.

Intravenous talc usually produces large, irregular nodular densities or consolidation in the upper portions of the midzones, which may rapidly progress into large masses or massive consolidation[35] (Fig. 7.9). Widespread irregular nodules may also occur and pulmonary volume loss may be permanent.[36] The large mass densities resemble those of pulmonary massive fibrosis in silicosis and coal worker's pneumoconosis, but may, however, appear far closer to the hilum than in the latter diseases.[37] The radiologic findings thus resemble sarcoid, apart from lymphadenopathy, which is far less common with talc. Hilar adenopathy may precede or be concurrent with the pulmonary manifestations of sarcoidosis. Intravenous talc may be differentiated from inhaled talc through histology and also because of the much larger size of the talc particles; the mean particle diameter in intravenous administration usually exceeds 10 μm as compared with 4 μm for inhalation particles.[38] Smaller particles of intravenous talc apparently traverse the capillaries without being trapped in the lungs and lodge in other organs.[35]

Kaolin

Kaolin is a clay that consists primarily of kaolinite, a nonfibrous silicate of aluminum found mostly in southeastern United States, England, Japan, Egypt, Czechoslovakia, and Germany.[1] Its use in ceramics has led to its common name, china clay. It is more recently being used, however, as a filler in plastics, rubber, paint, and adhesives; as a coating for high-quality paper; and in soaps and toothpastes.[39] Kaolin is often mined on the surface as a wet slurry and is probably innocuous in this form.[40] Dried kaolinite is documented as a cause of pulmonary disease when inhaled during bagging and on transportation.

Early reports of kaolin pneumoconiosis came from Cornwall, England, where kaolin is found with silica[41] and in reports of workers who also had tuberculosis. Recent reports have emphasized the distinction between earlier reports and inhalation of nearly pure kaolin, especially in Georgia.[42] However, kaolinite mined in Missouri for firebricks has a high free-silica content[43] and is more likely to lead to disease than is inhalation of pure kaolinite, especially in the absence of tuberculosis. Kaolin powder was used as treatment of pneumothorax in the 1950s.[44] In at least one case significant pulmonary disease occurred after kaolin particles entered the lung parenchyma.

Symptoms of pure kaolin exposure require prolonged inhalation of dried dust over a period of several years. Significant disease generally occurs only when there are also severe radiographic abnormalities[39] such as small nodules, which may become large and irregular anywhere in the lung (Fig. 7.10). Very large, well-defined masses may subsequently develop in any portion of the lung and may be more than 10 cm in diameter and generally bilateral; but unilateral and markedly asymmetric masses also occur. Peripheral emphysema is commonly associated with large masses. The appearance thus closely resemble typical findings in complicated coal worker's pneumoconiosis or complicated silicosis.

Pathologically, the nodules represent small regions of fibrosis, initially in peribronchial regions and generally associated with more diffuse interstitial inflammation and fibrosis. The large masses, usually colored blue or gray, show marked central coagulative necrosis and contain large quantities of dust. They are thus similar to the conglomerate lesions of coal worker's pneumoconiosis.[2] The mass lesions do not resemble the whorled, fibrotic masses of silicosis when kaolin is inhaled without silica,[39] indicating the fibrogenic effects of kaolin itself, although it clearly does not produce the same pathology as silica (Fig. 7.11).

Mica

Mica is a silicate of aluminum, and of its several forms, mined in India and the United States, the most important is muscovite. Mica is nonfibrous, splitting into thin sheets with a transparency and high resistance to heat and electricity that make it useful for windows in stoves and furnaces.[1] Muscovite, a potassium mica, was used for window glazing in the past and is now used as a lubricant, in

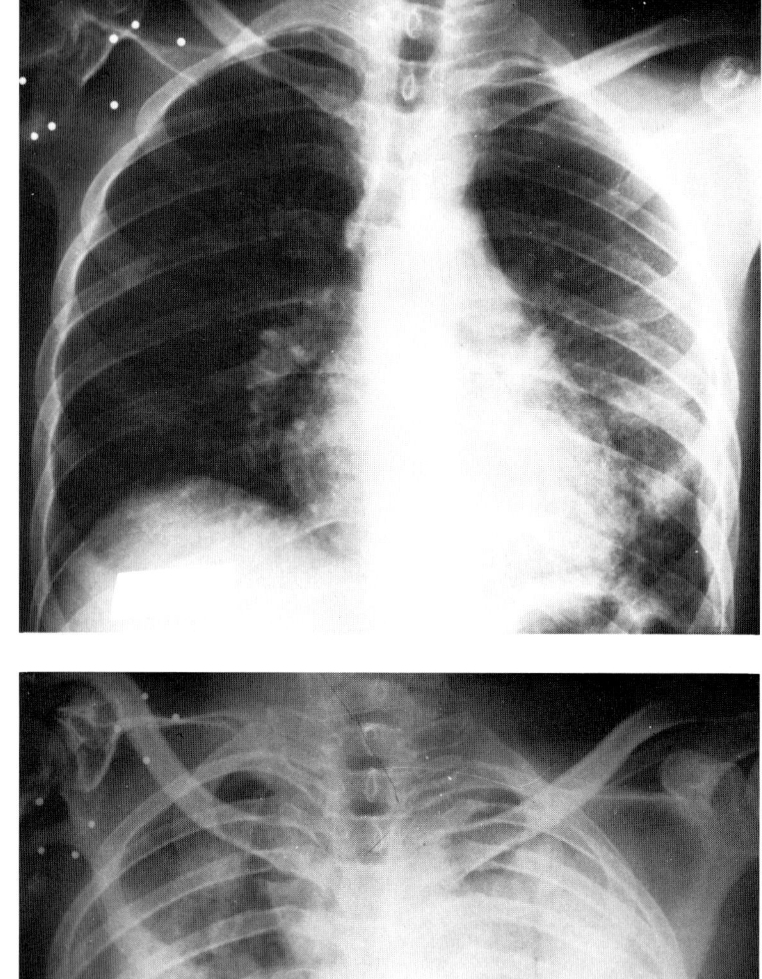

Figure 7.9

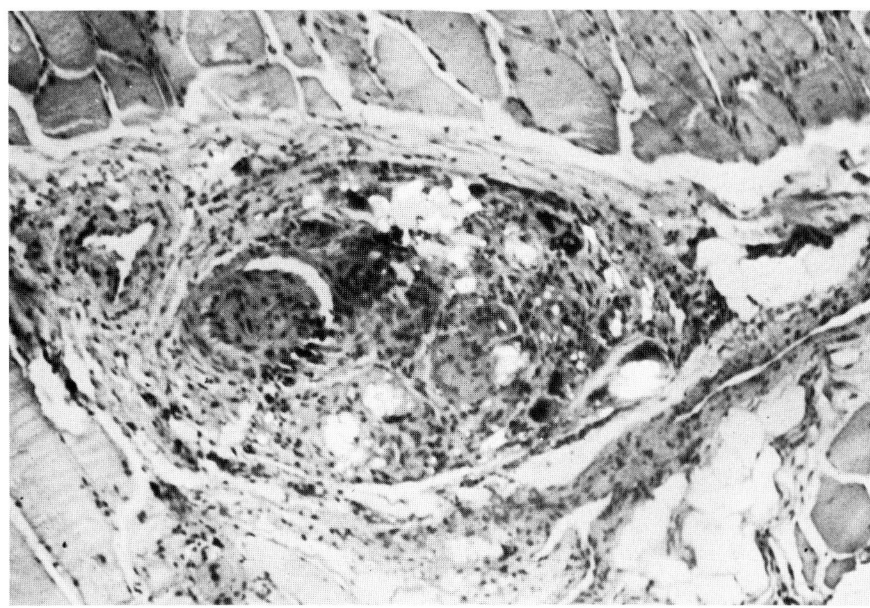

Figure 7.9. Talc disease due to self-administration of tablets intravenously. **A**. Initial chest film shows minimal consolidation of left lower lobe and interstitial infiltration elsewhere, especially on the left. A left pleural effusion is also present. (AFIP Negative No. 73-10492.) **B**. Film 7 months later on readmission demonstrates severe bilateral consolidation of the lungs with diffuse hypoventilation. (AFIP Negative No. 73-10492.) **C**. Histology of granuloma within muscle following intravenous injection. The granuloma contains numerous talc granules and inflammatory round cells. (AFIP Negative No. 73-10492.) From D.S. Feigin: TALC: Understanding its manifestations in the chest. AJR, 146: 295–301 February 1986, © by ARRS.

wallpaper and paint, and for appliances and lamps as an insulator.[45]

There have been many reports of disease related to inhalation of mica (especially muscovite), but in most, inhalation of other substances with mica, especially silica or asbestos or both, is mentioned. Definite disease related to pure mica inhalation is therefore not well established.[46] Pleural calcifications and thickening, for example, have not been shown to occur in mica exposure without asbestos contamination.

Radiographic findings in patients with significant mica exposure, usually to dried muscovite in ground form, consist of fine nodules diffused throughout both lungs in the lower zones (Fig. 7.12). Reticular interstitial infiltration may also occur, again favoring the lower zones (Fig. 7.13). Lymph-node enlargement probably does not occur unless silica has also be inhaled. Documented progress of lung lesions to honeycombing, both radiographically and pathologically, have been reported, but again it is not clear whether mica is the causative agent of fibrosis or pulmonary destruction.

Fuller's Earth

In "fulling," grease is removed from wool by an absorbent clay, hence "fuller's earth,"[24] an aluminum silicate; however, "fuller's earth" has also been used for other silicates such as bentonite. Today these clays are principally used in oil refining, as a binder in foundry molds, as a filter, and as a filler in cosmetics. The classification of fuller's earth as fibrous or nonfibrous is indefinite, although it is usually considered nonfibrous.

Clinical disease associated with fuller's earth is exceedingly mild and regarded as a benign form of pneumoconiosis.[1,2] Inhalation of dust from these clays may cause small nodules on the chest radiograph similar to those of simple silicosis and coal

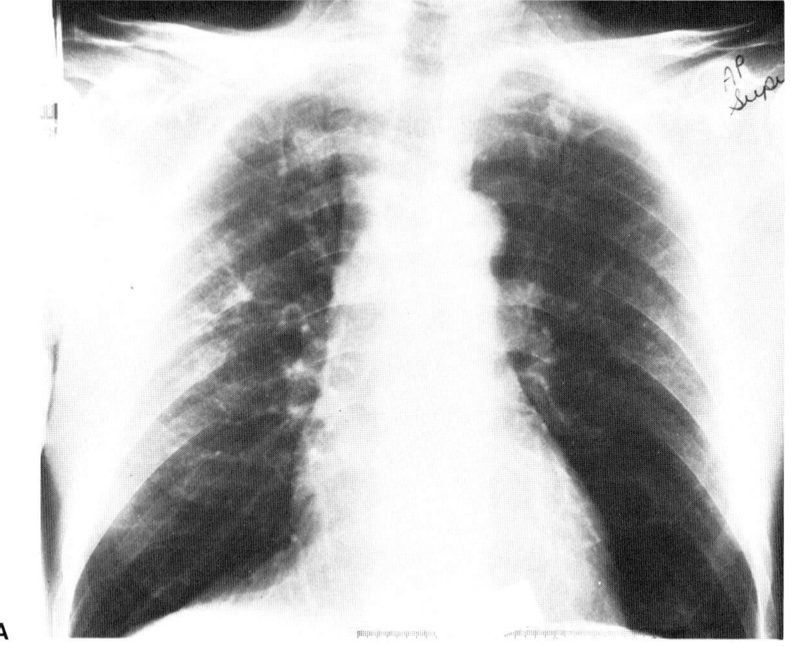

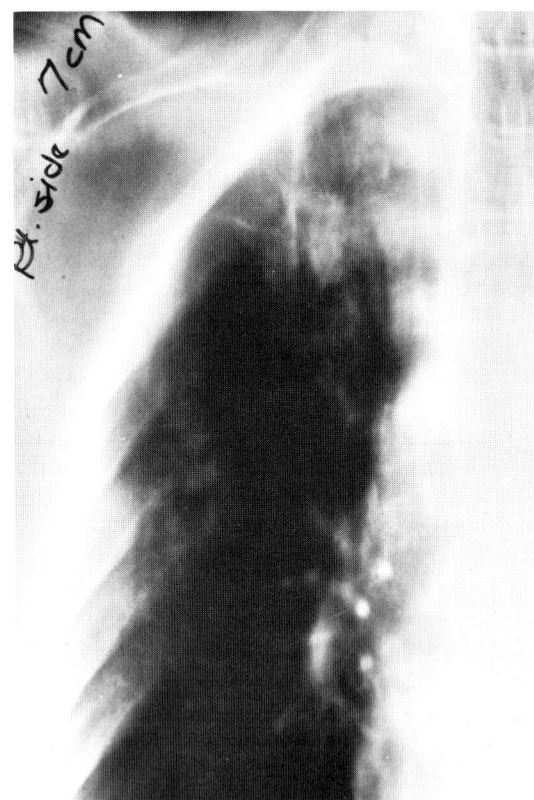

Figure 7.10. Kaolin pneumoconiosis in a construction worker. **A**. Film shows scattered nodules of varying sizes. (AFIP Negative No. 80-6334.) **B**. Tomogram of right upper lung demonstrates 2-cm benign mass among the nodules. (AFIP Negative No. 80-6334.)

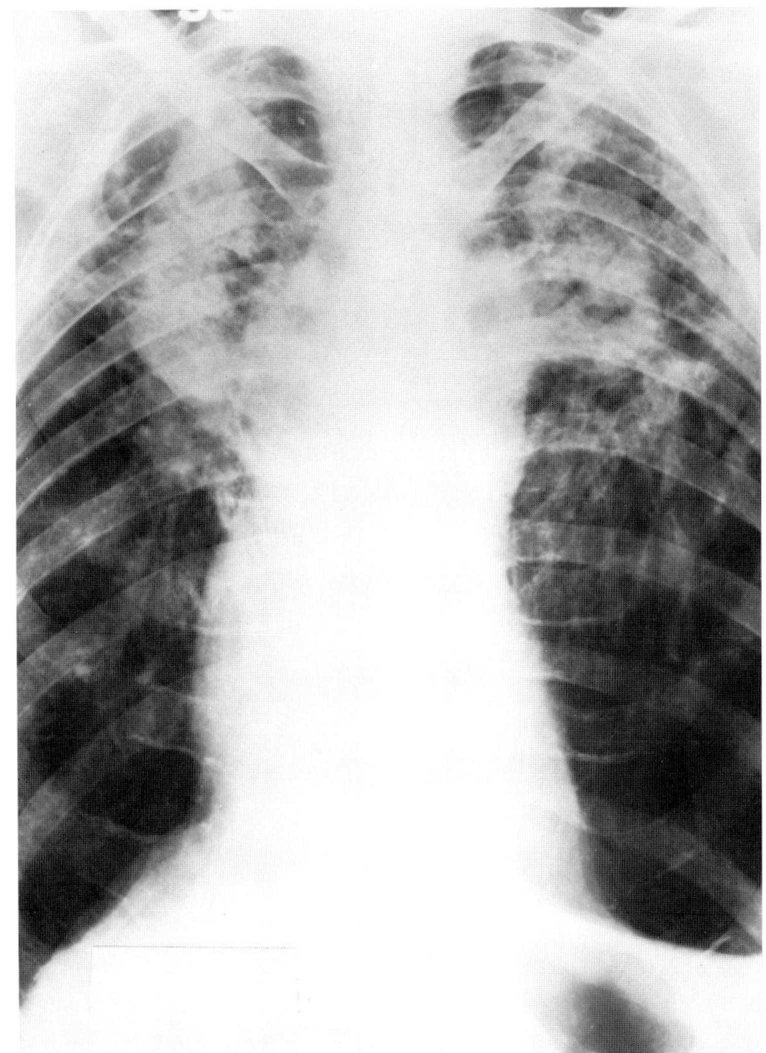

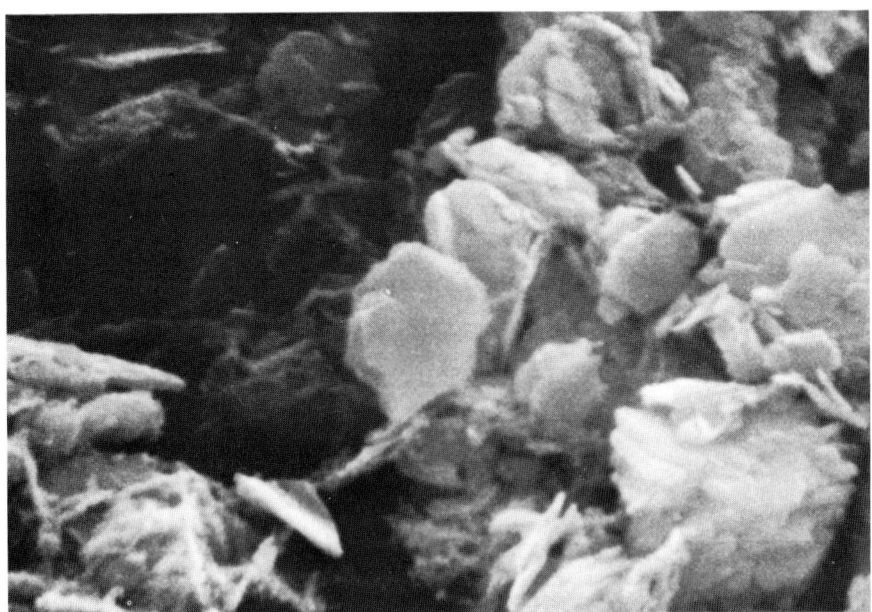

Figure 7.11. Advanced kaolin pneumoconiosis in a miner. **A**. Film shows bilateral large masses with peripheral emphysema and central hilar retraction as in complicated silicosis. (AFIP Negative No. 55-13046.) **B**. Scanning electron micrograph of lung sediment demonstrates wafer-shaped particles of kaolin (plus other substances). (AFIP Negative No. 67-9847.)

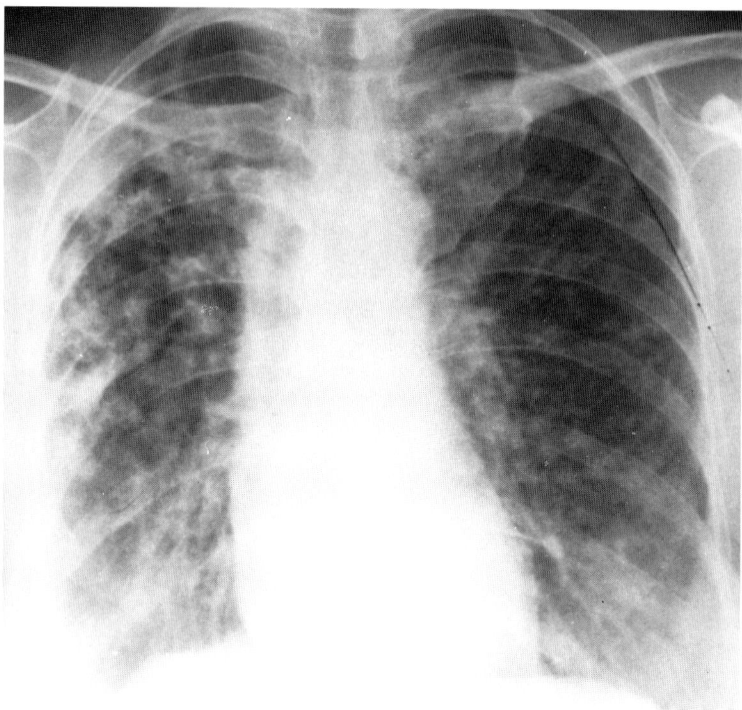

Figure 7.12. Mica inhalation in a muscovite worker from Kentucky. Irregular, unevenly distributed nodules are present throughout both lungs, especially in the right upper zone with some volume loss and pleural thickening. (AFIP Negative No. 66-8385.)

worker's pneumoconiosis; complicated disease with mass formation is only reported in patients also exposed to silica (Fig. 7.14). The few descriptions of pathologic changes emphasize the similarity to other benign forms of pneumoconiosis such as coal inhalation with deposits of dust forming black nodules containing macrophages with minimal adjacent fibrosis.[2]

Zeolite (Erionite)

Zeolites are hydrated aluminum silicates used as boiling stones[24] or as filters, especially molecular sieves in gas chromotography. Although most zeolites are nonfibrous, one fibrous form, erionite from central Turkey, has received considerable attention recently as a cause of malignant disease, especially mesthelioma.

The fibrous form of erionite is very similar to asbestos.[47] Pleural thickening and diaphragmatic plaques related to erionite exposure are well documented, as are bronchogenic carcinoma and pleural mesothelioma. The shape of the fiber is believed to be responsible, a theory supported by carcinoma occurring when synthetic fibers of similar dimensions are instilled into the pleural space of experimental animals.[48] Besides the dimensions of the fibers, their durability seems to play a part in producing the disease.

Man-Made Vitreous Fibers (Fiberglass)

In general, fibers with a diameter 3.5 to 200 μm are most often implicated in causing pulmonary disease,[24] but most synthetic fibers are too coarse to be pathogenic. Man-made fibers of appropriate diameter can be used for lightweight insulation and filters, usually of glass and ceramic fibers from molten kaolin, alumina, and silica. Ceramic filaments, necessary for high temperatures, are thought to be fibrogenic and may also play a role in provoking malignancies.[24] As previously mentioned, glass fibers have been shown to produce mesotheliomas when instilled in the pleural space of rats.[48]

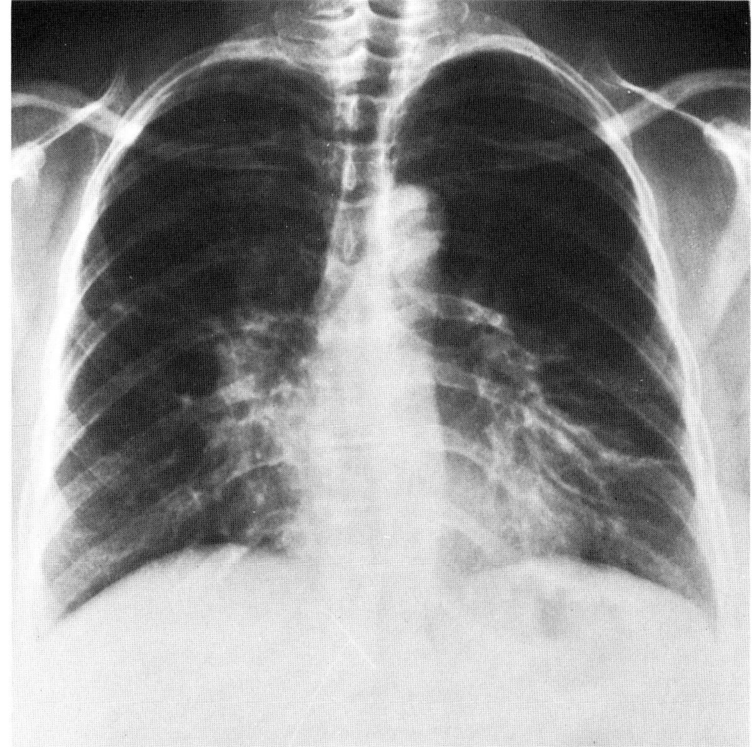

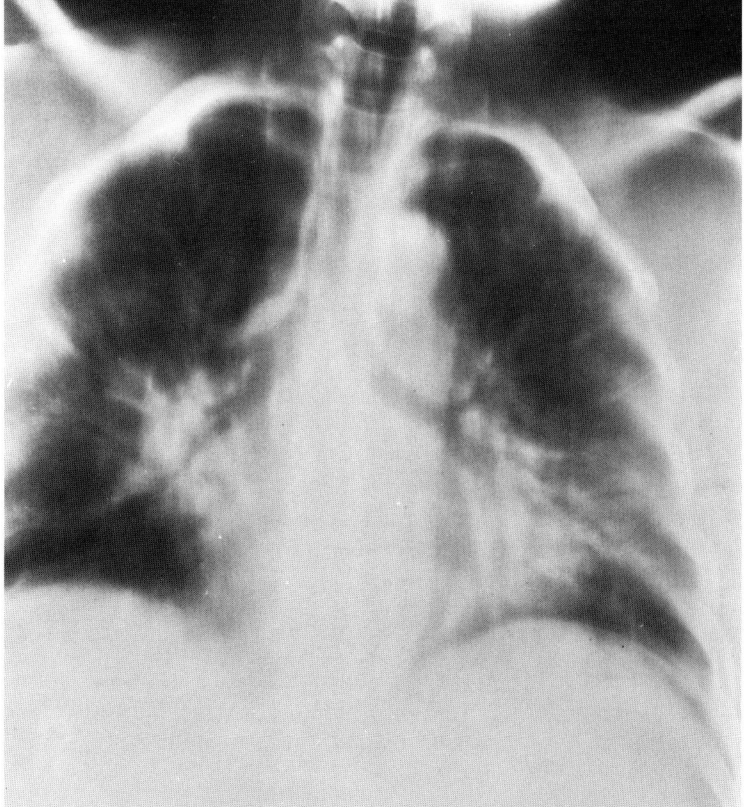

Figure 7.13. Mica inhalation in a miner reported as chronically exposed to silica. **A**. Frontal chest film demonstrates bilateral lower zone reticulations far more typical of mica inhalation than inhalation of silica. (AFIP Negative No. 81-1154.) **B**. Whole-lung tomogram emphasizes hilar enlargement with large lymph nodes bilaterally probably reflecting silica exposure. The reticulations, better seen on the plain film, are visible at the periphery. (AFIP Negative No. 81-1154.)

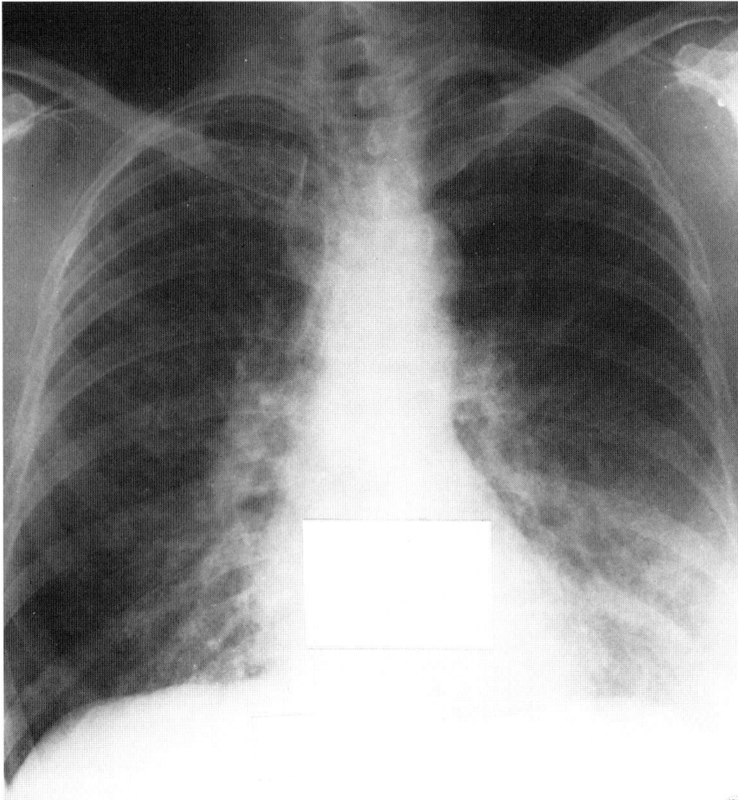

Figure 7.14. Fuller's earth pneumoconiosis in patient also exposed to silica. Numerous small nodules are present in both lungs, most obvious in the right midzone. Consolidation at the bases was probably unrelated and the bilateral hilar enlargement presumably reflects the silica exposure. (AFIP Negative No. 67-10335.)

Fibers of glass, including glass wool and rock wool, are known in some cases as a tracheobronchial tree irritant, but their effect on the lower respiratory tract is not well documented.[24] No distinct radiographic changes have been attributed to exposure to any man-made fibrous materials.

Miscellaneous Silicates

Wollastonite is a calcium silicate used to make ceramic tiles in the United States, Mexico, and Finland[49] and can have fiber dimensions similar to asbestos. Radiographic changes identical with those of asbestos have been reported from inhalation.

Vermiculite is another complex silicate reported as a cause of pulmonary disease similar to that caused by asbestos.[24] As it is usually found and used with mica or with asbestiform materials, vermiculite is not a proven independent cause of pulmonary disease or radiographic abnormalities.[50]

Cement is usually low in silica, consisting primarily of calcium silicates and aluminates; but when it is used, it is usually mixed with minerals, including silica and asbestos.[51] Cement may be responsible for radiographic abnormalities, consisting of small scattered nodules, following heavy and prolonged exposure.[1]

Acknowledgments. The author is grateful to the photographic branch of the Armed Forces Institute of Pathology, Washington, DC, for superb service in processing the illustrations and to Nancy Fletcher for excellent secretarial and administrative support. The guidance, advice, and logistic assistance of David S. Hartman, CDR, MC, USN, Chairman and Registrar of Radiologic Pathology at the AFIP, is also deeply appreciated.

References

1. Morgan WKC, Seaton A: Occupational Lung Diseases, ed 2. Philadelphia, WB Saunders Co, 1984.
2. Lapp NL: Lung disease secondary to inhalation of nonfibrous minerals. Clin Chest Med 1981; 2(2):219–233.
3. Gross P: The biologic classification of insoluble respirable dusts. J Occup Med 1979; 21(5):371–372.
4. Parkes WR: Occupational Lung Disorders, ed 2. London, Butterworth & Co Ltd, 1982.

4a. Churg A, Wright JL: Small-airway lesions in patients exposed to nonasbestos mineral dusts. Human Pathol 1983; 14(8):688–693.

5. Vallyathan NV, Green FHY, Craighead JE: Recent advances in the study of mineral pneumoconiosis. Pathol Annu 1980; 15(2):77–100.
6. Corn JK: Historical aspects of industrial hygiene–II. Silicosis. Am Ind Hyg Assoc J 1980; 41:125–133.
7. Ziskind M, Jones RN, Weill H: Silicosis. Am Rev Respir Dis 1986; 113:643.
8. Weill H: Occupational Lung Disease. Hosp Prac April 1981, pp 65–80.
9. Gong H Jr, Tashkin DP: Silicosis due to intentional inhalation of abrasive scouring powder. Am J Med 1979; 67:358–362.
10. Fletcher AC, Ades A: Lung cancer mortality in a cohort of English foundry workers. Scand J Work Environ Health 1984; 10:7–16.
11. Kawakami M, Sato S, Takishima T: Silicosis in workers dealing with tonoko. Chest 1977; 72(5):635–639.
12. Jain SM, Sepaha GC, Khare KC, et al: Silicosis in slate pencil workers. Chest 1977; 71(3):423–426.
13. Nelson AM, Rajhans GS, Morton S, et al: Silica four exposures in Ontario. Am Ind Hyg Assoc J 1978; 39:261–269.
14. Kolton R, Kichter ED, Israeli R: Occupational exposure to dust containing free silica in a ceramics factory. Isr J Med Sci 1981; 17(4):277–282.
15. Middleton EL: The present position of silicosis in industry in Britain. Br Med J 1929; 2:485.
16. Hughes JM, Jones RN, Gilson JC, et al: Determinants of progression in sandblasters silicosis. (Inhaled Particles). Ann Occup Hyg 1982; 26(1–4):701–712.
17. Craighead JE, Vallyathan NV: Cryptic pulmonary lesions in workers occupationally exposed to dust containing silica. J Am Med Assoc 1980; 244:1939–1941.
18. Cooper WC, Jacobson G: A 21-Year radiographic follow-up of workers in the diatomite industry. J Occup Med 1977; 19(8):563–566.
19. Bye E, Davies R, Griffiths DM, et al: In vitro cytotoxicity and quantitative silica analysis of diatomaceous earth products. Br J Ind Med 1984; 41:228–234.
20. Beskow R: Silicosis in diatomaceous earth factory workers in Sweden. Scand J Respir Dis 1978; 59:216–221.
21. Olscamp G, Herman SJ, Weisbrod GL: Nepheline rock dust pneumoconiosis. Diag Radiol 1982; 142(1):29–32.
22. Musk AW, Greville HW, Tribe AE: Pulmonary disease from occupational exposure to an artificial aluminum silicate used for cat litter. Br J Ind Med 1980; 37:367–372.
23. Gamble JF, Fellner W, Dimeo MJ: An epidemiologic study of a group of talc workers. Am Rev Respir Dis 1979; 119:741–753.
24. Feigin DS: Talc: Understanding its manifestations in the chest. AJR 1986; 146:295–301.
25. Tukiainen P, Nickels J, Taskinen E, et al: Pulmonary granulomatous reaction: Talc pneumoconiosis or chronic sarcoidosis? Br J Ind Med 1984; 41:84–87.
26. Smith AR: Pleural calcifications resulting from exposure to certain dusts. Am J Roentgen 1952; 67:375–382.
27. Ng TK: Talc and mesothelioma. Med J Aust April 1984, pp 452–453.
28. Vallyathan NV, Craighead JE: Pulmonary pathology in workers exposed to nonasbestiform talc. Human Pathol 1981; 12(1):28–35.
29. Scully RE, Mark EJ, McNeely BU: Case records of the Massachusetts General Hospital/Case 35-1982. N Engl J Med 1982; 307(10):605–614.
30. Wells IP, Dubbins PA, Whimster WF: Pulmonary disease caused by the inhalation of cosmetic talcum powder. Br J Radiol 1979; 52:586–588.
31. Moffenson HC, Greensher J, DiTomasso A, et al: Baby Powder–A Hazard! Pediatrics 1981; 68(2):265–266.
32. Rinaldo JE, Owens GR, Rogers RM: Adult respiratory distress syndrome following intrapleural instillation of talc. J Thorac Cardiovasc Surg 1983; 85:523–526.
33. Wegmen DH, Peters JM, Boundy MG, et al: Evaluation of respiratory effects in miners and millers exposed to talc free of asbestos of silica. Br J Ind Med 1982; 39:233–238.
34. Farber H, Fairman RP, Glauser FL: Talc granulomatosis: Laboratory findings similar to sarcoidosis. Am Rev Respir Dis 1982; 125:258–261.
35. Crouch E, Churg A: Progressive massive fibrosis of the lung secondary to intravenous injection of talc. A

pathologic and mineralogic analysis. Am J Clin Pathol 1983, pp 520–526.

36. Pare JAP, Fraser RG, Hogg JC, et al: Pulmonary "mainline" granulomatosis: Talcosis of intravenous methadone abuse. Medicine 1979; 58(3):229–239.

37. Sieniewitz DJ, Nidecker AC: Conglomerate pulmonary disease: A form of talcosis in intravenous methadone abusers. Am J Roentgenol 1980; 135:697–702.

38. Abraham JL, Brambilla C: Particle size for differentiation between inhalation and injection pulmonary talcosis. Environ Res 1980; 21:94–96.

39. Lapenas DJ, Gale PN, Kennedy R, et al: Kaolin pneumoconiosis–Radiologic, pathologic, and mineralogic findings. Am Rev Respir Dis 1984; 130: 282–288.

40. Lapenas DJ, Gale PN: Kaolin pneumoconiosis–A case report. Arch Pathol Lab Med 1983; 107:650–653.

41. Sheers G: Prevalence of pneumoconiosis in Cornish kaolin workers. Br J Ind Med 1964; 21:218–225.

42. Edenfield RW: A clinical and roentgenological study of kaolin workers. Arch Environ Health 1960; 5:392–403.

43. Lesser M, Zia M, Kilburn KH: Silicosis in kaolin workers and firebrick makers. South Med J 1978; 71(10):1242–1246.

44. Herman SJ, Olscamp GC, Weisbrod GL: Pulmonary kaolin granulomas. J Can Assoc Radiol 1982; 33: 279–280.

45. Davies D, Cotton R: Mica pneumoconiosis. Br J Ind Med 1983; 40:22–27.

46. Pimentel JC, Menezes AP: Pulmonary and hepatic granulomatous disorders due to the inhalation of cement and mica dusts. Thorax 1978; 33:219–227.

47. Lilis R: Fibrous zeolites and endemic mesothelioma in Cappadocia, Turkey. J Occup Med 1981; 23(8): 548–550.

48. Stanton MF, Layard M, Tegeris A, et al: Carcinogenicity of fibrous glass. J Natl Cancer Inst 1977; 58:587–603.

49. Huuskonnen MS, Tossavainen A, Koskinen H, et al: Wollastonite exposure and lung fibrosis. Environ Res 1983; 30:291–304.

50. Hurlbut CS: Dana's Manual of Mineralogy, ed 17. New York, John Wiley & Sons, 1961.

51. Mayer R: The Artist's Handbook of Materials and Techniques. New York, Viking Press, 1943.

8

Beryllium-Induced Disease

Howard Naidech, Robert M. Steiner, Jan Lieber, and Stephanie Flicker

Reaction of the lung to inhalation of dust depends on several factors, including the chemical nature of the dust, the size and concentration of the dust particles, the duration of exposure, and individual susceptibility. These factors are important in themselves and in combination, as they may be interdependent.[1]

Inhalation of beryllium—a rare element discovered by Vanquelin in 1791[2]—or its compounds is the cause of an important but less common pneumoconiosis. There are approximately 50 different minerals containing beryllium, and beryl, a beryllium aluminium silicate, is commercially the most important.

Uses of Beryllium

Because of its resilience, the most widespread industrial use of beryllium is as a copper alloy for springs and diaphragms. Since it does not spark, beryllium-copper alloys are useful for tools used by the oil industry. In addition, most x-ray tube windows contain beryllium, which readily transmits x-rays, and has a high melting point (1,285°C). It has been used in the aerospace industry as a rocket fuel and in manufactured parts for missile guidance and nose cones. The fluorescent phosphor, zinc beryllium manganese silicate was prepared by firing the individual metallic oxides of beryllium with silica. The solubility of the beryllium silicate decreases with increasing manganese content, leading to the potential for free beryllium inhalation.[3] Fluorescent lamp manufacturing plants in Massachusetts had a large number of cases of occupational beryllium disease. These employees were exposed to phosphors containing up to 12% beryllium oxide until 1942, when the American War Production Board controlled the use of beryllium, effectively reducing the oxide content of the phosphor to approximately 2%.[4]

Historical Perspective of Beryllium Disease

From 1945 to 1950, beryllium disease appeared in epidemic proportions in the United States, and illness appeared in workers in the fluorescent lamp and the neon sign industries, as well as in alloy production, and in laboratories using beryllium in the development of x-ray tubes and atomic energy.

It was first believed that only acute forms of beryllium disease occurred among workers, but by the end of 1947 it was clear that chronic cases also occurred, but were not previously recognized. By 1948 at least five cases of chronic disease in former plant workers and eight cases in nearby residents with no known occupational exposure had been identified in the United States.

Acute Beryllium Disease

Poisoning with beryllium may occur either in an acute or chronic form, the latter being the more common.[1] The acute syndrome occurs when workers are exposed to beryllium dust while working in refineries. The clinical presentation may be fulminating or insidious. In either case, the pathologic stages are nonspecific and are similar to those seen with chemical pneumonitis.

The disease affects the nasopharynx, tracheobronchial tree, and pulmonary parenchyma causing rhinitis, tracheitis, bronchitis, and pneumonitis. Clinical and epidemiological evidence suggests that the cause of severe chemical pneumonitis is usually a massive although brief exposure to beryllium compounds. Sulfate, fluoride, and chloride salts are particularly toxic. Fever is usually absent unless secondary infection occurs.

The fulminating variety of acute beryllium disease is characterized by the clinical manifestations of acute pulmonary edema and may be rapidly fatal.[5] Pathologically, proteinaceous edema of the lungs is present without associated interstitial fibrosis. Radiological findings include bilateral diffuse air-space disease that varies with the severity of the inhalation process. Asymmetrical alveolar infiltrates and discrete bilateral large or small nodules may appear on the chest radiograph.[6]

The insidious or gradual development of acute berylliosis can produce a clinical syndrome occurring weeks after the initial exposure. Clincally, there is initially dry cough, substernal pain, shortness of breath with exertion, anorexia, weakness, and weight loss. Hyaline membranes in the alveoli and an organized pneumonitis similar to that seen in viral or uremic pneumonitis may occur. Rales and rhonchi suggesting asthma may be present.

Radiology

Chest radiographs are usually normal initially, but within 1 to 4 weeks symmetrical bilateral diffuse pulmonary parenchymal infiltrates are seen. The air-space pattern may be lobar or segmental and may or may not be accompanied by peribronchial thickening. This acute process is a form of chemical pneumonitis and will progress either to complete recovery or to death, depending on the severity of the disease.[7] Those who survive show complete resolution of the infiltrates and the subsequent appearance of discrete large or small conglomerate nodules scattered throughout both lungs, or there will be complete clearance within 1 to 4 months. Such individuals do not usually have any sequelae. Those few cases that have been available for pathological study have shown alveolar septal widening due to edema with distortion of the alveolar spaces.[7,8] Foamy desquamated cells and proteinaceous fluid are found within the interalveolar septa. Granulomas and inclusions are absent (Fig. 8.6).

Chronic Beryllium Disease

Chronic beryllium disease is more common than the acute syndrome. Most patients with chronic beryllium disease have a history of exposure to beryllium oxides, salts, or alloys of two or more years' duration. Although some patients may remain asymptomatic, in most case a clinical syndrome develops gradually, following a symptom-free interval of up to 15 years after the last exposure to dust.[1] Symptoms include fatigue, weight loss, shortness of breath on exertion, a migratory arthralgia, and cough. The liver and spleen may be palpable, and in up to 10% of the patients renal calculi develop.[1] With progression, cyanosis and clubbing of the fingers and toes occur, and later, possibly cor pulmonale. Hypergammaglobulinemia and polycythemia have been reported. The diagnosis of chronic beryllium disease is suspected from a history of exposure to dust and a chest roentgenogram showing diffuse infiltrative disease.[9]

Radiology

Radiographs obtained following chronic exposure show evidence of granulomatous formation in the lungs (Fig. 8.1 to 8.6). Radiologic changes may precede the development of the clinical syndrome by several years. Reticular, nodular, fine or coarse densities, and air-space infiltrates are present on radiographs (Fig. 8.1), and the majority of patients show evidence of hilar adenopathy, which may be bilateral and accompanied by paratracheal and ductal adenopathy (Fig. 8.1). The presence of adenopathy suggests a differential diagnosis of sarcoidosis, tuberculosis, and silicosis. Lung volumes may be small, and extensive honeycombing and bullous formation may be seen. Ten percent of the patients developed pneumothorax. Pneumothorax may develop due to rupture of blebs and is often

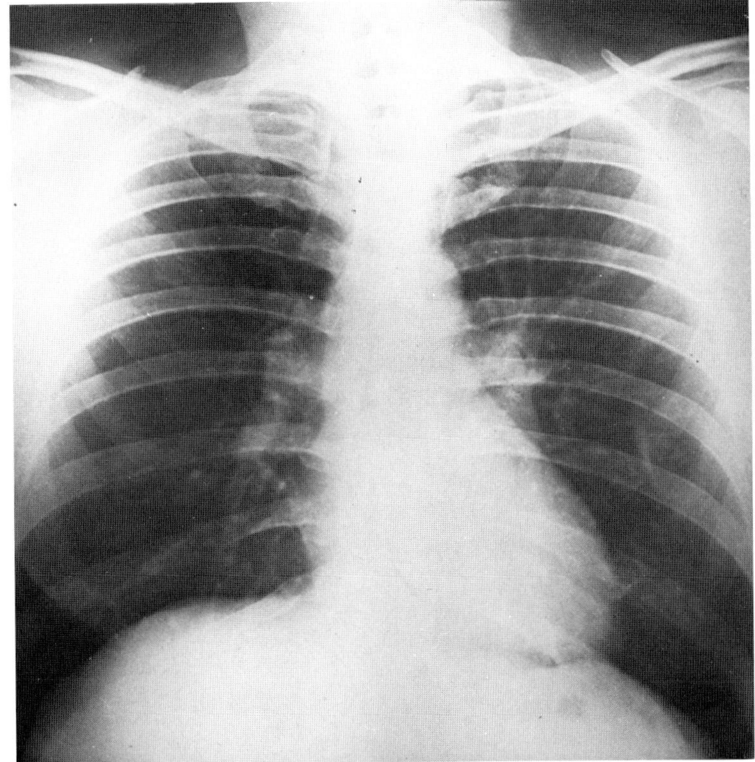

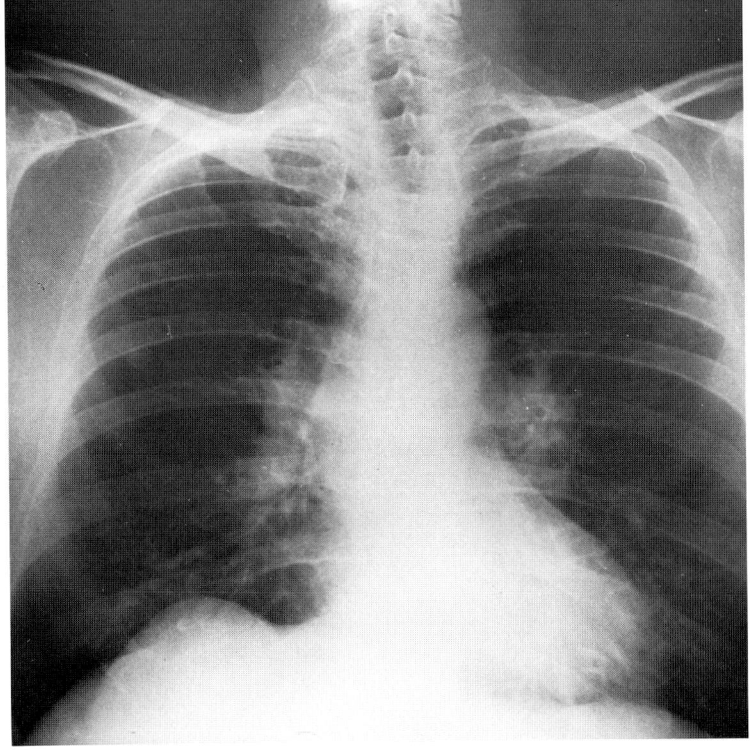

Figure 8.1. Chronic beryllium disease. **A**. A 32-year-old new worker in a beryllium plant with a normal chest radiograph. **B**. Sixteen years later films show diffuse interstitial changes and bilateral hilar adenopathy. Biopsy showed interstitial granulomatosis compatible with chronic beryllium disease.

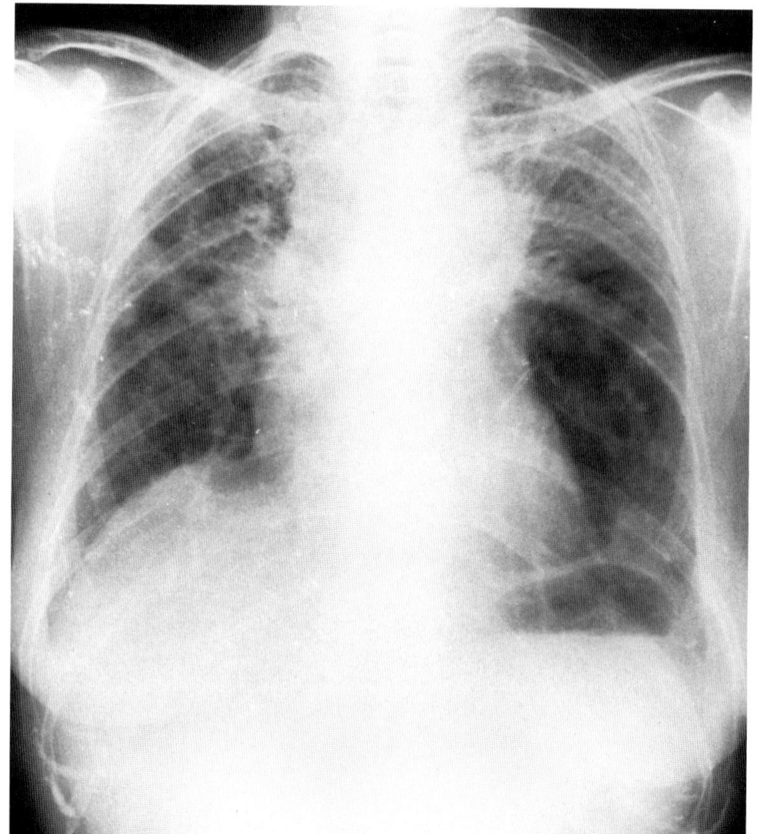
A

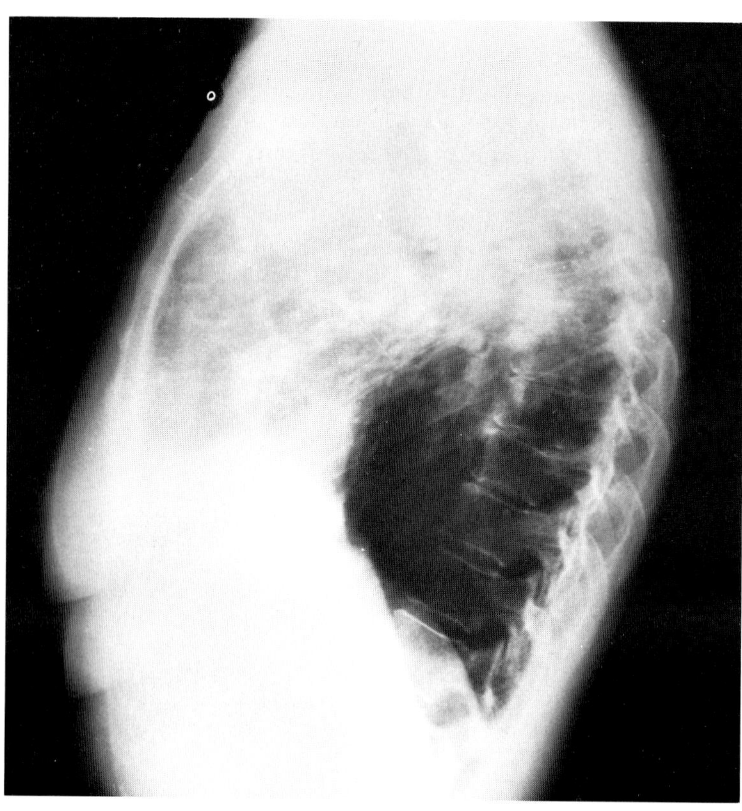
B

Figure 8.2. Chronic beryllium disease. Postero-anterior (**A**) and lateral (**B**) films of the chest in a 59-year-old female beryllium worker showing marked bilateral interstitial fibrosis and obstructive emphysema in both lower lobes.

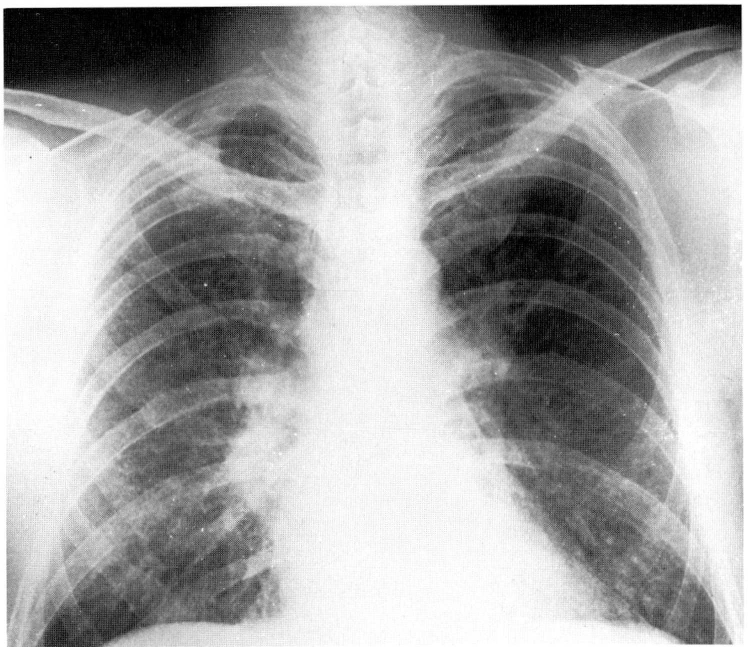

Figure 8.3. Man aged 42 years. Radiograph 20 years after initial employment. On lung function test there was normal lung volume, but marked decreased diffusion capacity. The film shows diffuse pulmonary interstitial fibrosis and hilar adenopathy compatible with the diagnosis of chronic beryllium disease.

difficult to manage. Right-sided heart enlargement and pulmonary hypertension occur late in the disease (Fig. 8.4).

Pathology

The chronic form of berylliosis demonstrates typical histopathological characteristics.[8] These include the presence of focal calcifications in the lungs, often described as shell-like bodies, in 64% of patients.[8] Calcospherites or Schaumann bodies also described in sarcoidosis have been reported.[10] Calcifications varying from small scattered inclusions to large and complex bodies may be widely scattered about the lungs and hilar nodes. The presence of large numbers of calcific bodies is a useful diagnostic feature in the recognition of chronic beryllium disease. In 20% of the patients asteroid bodies occur within giant cells.[8] These are spiculated inclusions associated with vacuoles. They occur in sarcoidosis and foreign-body granuloma in addition to beryllium disease. Partially or completely hyalinized sharply marginated nodules are found in 40% of the cases.[8] These nodules are inactive, and they may calcify or be accompanied by granuloma. Interstitial fibrosis is present in most chronic cases and varies considerably in degree in different portions of the lung or even in a single lobe. With increasing severity and time, bronchiectasis and emphysema may develop. In those patients who develope pulmonary hypertension, peripheral venous thrombosis and embolism are likely to occur. Episodes of embolism will further compromise the pulmonary arterial vascular bed, increasing pulmonary arterial pressure. Cor pulmonale superimposed on severe respiratory insufficiency is the usual cause of death in these patients.[8]

Laboratory Diagnosis

Early spectrographic methods of tissue analysis for beryllium have been replaced by chemical methods sensitive enough to detect 0.002 μg of beryllium per sample. Unfortunately, such methods cannot differentiate beryllium compounds from the inert beryllium silicate that is present in some fuels and dusts and that may be found in lungs and hilar lymph nodes. The finding of beryllium in autopsy or biopsy specimens of the lungs or its excretion in

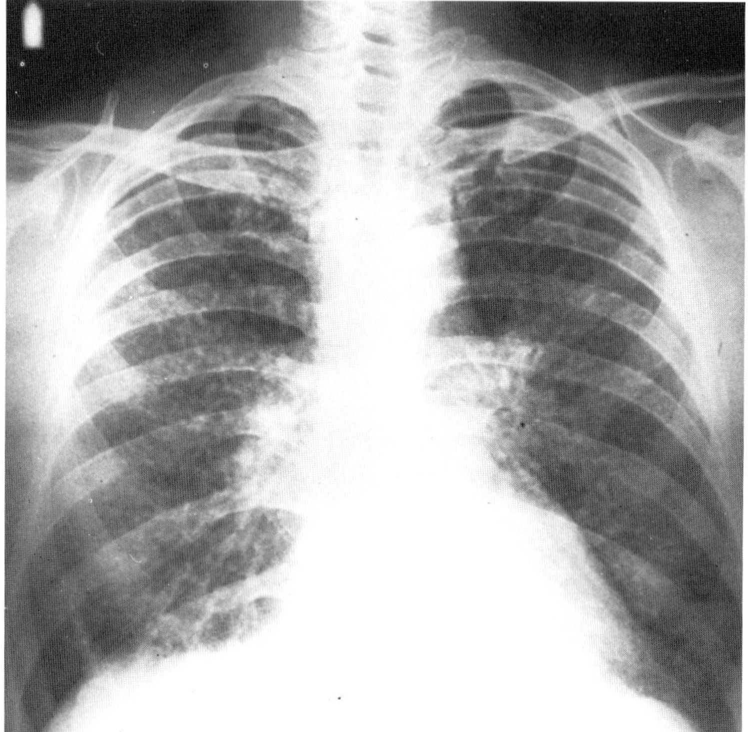

Figure 8.4. A 44-year-old man with a 5-year history as a beryllium plant employee. There has been moderate dyspnea for the last 5 years. Chest films show moderate diffuse reticular nodule disease and hilar adenopathy.

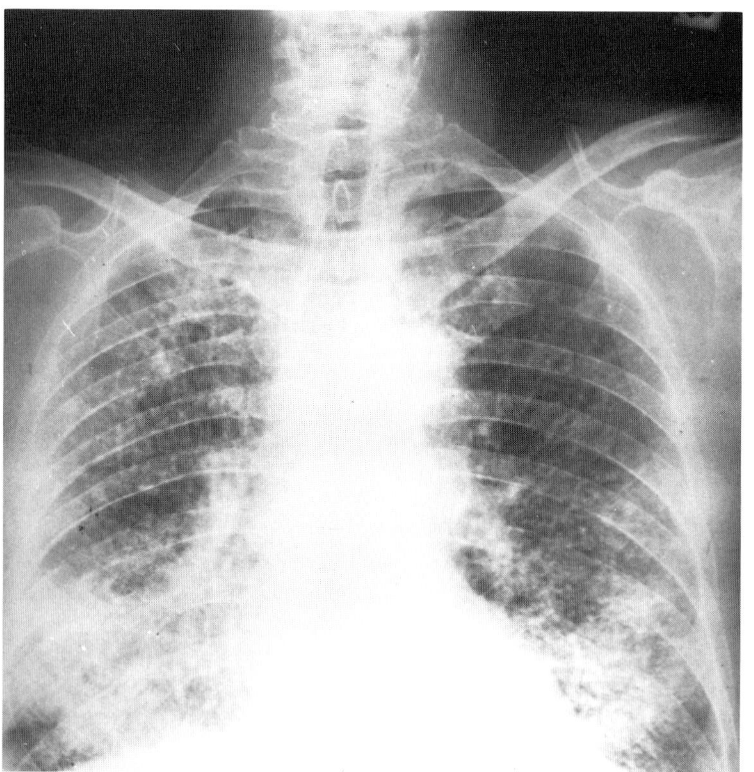

Figure 8.5. A 67-year-old man initially had acute pneumonitis after handling drums of beryllium-aluminium alloy. Films 4 years after the acute event show diffuse nodular disease with coalescence at the right base. An infiltrate in the right upper lobe represents superimposed infection in this patient with chronic beryllium disease.

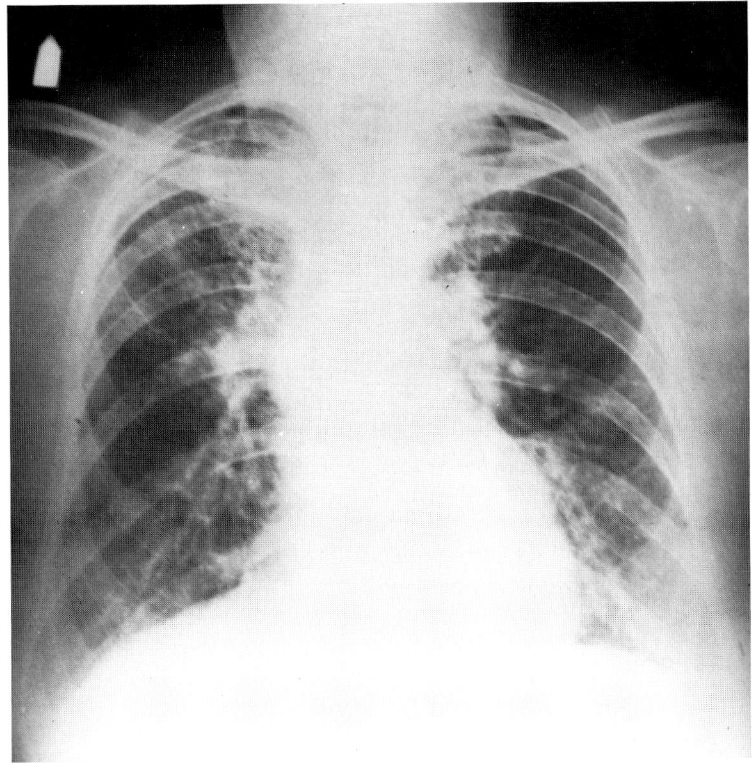

Figure 8.6. A 47-year-old woman with shortness of breath and weight loss. Bilateral diffuse interstitial disease compatible with chronic granulomatous disease due to chronic beryllium exposure is seen on the chest radiograph.

the urine is merely evidence of exposure and does not produce illness in the majority of beryllium workers. The amounts of beryllium measured in various parts of the lung may differ as much as tenfold and on occasion may even be reported as negative. On the other hand, a negative report of a single beryllium assay should not be used to rule out beryllium disease, nor should a positive or high beryllium assay without clinical findings be used as the sole criterion for the diagnosis of the disease.[10] Latterly, a technique for harvesting bronchoalveolar lymphocytes and inducing lymphocyte proliferation to in vitro beryllium exposure has shown a specificity and sensitivity approaching 100%.[9]

Carcinogenicity

The question of whether beryllium is a carcinogen has not been satisfactorily resolved. Lung cancer was recorded in rats and monkeys following experimental introduction of beryllium salts, usually beryllium sulfate or oxide. The introduction of some beryllium compounds intravenously or directly into the bone produced osteogenic sarcoma in rats and mice.

Epidemiological evidence suggests that beryllium may be a human carcinogen, but the studies produced up to this time have been challenged because of unsatisfactory sample size and insufficient controls.[11]

The commonly used term berylliosis is misleading because it not only implies that beryl, a naturally occurring silicated beryllium, is harmful but it also suggests that beryllium toxicity is a dust disease, similar to other forms of pneumoconiosis. Although pulmonary involvement dominates the clinical picture, it has been clearly established that a number of other organs and biochemical systems are affected. In the absence of satisfactory treatment, control of the disease is directed toward the prevention of beryllium inhalation through engineering control and personal hygiene. Effective prevention has been measured by monitoring of cases through the Beryllium Registry.

Treatment

The role of steroids in modifying the clinical course in many patients is difficult to evaluate. Steroids were often given to workers who were likely to be exposed to heavy doses of beryllium. Some relationship has been found between the length and severity of the clinical course and the use of steroids, as many patients did show distinct clinical improvement following the use of steroids.[12,13] However, there was no clear relationship between the effect of steroids and the histological appearance of the lungs reported. In addition, there is no clear relationship between the histological pattern and the nature of industrial exposure or the length of the latency period following either the earliest initial exposure or the onset of clinical symptoms. Several chelating agents have been tried, but none were found successful.

References

1. Fraser RG, Pare JAP: Diagnosis of Disease of the Chest. ed 2. Philadelphia, WB Saunders Co, 1979.
2. Hardy HL, Tabersham IR: Delayed chemical pneumonitis occurring in workers exposed to beryllium compounds. J Ind Hyg Toxicol 1946; 28:197–211.
3. Fonda GR: The constitution of zinc beryllium silicate phosphors. J Phys Chem 1941; 45:282–288.
4. Morse GE: In Vowald AJ (ed): Pneumoconiosis. New York, Harper Bros, 1950, pp. 147–149.
5. De Nardi JM, Van Ordstrand HS, Curtis GH: Berylliosis, summary and survey of all clinical types in a ten year period. Cleve Clin Q 1952; 19:171–193.
6. Van Ordstrand HS, Hughes R, Carmody MG: Chemical pneumonia in workers extracting beryllium oxide. Report of three cases. Cleve Clin Q 1943; 10:10–18.
7. Van Ordstrand HS, Hughes, R, De Nardi JM et al: Beryllium poisoning. JAMA 1945; 129:1084–1090.
8. Frieman DG, Hardy HL: Beryllium disease. The relation of pulmonary pathology to clinical course and prognosis based on a study of 130 cases from the U.S. Beryllium Case Registry. Human Pathol 1970; 1:25–44.
9. Aronchik JM, Rossman MD, Miller WT: Chronic beryllium disease: diagnosis, radiographic findings, and correlation with pulmonary function tests. Radiology 1987; 163:677–682.
10. Lieben J, Dattoli JA: Quantitative beryllilum studies in postmortem lungs. Arch Environ Health 1963; 7:183–187.
11. Disher DP: Letter to WH Foege. Printed in Speaking Out, a Cabuto Berylco commercial publication, 1981.
12. Fabroni SM: Pathologia pulmonare da polveri di berillio. Med Lav 1935; 26:297–312.
13. Eisenbud M, Wanta RC, Dustan C, et al: Non-occupational berylliosis. J Ind Hyg Toxicol 1949; 31:282–294.

9

Occupational Diseases Due to Organic and Metallic Inhalants

C. Molina and D. Caillaud

Pulmonary disease due to organic and metallic inhalants is rare, producing a variety of tissue responses. These responses range from benign pulmonary reaction with simple pulmonary pigmentation and minimal stroma to pulmonary fibrosis with macrophages or pulmonary lesions due to immune mechanisms, leading to granulomas or fibrosis. Toxic reactions causing pulmonary edema also occur.

All these respiratory diseases have very similar radiographic patterns, precluding a precise etiological diagnosis from the film appearances. Therefore the essential information as to the patient's occupation and duration of exposure to organic or metallic inhalants must be elicited as well as a thorough clinical history, particularly whether the onset of the disease was insidious or rapid, and its temporal relationship to the individual's work.

Other diagnostic tests, including those of lung function, immunological studies such as skin tests and total and specific IgE, bronchoalveolar lavage with mineral analysis of the fluid and lung biopsy (especially for metals and microorganisms) are also essential.

Part 1: Pulmonary Disease Due to Organic Inhalants

Organic dusts from animals, vegetables, microbial, or chemical sources can act as antigens to trigger an immune response. Whereas large particles (5 to 50 μm) do not usually pass beyond the level of the upper airways or bronchi – more often causing rhinitis or asthma, especially in atopic persons – small particles of organic dusts reach the alveoli, resulting in extrinsic allergic alveolitis (EAA) or hypersensitivity pneumonitis (HP) characterized by inflammation of the peripheral gas-exchanging terminal bronchioles.

A great number of agents have been identified in occupational environments as producing similar pathological changes and immunological reactions. The first and most important of these diseases to be recognized was farmer's lung[1,2] due to inhalation of the dust of moldy hay. Many other dusts can induce similar reactions either in rural or industrial occupations.

All these diseases may be recognized by a combination of their clinical, radiographic, functional, pathological, and immunological findings. *Clinical features* include diffuse pneumonitis with dyspnea, fever, loss of weight, and rales or crackles on auscultation. Some of these symptoms and signs often occur acutely, four to six hours after contact with the causal dust. The radiographic signs of diffuse bilateral pulmonary infiltration occur with a micronodular or nodular pattern. Functional tests show a restrictive ventilatory pattern with impairment of alveolar capillary gas-exchange and early decrease of compliance, sometimes with evidence of small airway disease.[3] Pathological changes characteristically affect the distal structures of the lung, at first exudative and inflammatory with lymphocytes predominating, followed by an alveolar and interstitial pseudotuberculoid type of granulomatosis. Immune reactions, including precipitins to organic dusts mediating Arthus-type hypersensitivity states (type III) and evidence of delayed-type (IV) reactions, are well documented by cellular immunological tests and bronchoalveolar lavage.[4]

During the 1970s there were many reports on the etiology, clinical features, and pathogenesis of the most frequent EAA due to occupational factors. A whole group of similar conditions were observed in industrial and urban areas. Many of these diseases identified throughout the world depend on climatic and geographical factors, various exotic habits, or traditional occupations such as sericulture in Japan and coffee workers in South America.

Allergen Sources and Causal Agents

In most cases the clinical features of EAA have been identified in association with a particular crude inhalant, for example, dusts of moldy hay, bird droppings, and rat urine. In certain instances a specific agent, proven immunologically or by challenge tests, has been isolated. Three main types of causal agents have been described: thermophilic actinomycetes, animal serum proteins, and fungi.

Thermophilic actinomycetes are found in moldy hay, in bagasse extracts, and in air-conditioning systems. An agricultural worker, handling moldy hay, can inhale up to 750,000 spores per minute.

Proteins have been isolated as the active antigens in bird droppings, namely, serum immunoglobulins (IgA) as the species-specific antigen of pigeons.[5] The proteolytic enzymes obtained from *Bacillus subtilis*, known to be made of 76 amino acids, are also antigenic, found in the detergent industry and in air-conditioning filters. There can be as many as 3 million spores in 1 g of detergent powder.

Fungi, particularly the *Aspergillus* and *Penicillium* species, are the most common molds found in damp interiors. Agricultural workers may develop allergic bronchopulmonary aspergillosis associated with *Aspergillus fumigatus*; typical alveolitis occurs in malthouse workers exposed to the inhalation of spores of *Aspergillus clavatus*, and respiratory disorders are found in cheese workers who use a blue powder rich in *Penicillium casei*. Other species may proliferate in air-conditioning systems and in cork factories.

Miscellaneous allergens including vegetable particles, such as wood dust, flour, coffee, and sisal, may be responsible for cases of alveolitis. Mites (*Acarus siro*, *Tyrophagus casei*) were discovered on the rind of certain cheeses in local dairies and are the cause of respiratory problems among cheese washers. Parasites may provoke alveolitis in bakers and grain workers. Last but not least, aerosols (*isocyanates*, *fumes*) may induce hypersensitivity reactions involving alveoli and the interstitium.

Farmer's Lung

Etiology

There is a marked seasonal variation of the disease and a very variable incidence in different regions. The largest number of cases occurs in autumn and winter when the preceding summer has been rainy. Cold and humid regions are particularly affected. The disease is seen in mountainous or semimountainous regions of northern Europe such as Finland, Wales, and Scotland, in the Massif Central in France, The Great Lakes in the United States, and Quebec. In poorly equipped farms the workers are often exposed by threshing and collecting moldy hay to feed animals, but "farmer's lung" also occurs in modern farms with automatic agricultural machinery, the hay being stored in enormous silos. Moldy hay is the most important causal agent, but all moldy vegetable dusts may be responsible. The disease has also been observed among grain-elevator operators and workers in the wooden-ship industry.

Radiographic Signs

Recent and Acute Forms. A normal radiograph, especially one taken some time after an acute attack, does not exclude the diagnosis as radiologic manifestations may be delayed.

In a recent attack or if progressive, as in 66% of our cases, miliary or reticular/micronodular changes are encountered most frequently (Figs. 9.1, 9.2). These changes consist of very fine micronodulations evenly distributed through both lungs, sometimes almost at the limit of visibility. Less penetrated films or direct enlargements may be necessary for their demonstration (Figs. 9.3, 9.4). At times, there is an alveolar pattern producing nodules with indefinite margins, often confluent at the apices of the lung, but occasionally also

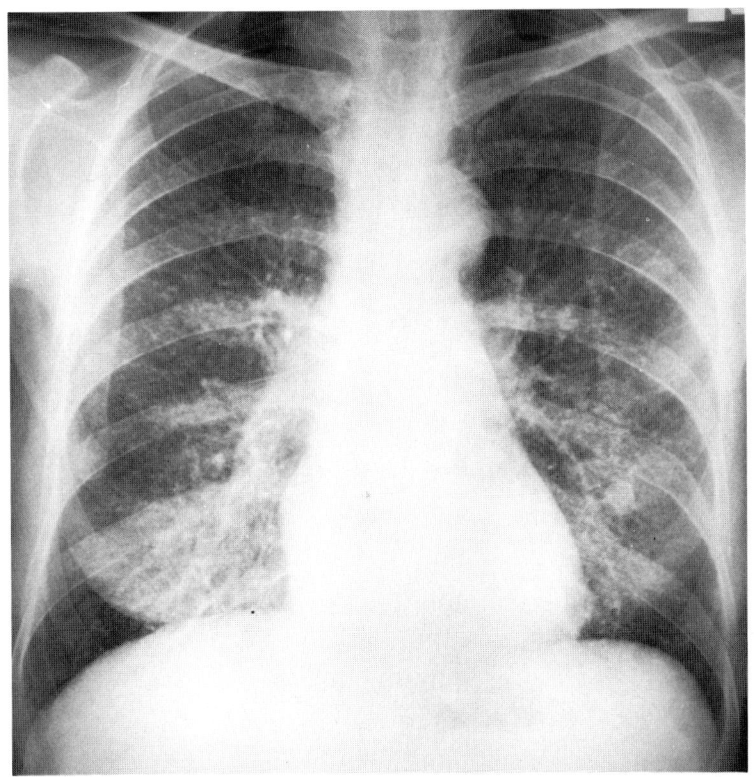

Figure 9.1. Farmer's lung: a reticular form.

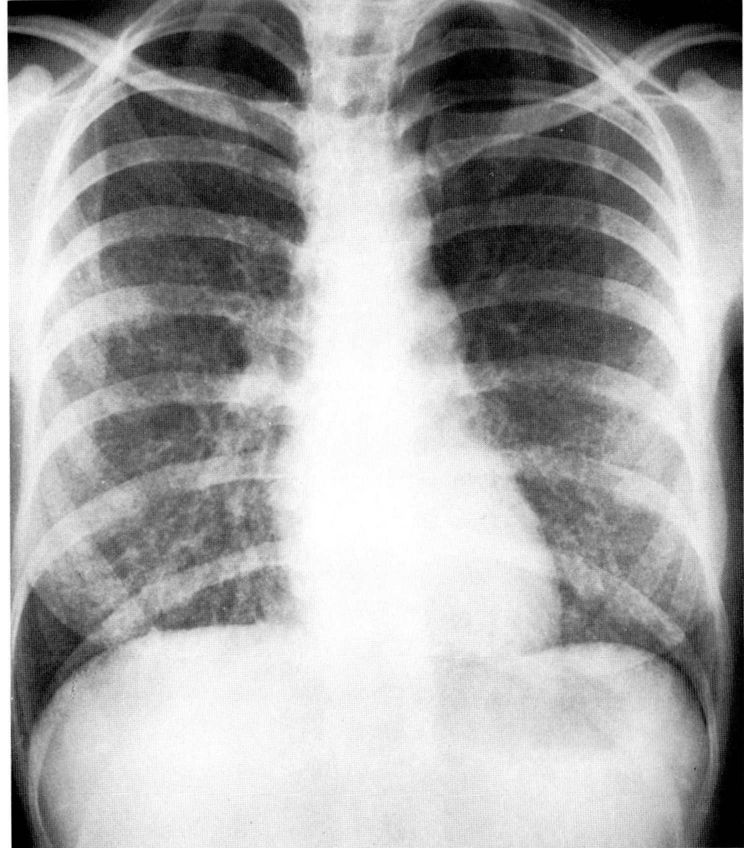

Figure 9.2. Farmer's lung: very fine micronodulation.

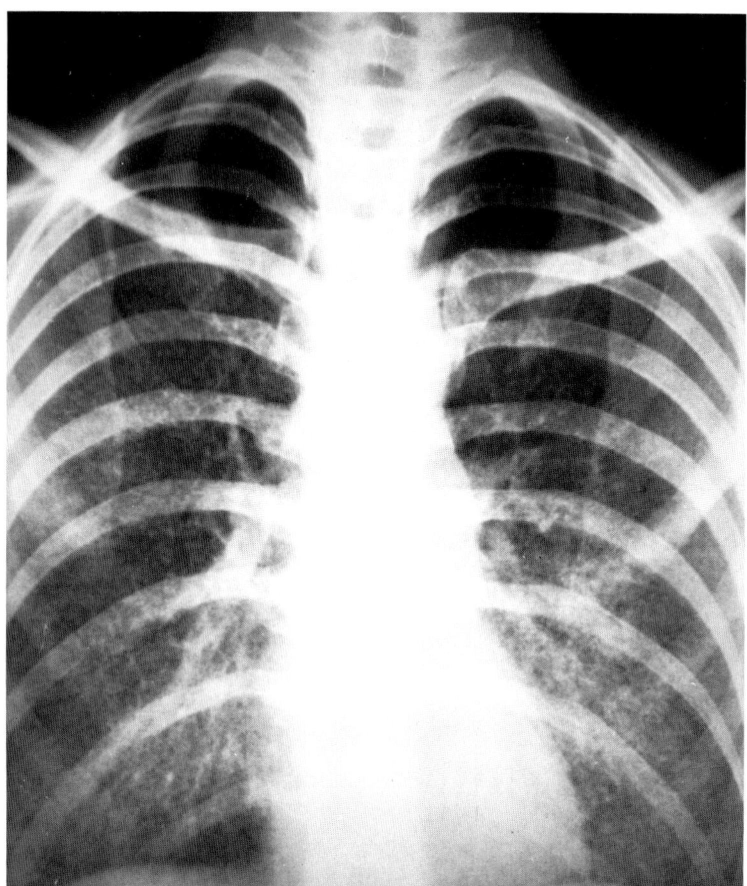

Figure 9.3. Farmer's lung: an enlarged radiograph to demonstrate the fine micronodular changes that are present.

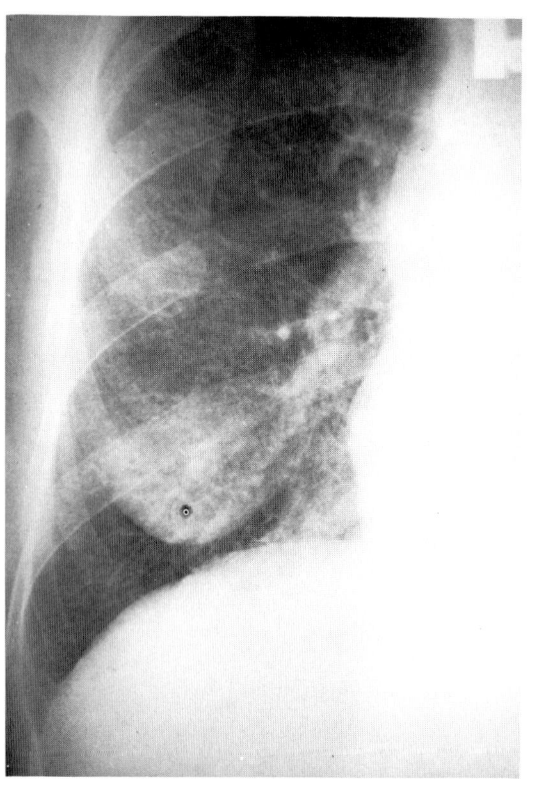

Figure 9.4. Farmer's lung: a magnified right chest radiograph to show profuse micronodules throughout the lung field.

at the bases, having a ground-glass appearance (Fig. 9.5).

In very acute forms the picture may be that of pulmonary edema or adult respiratory distress syndrome, with extensive infiltration of both lungs (Fig. 9.6), but occasional cases with predominantly unilateral changes have also been described (Fig. 9.7).

These changes usually disappear in two to three weeks but rarely are complicated by pneumothorax or pericarditis.

Three important negative features should be stressed in these cases: the absence of hilar adenopathy, the absence of pleural changes (an extremely important differential sign), and the absence of cavities.

Computed tomography (CT) performed in several cases of allergic alveolitis[6,7] showed interstitial densities very different from nodular densities observed in other interstitial diseases such as silicosis, sarcoidosis, or lymphangitic malignancy. Moreover, these interstitial densities have a marked *central distribution*[3] (Fig. 9.8) in allergic alveolitis, seen both on plain films and CT scans, whereas in fibrosing alveolitis and rheumatoid lung disease these densities showed a striking *peripheral* predominance.

McLoud et al[8] suggest the use of a modified International Labour Office (ILO) classification for a description of these infiltrative and diffuse lung diseases. According to this classification, allergic alveolitis belongs to the group of *reticulonodular* opacities (x,y,z) (which are predominant lesions in 57% of their cases) like other granulomatous diseases (sarcoidosis, 40%); whereas in silicosis small round opacities (p,q,r) predominate, and in asbestosis the small irregular linear opacities (s,t,u) are more frequent.

Chronic Forms. In the chronic forms of farmer's lung, the films show diffuse interstitial fibrosis with retraction of a hemithorax, a high diaphragm, or a reticulonodular pattern (Fig. 9.9), and sometimes microcystic changes producing a honeycomb pattern (Fig. 9.10) indistinguishable from that of the late stages of fibrosing alveolitis.

In late cases the picture is less clear. One can see evidence of emphysema with increased transradiancy at the bases, a paucity of pulmonary vessels (Fig. 9.11), and enlargement of the heart and pulmonary arteries indicating pulmonary hypertension.

Corticosteroids will not prevent irreversible pulmonary fibrosis if exposure to moldy dust continues (Fig. 9.12).

Farmer's lung has been regarded as an occupational disease in England since 1964, in France since 1973, and now in almost all European countries.

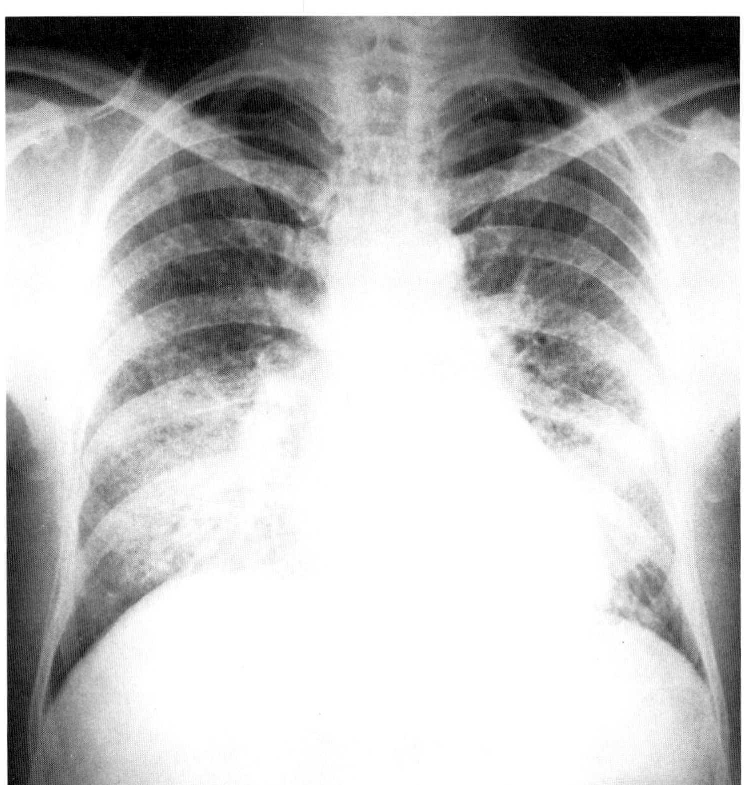

Figure 9.5. Diffuse infiltration producing a ground-glass appearance. The change was attributed to the patient's occupation, ie, "farmer's lung."

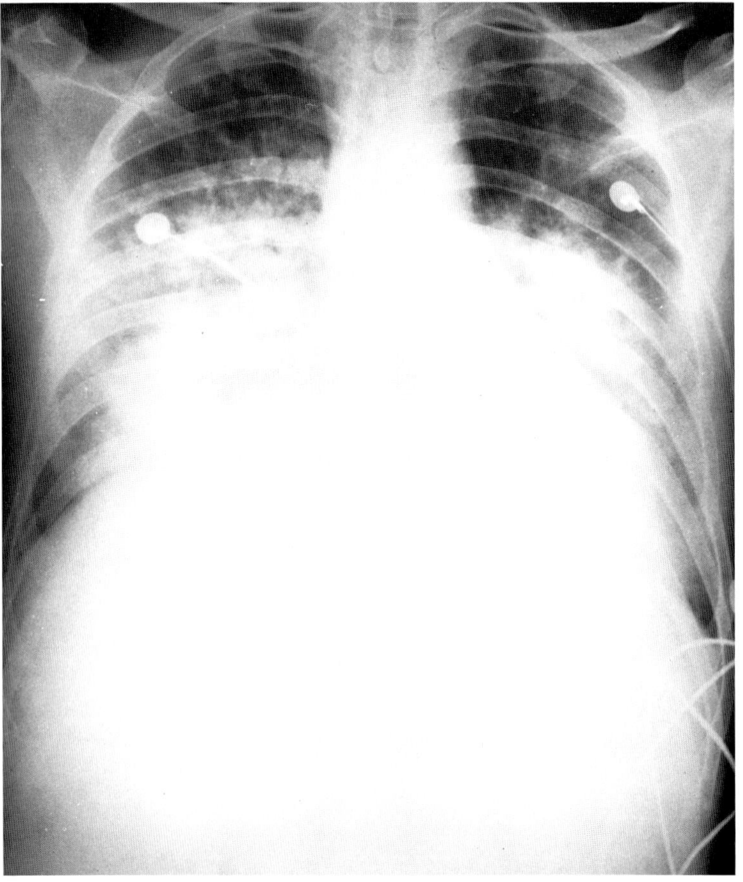

Figure 9.6. Demonstrating farmer's lung that presented with an acute respiratory distress syndrome. This is considered a less usual presentation.

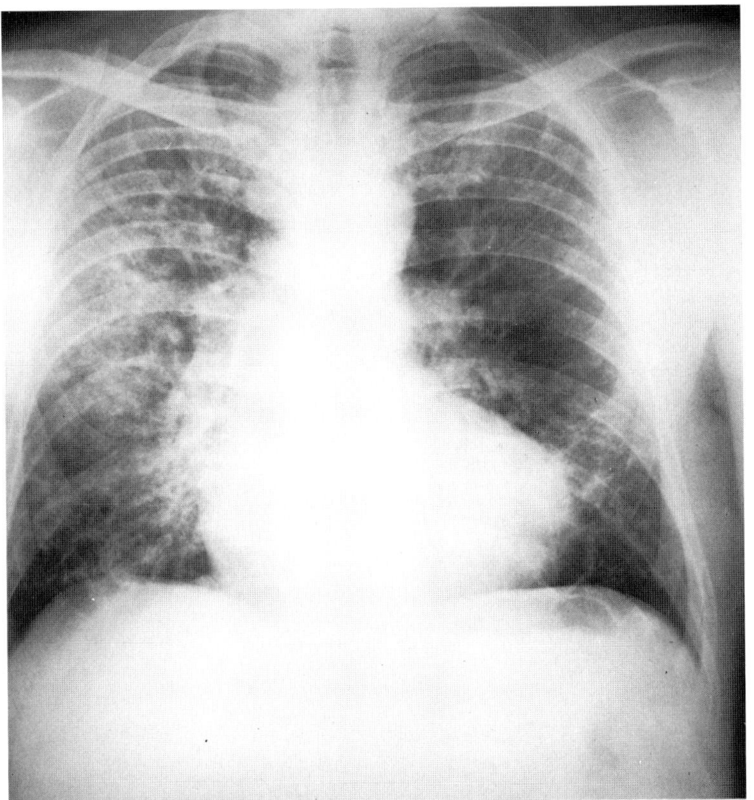

Figure 9.7. Farmer's lung: coarse infiltrations in both lungs, but more predominant on the right side.

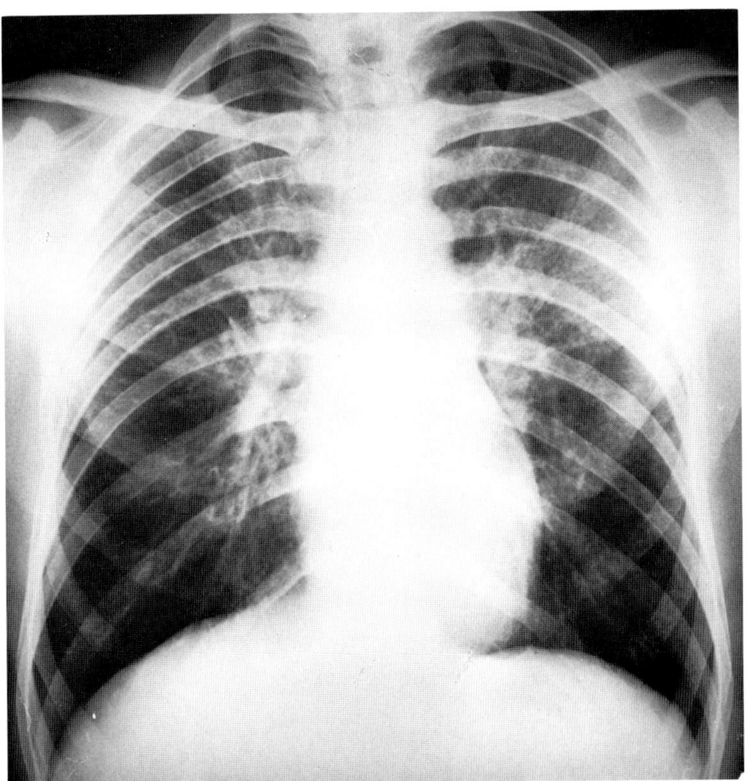

Figure 9.8. Farmer's lung demonstrating perihilar infiltrates.

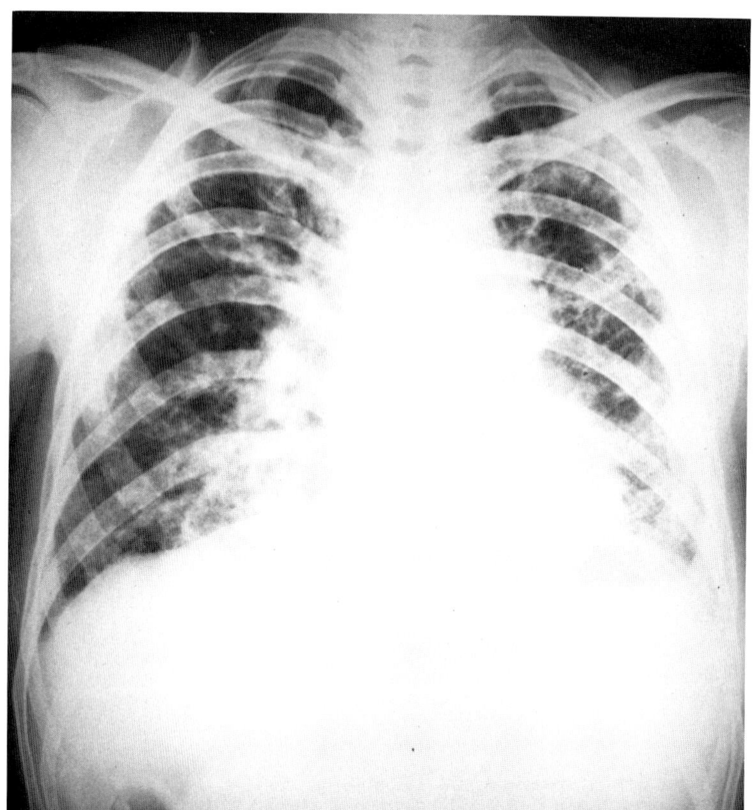

Figure 9.9. Chronic form of farmer's lung with well-established "fibrotic changes."

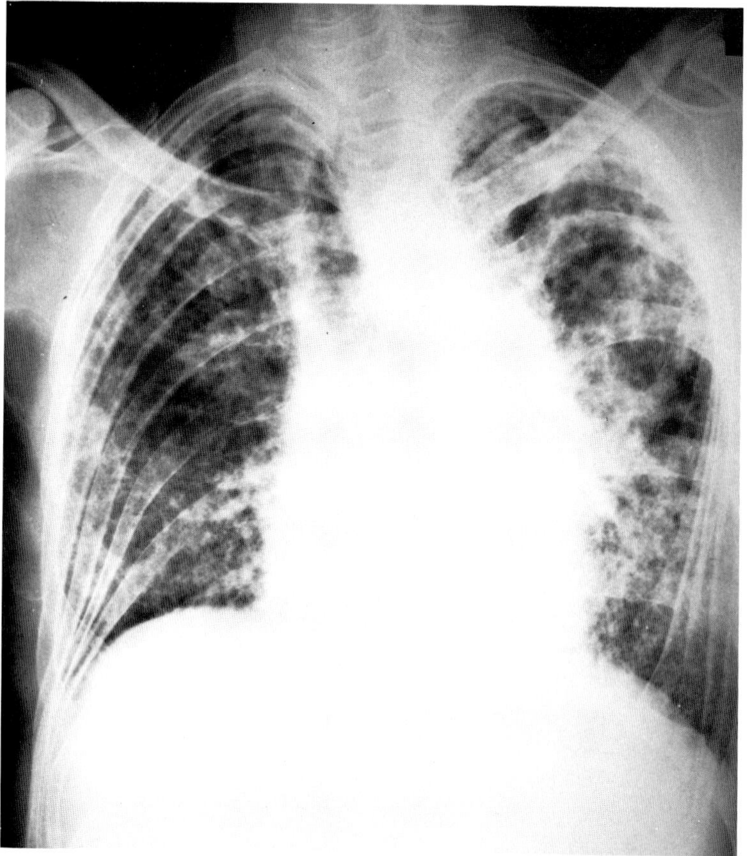

Figure 9.10. Farmer's lung: advanced infiltrative lung pathology giving rise to "honey-comb" lung.

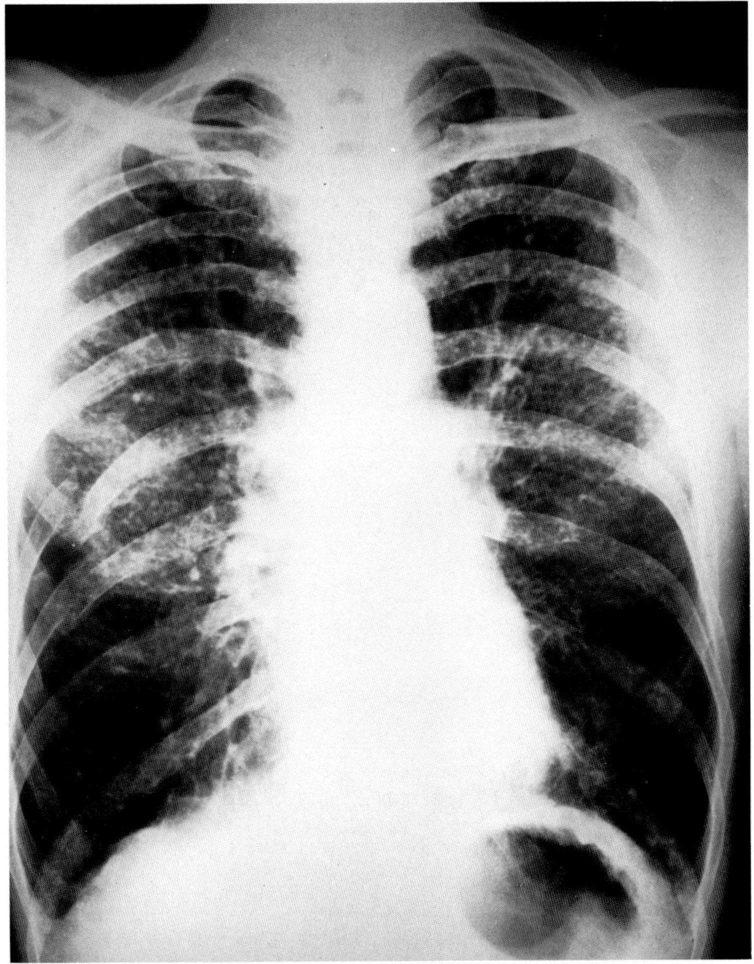

Figure 9.11. Farmer's lung: chronic form with diffuse nodular infiltration of the lungs and associated basal emphysema.

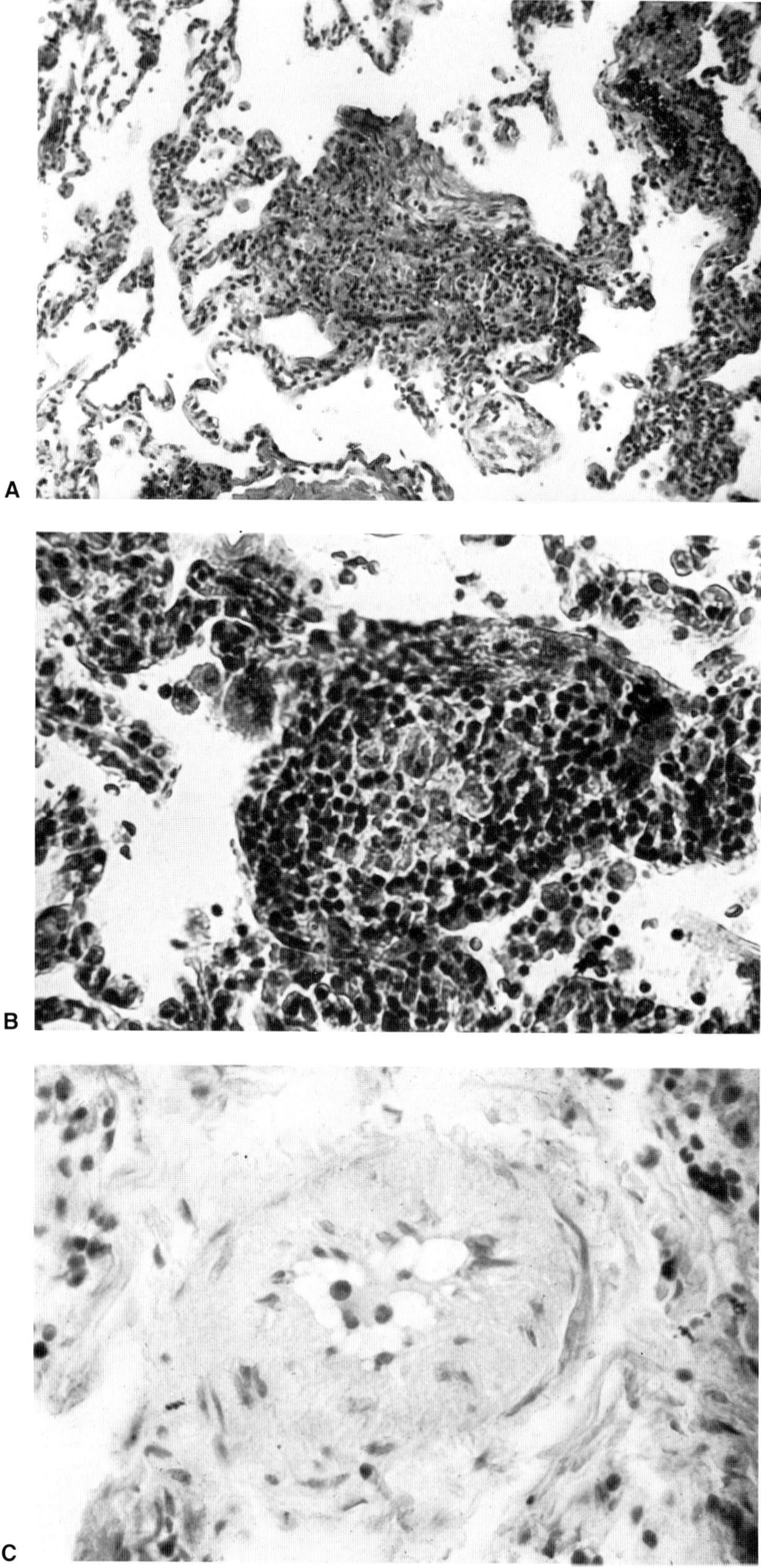
A
B
C

Bird Breeder's Disease

Bird breeder's disease (BBD) is another major form of EAA. The first case described in pigeon breeders was quite different from ornithosis and is considered to be a hypersensitive reaction to protein antigens contained in the droppings of pigeons. The budgerigar, a common household bird in the United Kingdom, was later implicated, and we reported the first French case in 1969.

Etiology

Although a large number of cases have been observed in pigeon fanciers and pigeon breeders, the disease is sometimes occupational, being found in all sorts of industrial and agricultural circumstances, and provoked by birds other than pigeons.[5] Unlike farmer's lung, BBD can be observed in all climates and at all latitudes, particularly where bird breeding is widespread, as in Belgium, England, France, and the United States. In many areas the disease occurs in poultry breeders and workers caring for birds and poultry, but even a single budgerigar or dove may provoke the disease. Although pigeons, doves, and parakeets are the main culprits, ducks, turkeys, pheasants, geese, and chicken can also induce the various forms of the disease.

The dust of bird droppings is essentially the cause and explains the frequency of the disease, but the feathers and the serum can also provide the antigens responsible for BBD (eg, pigeon IgA).

Symptoms and Radiographic Signs

The symptoms of BBD are similar to that of farmer's lung. Acute forms are more frequent with either rapid or insidious onset and with typical clinical, radiographic, and pulmonary signs and symptoms of alveolitis (Figs. 9.13 and 9.14). Chronic forms, with diffuse interstitial fibrosis, may be observed as occupational diseases, depending on the duration of the exposure. Our first patient was exposed to birds for 19 years and was thought initially to have tuberculosis, ornithosis, or sarcoidosis. Her condition was finally diagnosed as cryptogenic interstitial fibrosis (Fig. 9.15).

Mushroom Workers' Lung

The actinomycetes molds or parasites contained in mushroom compost are responsible for acute and chronic forms of alveolitis in the western regions of France. It is characterized by an early decrease of diffusing capacity of the lung for carbon monoxide (DLCO), the frequent presence of precipitins to the responsible antigen (*Actinobifida dichotomica*, *Aspergillus* species, or parasitic insects), a positive challenge test at the workplace, and lymphocytes in bronchoalveolar lavage. Measures of control are straightforward. The disease in France is regarded as an occupational illness.

Bagassosis

The fibrous residue of sugar cane is called bagasse. Previously used as a combustible material, bagasse is now treated industrially for the manufacture of paper, insulation panels, and explosives.

Radiographic changes are negligible during the reversible stages of the disease, but later there are signs of chronic bronchitis and emphysema, or pulmonary fibrosis.

Thermoactinomyces sacchari is the most frequent causal agent identified in bagasse extracts, and precipitins to these agents have been found in exposed workers.

◄ **Figure 9.12.A.** Interstitial granulomata with thickening of interalveolar walls. (Pulmonary biopsy: Farmer's lung.) **B.** Granulomatous nodule of a pseudotuberculoid type, centered around multinucleated macrophages (high magnification) explaining the micronodular radiographic images. **C.** Early changes of collagen and precollagen fibers with vascular alteration. (Biopsy: Farmer's lung.)

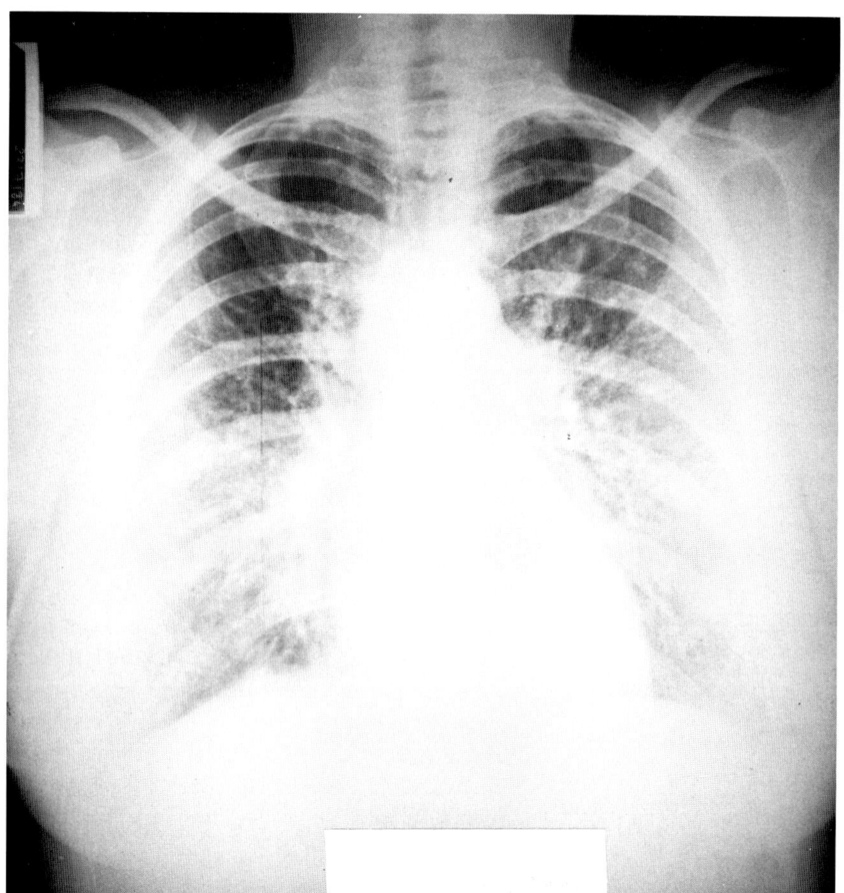

Figure 9.13. Bird breeder's disease: recent onset: upper zone (left) nodulations and perihilar infiltrates present.

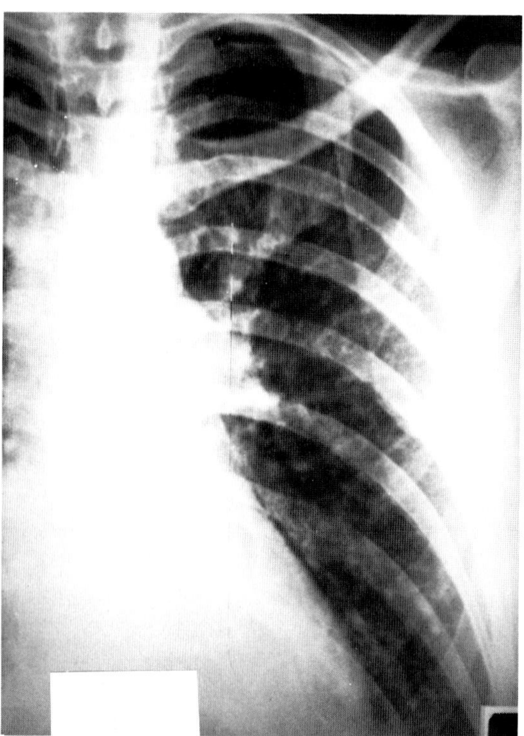

Figure 9.14. A magnified view of the left lung to show nodular infiltration of the lower two thirds of the lung. Recent onset of Bird breeder's disease.

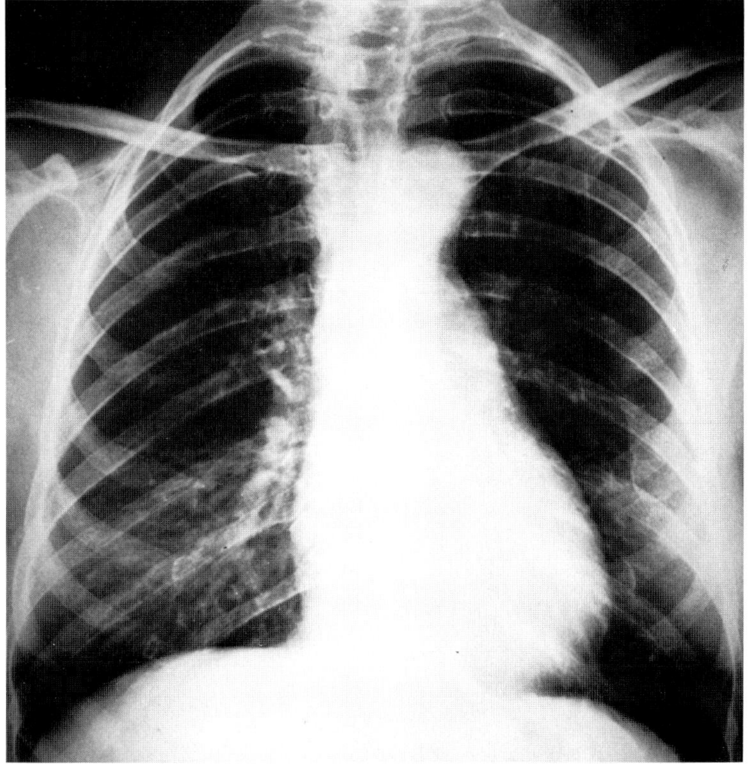

Figure 9.15. Bird breeder's disease with evidence of basal linear infiltrates.

Other Occupational EEA

Cheese Washers' Lung. Reported in workers exposed to dusts of *Penicillium* and also of mites (*Tyrophogus casei*, *Acarus siro*) found on the surface of cheese. In epidemiological studies there was a 10% to 15% incidence of alveolitis among exposed workers; similar cases having been recorded in Switzerland.

Wheat Weevil Lung. Due to an insect (*Sitophilus granarius*) responsible for alveolitis among millers, bakers, and handlers of flour.

Maple Bark Disease. Described in workers handling and producing railway sleepers from maple trees. Numerous molds developing between the dead wood and the cork are inhaled by the worker.

Wood Dust Diseases. Either red wood or exotic woods (iroko, okoume) or lumber handling can provoke not only asthmatic attacks but also alveolitis and fibrosis (Fig. 9.16).

Suberosis. Described in Portugal in cork factories; due to inhalation of particles of cork contaminated by *Penicillium frequentans*. Cork is used for the production of bottle corks, disks, and insulating sheets.

Byssinosis. Often regarded as an immune disease, occurs in workers engaged in processing cotton flax and hemp fibers and is characterized by the onset of dyspnea and malaise during the first day back at work, ("Monday fever"), increasing in severity during the working week, with respite of symptoms at the weekend. In the later stages the clinical and roentgenological picture is that of chronic bronchitis and emphysema, possibly terminating in cor pulmonale.

Ventilation pneumonitis. Includes two similar but distinct diseases: *Hypersensitivity pneumonitis* with mild symptoms and with a typical radiographic pattern of alveolitis (due to *Thermoactinomycetes*); *Humidifier fever*, which occurs in factories with wood paper printing where hot humidifier systems are in use and where stagnant water and poor maintenance result in the development of a large number of microorganisms (actinomycetes, amoeba, bacteria, and fungi like *Alternaria, Penicillium*).

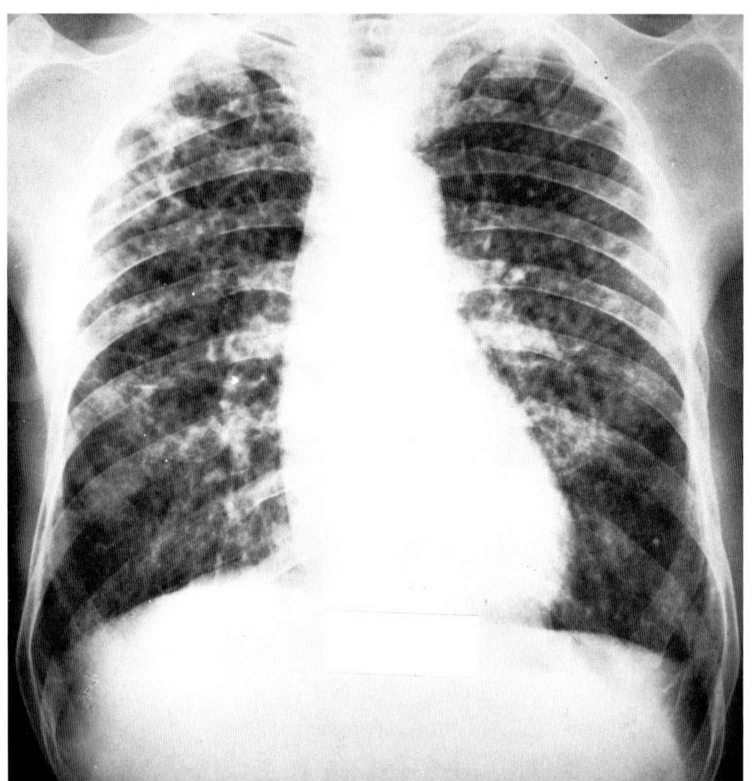

Figure 9.16. Wood dust disease – chronic type with diffuse linear and nodular changes in both lungs.

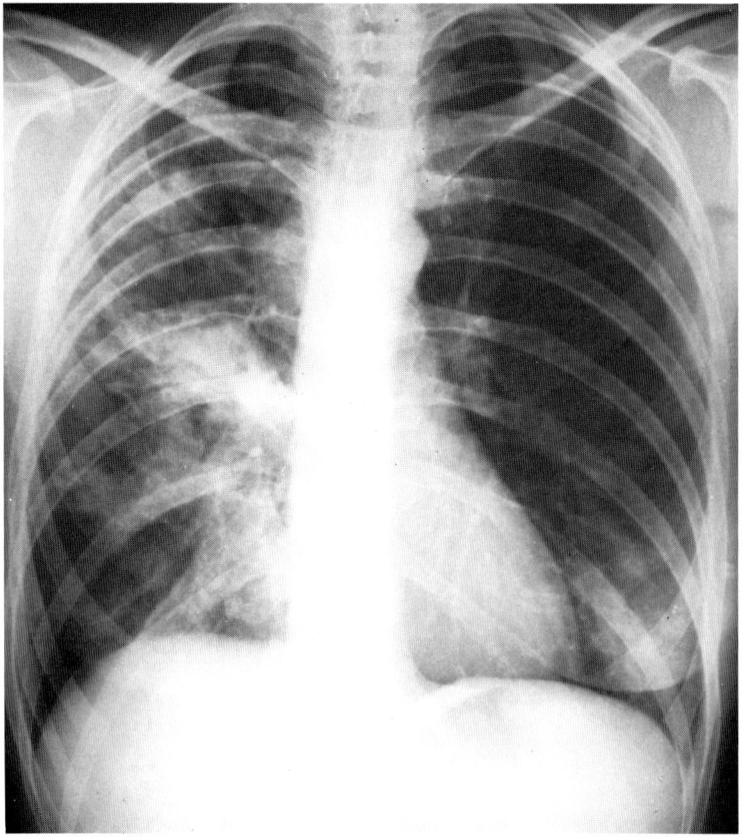

Figure 9.17. Unilateral allergic bronchopulmonary aspergillosis. The major infiltration is in the right perihilar and midzone.

It is often a "Monday fever," which improves during weekends and holidays, producing no significant or specific signs on the chest radiograph. The most important differential diagnosis is pneumonia due to *Legionella pneumoniae*.

There are a large number of reports of HP following exposure to various agents including malt workers (*Aspergillus*), detergent factory workers (proteolytic enzymes, *B subtilis*), rat handler's lung (rat urine protein), sericultural workers in Japan (ripe larva urine), furrier's lung, coffee workers, and sisal workers.

Allergic Bronchopulmonary Aspergillosis (A.B.P.A.)

Sometimes observed among farmers ABPA may be regarded, in such cases, as an occupational bronchopulmonary disease. This immune-related condition is due to a combination of two types of hypersensitivity: IgE immediate type hypersensitivity with asthma and late, semidelayed pulmonary hypersensitivity with the presence of precipitating antibodies. Pepys in the United Kingdom[1] provided the first description of allergic bronchopulmonary aspergillosis. In the United States, this disorder was thought to be very rare up to the last few years, while in France the disease seems to be uncommon.

Clinical Studies

In 95% of cases the disease develops in asthmatic or atopic subjects, on average 18 years after the first symptoms. Seasonal factors play an important role. Thus, in 75% of cases, the disease is observed in autumn and winter, consisting of repeated febrile episodes with transitory or widespread pulmonary shadows, blood eosinophilia, and mucoid plugs containing *Aspergillus* spores in the sputum, in subjects with asthma, eczema, or hay fever.

The eosinophilic infiltrations on chest radiographs are unilateral or bilateral (Fig. 9.17), sometimes as *fluffy* migratory pulmonary opacities (Fig. 9.18). The opacities, usually due to bronchial obstruction by mucous plugs (mucoid obstruction) (Fig. 9.19), are often confused with malignant metastases or patchy atelectasis. Perihilar tubular shadows due to proximal bronchial dilations are seen in 40% of cases.

Sputum plugs, present in half the cases, are found on bronchoscopy or in sputum followed by reaeration of the segmental or lobar collapse as the bronchus is reopened but often revealing *proximal bronchiectasis* (Figs. 9.20 and 9.21). However, removal by bronchial aspiration of the mucoid plug is not necessarily followed by immediate clearing of the radiographic changes.

The bronchial casts contain fibrin, mucus, Charcot-Leyden crystals, and Curschmann spirals, together with eosinophils, spores, and mycelial hyphae. However, isolation of *Aspergillus* from the sputum is not pathognomonic of disease and, conversely, *Aspergillus* may be absent from the sputum of typical cases of aspergillosis.

Immunological Studies. These are essential for the diagnosis of aspergillosis and to eliminate other conditions accompanied by eosinophilia and pulmonary shadows like Loeffler's syndrome due to parasitic infiltration or to periarteritis nodosa.

Skin tests with *Aspergillus* extracts are always positive, whether the test is done by scarification, pricking, or intracutaneous injection. The intracutaneous test, when made with a solution of *A fumigatus* (1/1,000), leads to a dual, immediate, and late (semidelayed) reaction four to eight hours later.

Challenge Tests. Inhalation of a solution of *Aspergillus* extract also causes a dual reaction, immediately followed by a late (semidelayed) reaction, with a febrile response together with dyspnea and a fall in the forced expiratory volume$_1$ (FEV_1). Pepys[1] even noted a general reaction as well as alveolar and asthmatic responses. Reports indicate inhibition of the late reaction by corticosteroids and partially by isoprenaline or sodium cromoglycate. However, in our patients these therapeutic agents were not effective.

Serological Tests. They usually show high levels of total serum IgE, specific IgE, and IgG antibodies. Total serum IgE decreases during steroid treatment

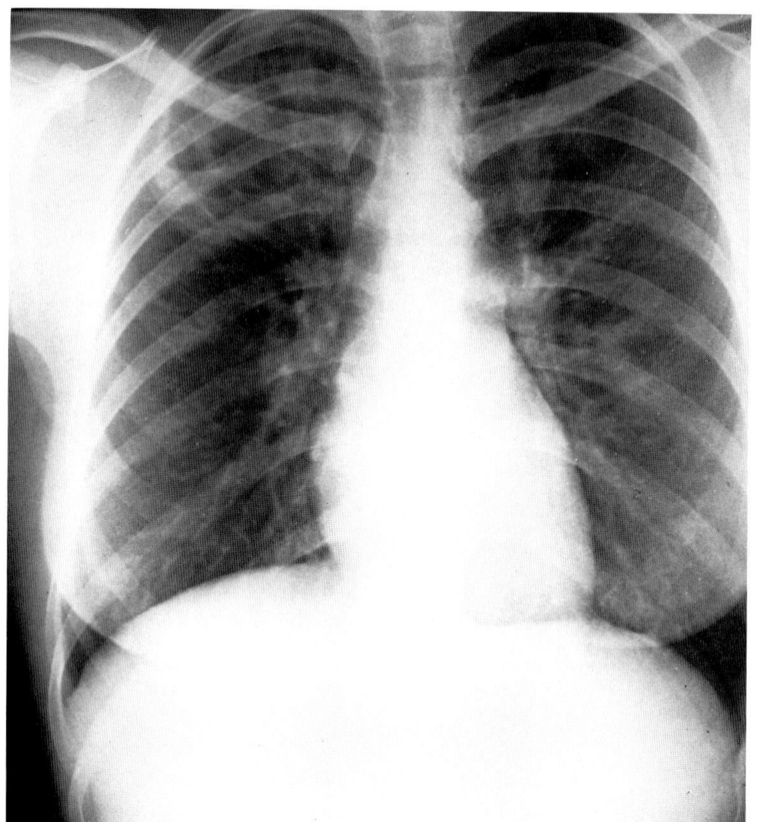

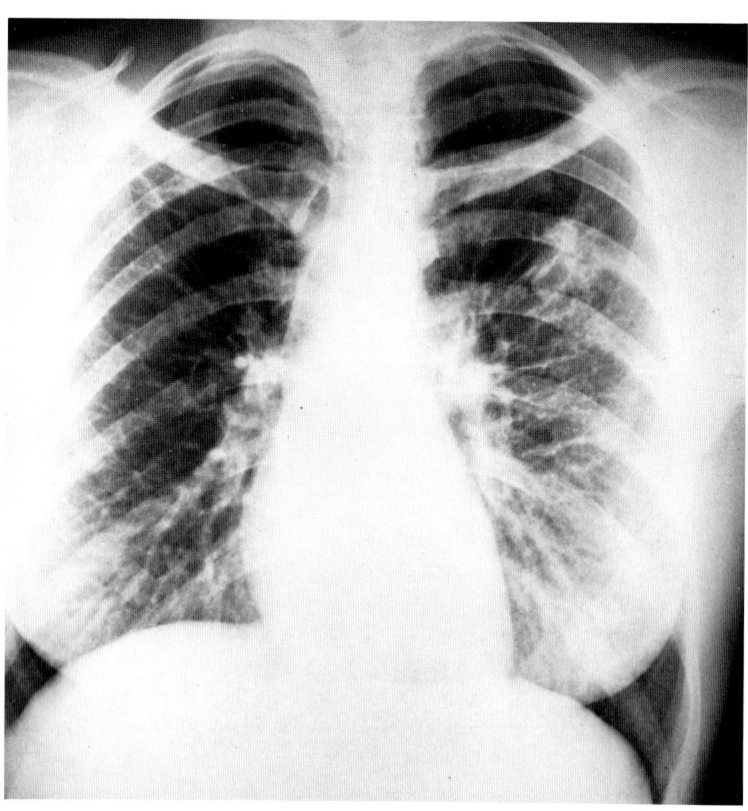

Figure 9.18.A. Migratory form of allergic bronchopulmonary aspergillosis showing right upper lobe infiltrate. **B**. Allergic bronchopulmonary aspergillosis: a left upper lobe infiltrate has replaced the previous right upper lobe change.

Figure 9.19.A. Mucoid impaction in bronchopulmonary aspergillosis resulting in collapse at the right upper lobe and hilar shadowing. **B**. Posttreatment of mucoid impaction in bronchopulmonary aspergillosis. Small opacities still present in the lung; however, the areas of opacification and collapse are markedly improved.

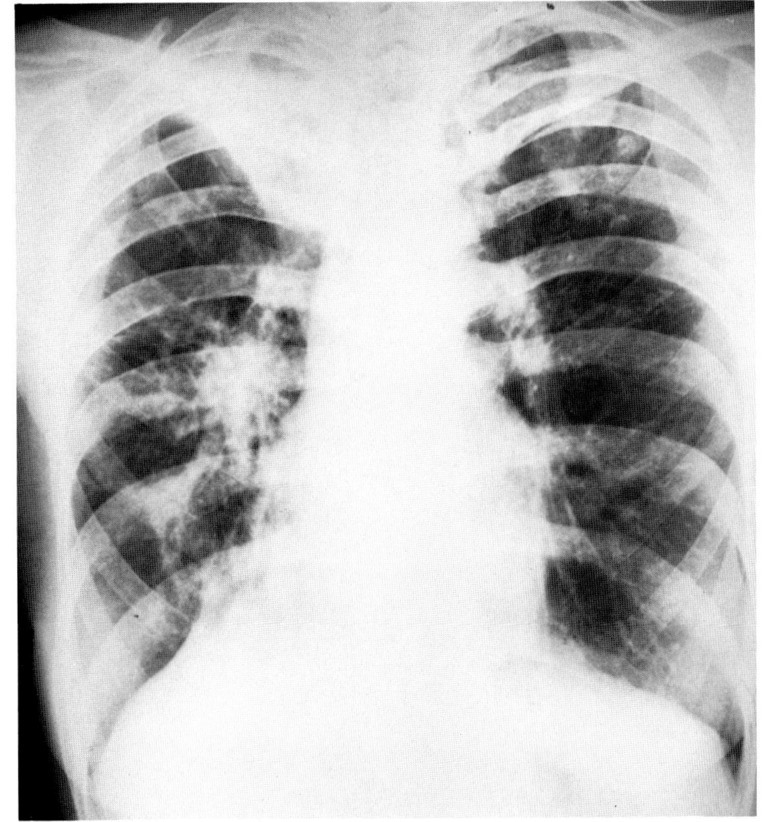

A

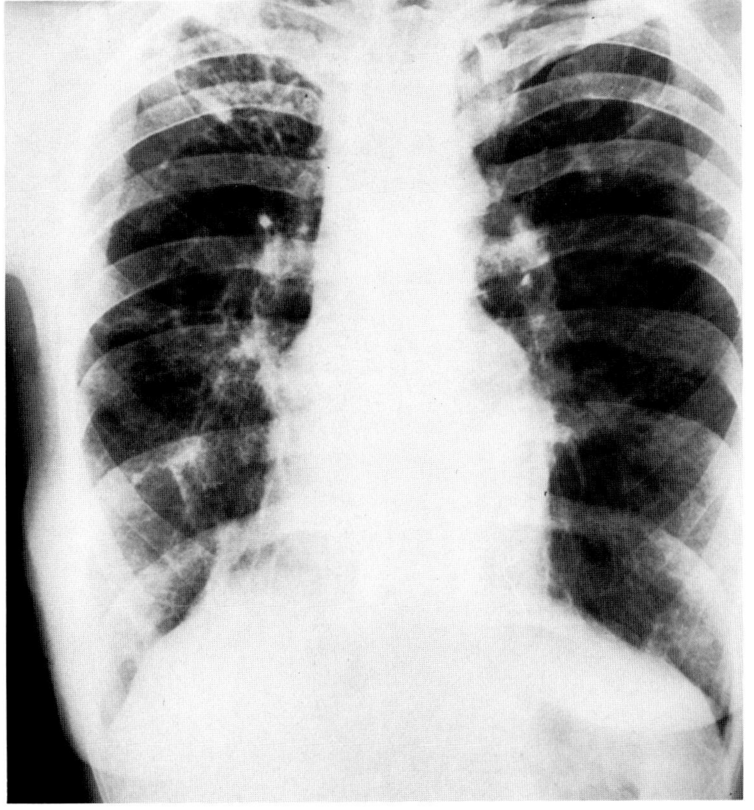

B

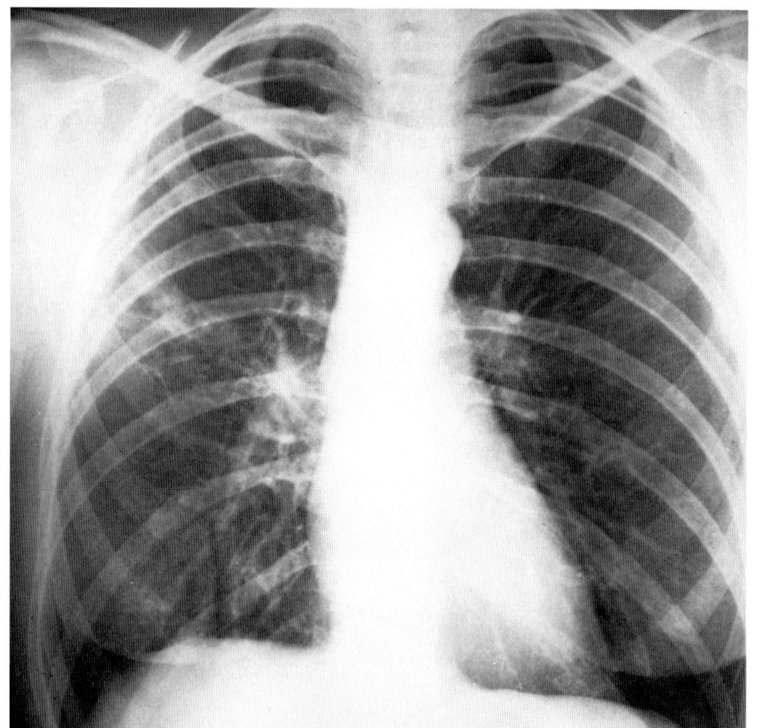

A

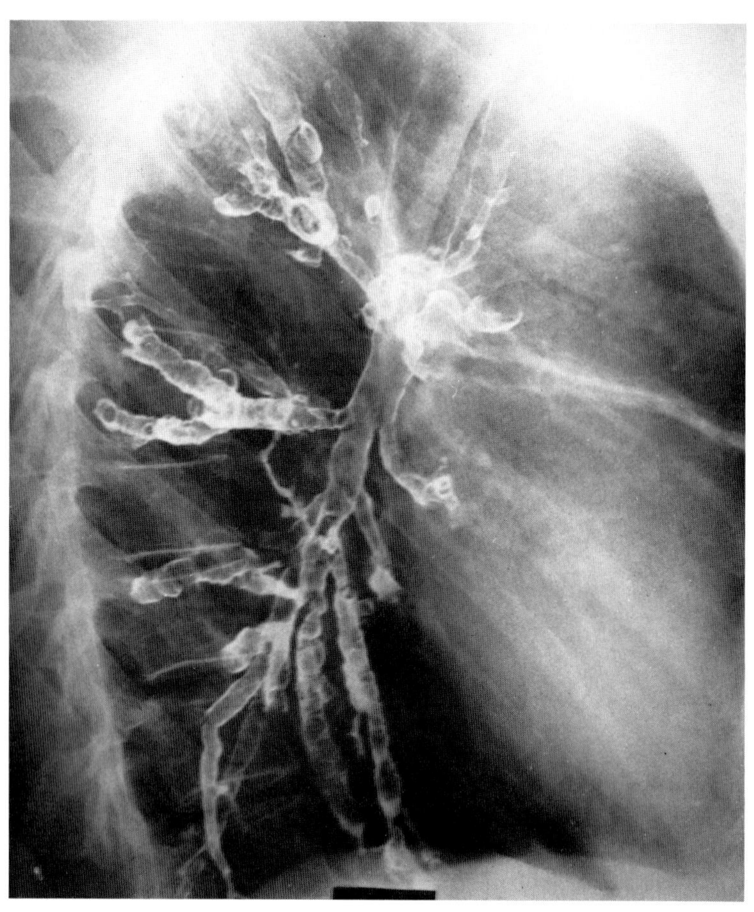

B

Figure 9.20.A. Treated allergic bronchopulmonary aspergillosis with right perihilar ring shadows and slight infiltrates. **B**. Bronchogram to illustrate the extent of proximal bronchiectasis present in **A**.

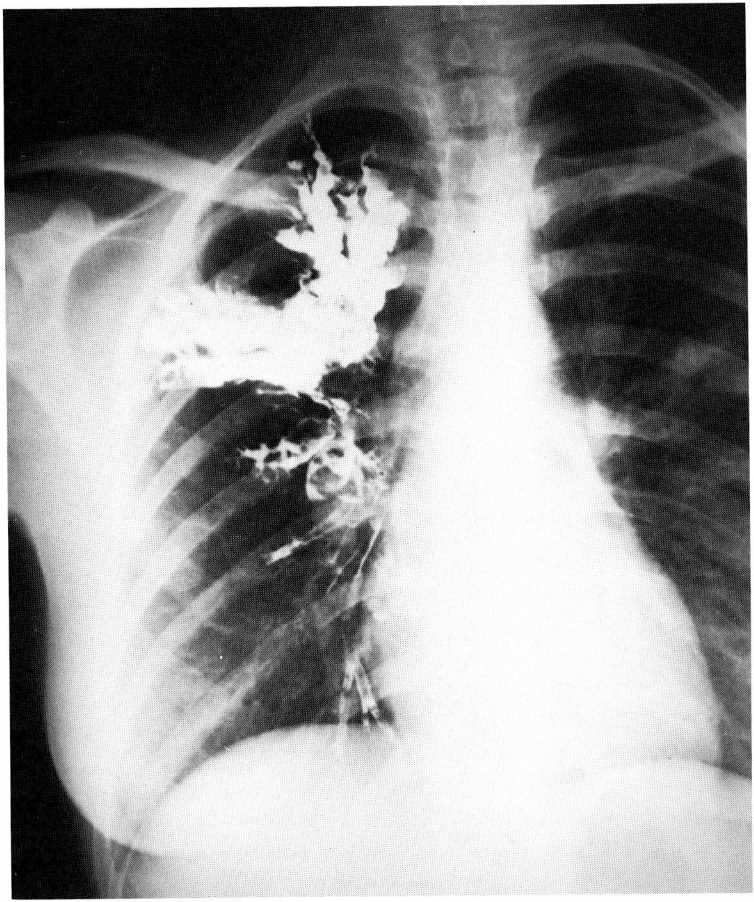

Figure 9.21. Severe proximal bronchiectasis in bronchopulmonary aspergillosis shown on a bronchogram (Fig. 9.20B).

and may be used, together with chest films, to monitor treatment. In 90% of cases, immunoelectrophoresis in agar gel or agarose with double diffusion by Ouchterlony's test, provides evidence of anti-*Aspergillus* precipitating antibodies.[2] In our patients, up to 13 arcs were observed. The intensity of the reactions seems to be linked to the presence of sputum plugs.

The presence of precipitins, the semidelayed reactions to skin and inhalation tests, and the perivascular deposition of antibodies of the IgG and IgM classes favor an Arthus-type reaction. Type I hypersensitivity reaction is proved by the immediate response to skin and inhalation tests.

Pathological Anatomy and Pathogenesis

Bronchial lesions are common and are characterized by glandular hypersecretion leading to the development of mucoid impaction. Pulmonary ventilation disturbances caused by mucus plugs are associated with peribronchiolar and alveolar infiltration by plasma cells, eosinophils, and monocytes and disappear during corticosteroid treatment. Vasculitis and thickening of the arterioles may also occur and can result in allergic bronchocentric granulomatosis.[1]

Aspergillus can also infect pulmonary cavities in long-standing healed tuberculosis but also can occur in bullae and cavities due to infarcts or hematomas. A mycetoma form consisting of a fungal nodule or mass lying free within the cavity frequently manifests as hemoptysis when the original disease is quiescent. The radiographs are characteristic. There is a clearly defined crescent of air between the mycetoma and the wall of cavity, moving freely as the subject changes position from erect to supine or prone. The signs are demonstrable on plain films but best shown on tomography or CT.

In conclusion, in spite of new imaging modalities, the radiologist encountering alveolar and interstitial disease usually only provides a description of the changes and not a definitive final diagnosis, which is invariably determined by other methods such as immunological techniques, bronchoalveolar lavage, transbronchial biopsy, or open-lung biopsy.

PART 2: PULMONARY DISEASES DUE TO METALLIC INHALANTS

The lung can react to chemical exposure in several ways including direct toxicity and delayed tissue reactions to dust accumulation. The first pulmonary effect of acute toxic damage to the bronchial and alveolar epithelium is of two types: a severe form consisting of chemical pneumonitis manifesting as delayed, noncardiogenic pulmonary edema, and a minor form consisting of metal fume fever.

A second response shown by the lung to metal exposure may lead to pneumoconiosis redefined by the Fourth International Conference held in Bucharest in 1971 as "the accumulation of dust in the lungs, and the tissue reaction to its presence." The tissues react to dust in three different ways. The first is a minimal stromal reaction—the nonfibrogenic or benign pneumoconiosis due to iron, antimony, barium, rare earth, and tin. The second is a reaction resulting in permanent scarring—the fibrogenic pneumoconiosis such as silicosis and asbestosis and an interstitial pneumonia and fibrosis due to berylliosis and hard metal disease. The third reaction is the possibility of carcinogenic effect from exposure to metals. The greatest danger arises in workers exposed to radioactive metals (uranium, thorium); however, the incidence of bronchial carcinoma arising from exposure to chromate, nickel, arsenic, iron dusts, and fumes is greater than expected in the general population. Minerals in the lungs may be identified by electron probe analysis and X-ray diffraction in lung-biopsy specimens or fluid after bronchoalveolar lavage. The concentration of one or more elements may also be estimated by the magnitude of X-ray emission.

Metal Fumes

Metal fume fever is a fairly common syndrome with a short incubation of four to eight hours after exposure. Symptoms resemble the onset of a viral "influenza" or bacterial infection with sudden onset of malaise, fever of 39°C, chills, profuse sweating, headache, joint pains, myalgia, and nausea but followed by a metallic taste in the mouth, irritation of the nose and the throat, cough and tightness of the chest often aggravated by deep inspiration. On physical examination there may be fine, moist rales at the lung bases. The chest radiograph is usually normal, but inhalation challenge provokes a reduction of lung volumes, often with a significant decrease in vital capacity and an associated polymorphonuclear leukocytosis. The symptoms subside within 24 hours. It is a benign and self-limiting disease; no complications or sequelae occur.[9] The most important diagnostic clues to "metal fume fever" are a history of recent fume exposure and complaints of nasal irritation and a metallic taste. Individuals who work continuously with metal seem to acquire a tolerance, but quickly lose it after being off work for a short period, even the weekend, hence "Monday fever." The metals incriminated are zinc (the first to be recognized), iron, antimony, tin, selenium, aluminium, nickel, manganese, magnesium, silver, and copper—all being encountered in fresh metal oxide fumes in welding, smelting, and galvanizing operations.[10,10a] The pathogenesis of the syndrome is unknown, but some features suggest an immunological reaction, or an endotoxin-like response.

Chemical Pneumonitis

Delayed noncardiogenic pulmonary edema or chemical pneumonitis is an uncommon syndrome, resembling adult respiratory distress syndrome.[9] There is a complete absence of immediate symptoms to warn workers that they are receiving a hazardous exposure. After a latent period of four to ten hours, the first premonitory symptoms, similar to metal-fume fever, occur. Two factors are of value in early differentiation between the two

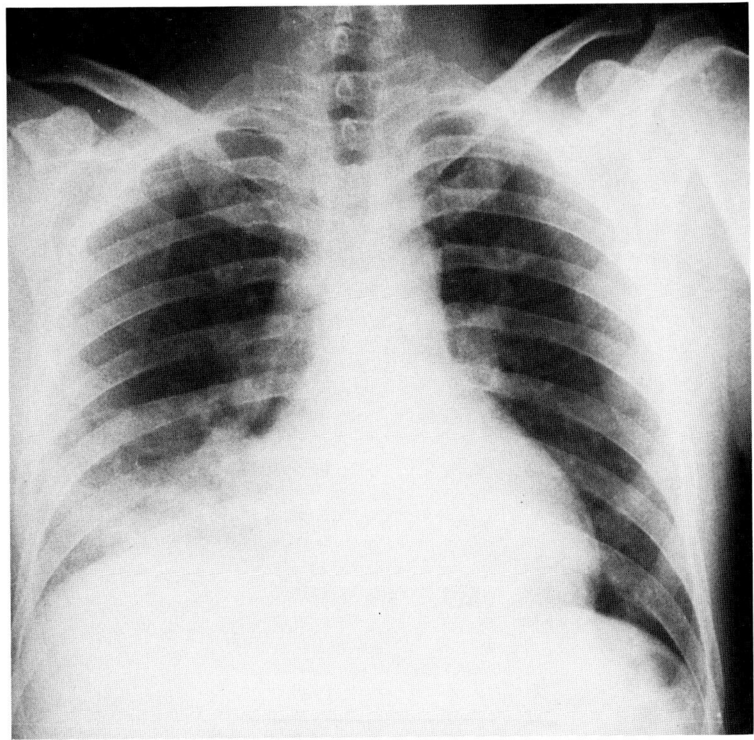

Figure 9.22. Chemical pneumonitis: Kerosene pneumonia with confluent opacity of lower right lung field.

disorders: (1) the onset of chest pain, often delayed 14 to 36 hours after exposure, and (2) an ashen-grey cyanosis without dyspnea. At this stage the physical examination of the chest is negative, but a chest film usually reveals numerous scattered patchy bronchopulmonary infiltrates probably due to interstitial edema.[11] Later the clinical manifestations are those of acute alveolar edema, with the onset of dyspnea, cough, and hemoptysis. Moist rales and rhonci are evident on physical examination. The chest radiograph reveals typical noncardiogenic pulmonary edema. The prognosis should be guarded because chemical pneumonitis is a potentially lethal syndrome, the case fatality ranging between 15% and 20% in cases of cadmium pneumonitis.[12]

If the patient survives the acute exposure, there may be a persistent restrictive ventilatory defect.[13] The metals responsible are the same as those in metal-fume fever, but particularly beryllium,[14] cadmium, nickel, carbonyl,[15] and manganese.[16] *Pathologically*, there is interstitial edema, then alveolae fill with proteinaceous fluid, and intra-alveolar hemorrhage occurs. The epithelium is infiltrated by inflammatory cells, and there is a complete separation of entire intact sheets of pulmonary epithelium from its underlying stroma. Determining the causes of pneumonitis can be difficult. Oxidizing agents need to be considered, eg, oxides of metals, and also gases such as phosgene, nitrogen dioxide, and ozone. Blood levels of the metal correlate best with acute exposure, and urine levels are a better reflection of the total-body burden. To substantiate the diagnosis, analysis of the fumes, from possible offending materials being used, is necessary[17] (Fig. 9.22).

Nonfibrogenic Pneumoconiosis (Benign Pneumoconiosis)

Until the 1930s, nonfibrotic forms of pneumoconiosis were unknown. Harding et al.,[18] who described siderosis of welders, were the first to postulate that some dusts might lie inertly in pulmonary tissues without provoking fibrosis, although producing

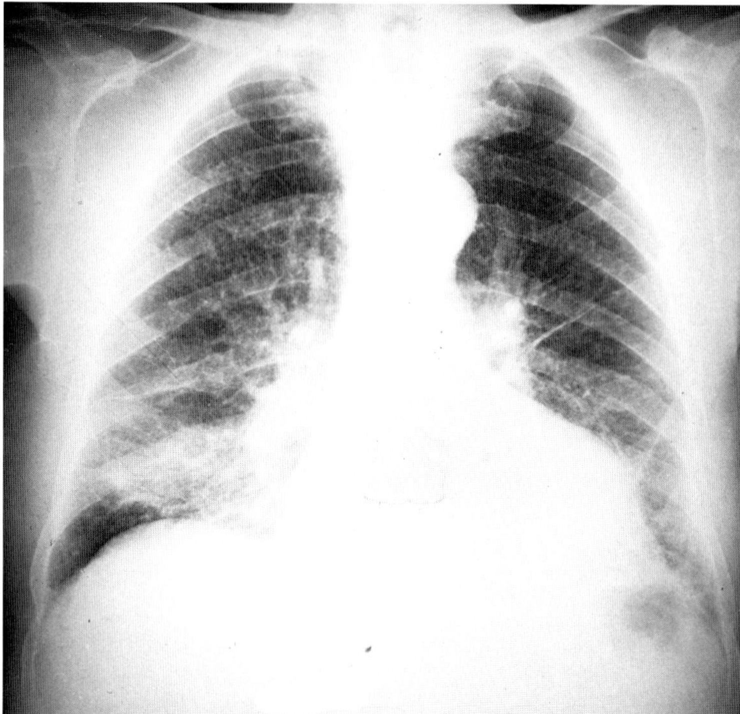

Figure 9.23. Siderosis: the lungs are infiltrated with fine, widely disseminated reticulonodular opacities. (Courtesy of Professor P. Lamy and Professor D. Anthoine, Nancy, France.)

radiographic opacities. Inhaled particulate matter can remain in the lungs for years, without symptoms, abnormal physical signs or incapacity for work and associated with normal lung function tests—all of which emphasize the discrepancy between the severity of the radiographic changes and the clinical picture.[18]

Chest films typically show small opacities ranging in size from a pinhead or miliary to a millet seed (p-q), which do not tend to conglomerate. The hilar lymph nodes are not calcified and in particular have no shell-like calcifications characteristic of advanced silicosis. The opacities are often uniformly distributed, with a variable profusion ranging from 1/1 to 3/3 (ILO). The nodules are denser than those of silicosis or coal worker's pneumoconiosis, but vary with the atomic weight of the element; the density is greatest for rare earths, lowest for siderosis, and intermediate for antimony, tin,[19] and barium.[20] When only minimal changes are present, they may be shown by special techniques such as macroradiography or xeroradiography. When exposure to dust ceases, the opacities slowly begin to disappear, in contrast to silicosis, and may, with time, resolve almost completely after exposure ceases.[21]

Siderosis

Siderosis is the most frequent of benign pneumoconiosis, caused by the inhalation of ferric acid ($Fe_2 O_3$) and iron, usually in the form of hematite. The main occupations producing siderosis are electric arc and oxyacetylene welders (arc welder's siderosis),[18] workers polishing metals and optical lenses with iron oxide powders, and iron miners.[22] The typical form is identical to other benign pneumoconioses (simple siderosis) in symptomless workers. Chest films show reticulonodular opacities, widely disseminated in both lungs (Fig. 9.23). The density of individual nodules appears to be lower than those of silicosis. Macroscopically, the lungs are black, while microscopically, there is a peribronchial and perivascular concentration of numerous macrophages laden with coarse black granules without accompanying fibrosis. This has been confirmed experimentally where iron oxides have also been shown not to cause fibrosis in the lungs of animals.[9]

French workers have described a complicated siderosis in welders, diffuse interstitial fibrosis proceeding to "honeycombing," and a conglomerative form resembling progressive massive fibrosis due to the combined exposure to iron oxide particles and other more toxic constituents of welding fumes and gases.[23] The constituents of the gases and fumes inhaled will depend upon the composition of the metals welded, eg, steel, aluminium, and the reactions of substances in the working atmosphere, especially in an enclosed space without natural ventilation (eg, nitrogen dioxide, ozone, nitric oxide).[24]

Stannosis

This pneumoconiosis is caused by the inhalation of oxides of tin (atomic number 50). Industrial exposure most commonly occurs during the mining, particularly of cassiterite (mainly in the dioxide),[22] smelting and refining of ore, and in industries where fumes of tin oxide form.

Pathologically, black or dark grey foci, 2 to 5 mm in size, are distributed uniformly throughout the lungs. Histological staining shows dense aggregates of dust-laden macrophages surrounding respiratory bronchioles, but focal emphysema seen in association with dust foci in coal worker's lung is not a feature observed in these tin workers.[19]

Antimony Pneumoconiosis

Similarly, exposure to antimony (atomic number 51) during the mining, smelting, and refining of the ore leads to antimony pneumoconiosis. It is also described in stibnite workers and in the production of alloys where antimony is combined with other metals (tin, lead, and copper), such as in the manufacture of abrasives, and in typesetting in the printing industry. Some of the workers are affected by exposure to antimony oxides, sulfides and powder ore. The duration of exposure is from 1 to 15 years.[25] Data on lung histology in humans are lacking, owing to its benignity.[26]

Baritosis Pneumoconiosis

The two chief ores of barium (atomic number 56) are barytes ($BaSo_4$) and whiterite ($BaCo_3$). In industry, they are used in paint making (lithopone), as an extender of filler for paper, textiles, leather, soap, rubber, and linoleum. In medicine, barium sulfate, characterized by its extreme insolubility and its high radiopacity, is used as an opaque medium in radiographic examination of the gastrointestinal tract. Histological examinations of the lung in animal experiments show only a mild foreign body reaction to barium sulfate and no evidence of fibrosis.[21]

Rare Earth Pneumoconiosis

The rare earths are a group of 14 elements. Their atomic numbers range from 58 to 71. Cerium (atomic number 58) is quantitatively the most important component of rare earth metals. Cerium, mixed with other metals, is of great value in metallurgic industry for preparation of special alloys and doxidiser agents, in the lithographic industry, as arc stabilizer in carbon arch lamps in the gas mantle industry, and in various pyrotechnics in the electronic industry, such as in color television tubes, and for mercury vapor and fluorescent lamps. These dusts are practically inert, inducing only small agglomerations of histiocytes around the dust deposits in animal experiments. In later stages, perifocal emphysema and a slight fibrosis of the lungs are noted.[27,28]

Hard Metal Pneumoconiosis

Hard metal is an alloy of tungsten carbide, cobalt, and occasionally other metals such as titanium and tantalum. Hard metals are used whenever strength, rigidity, and resistance to heat and wear are needed. Major uses are for cutting tools, drilling equipment, alloys, and ceramics. To produce tungsten carbide, a process of powdered metallurgy is used to blend and heat tungsten and carbon, using cobalt as a binder. Both those who make the alloys (by sintering or pressure melting of metal powder) and those who grind the alloy, appear to

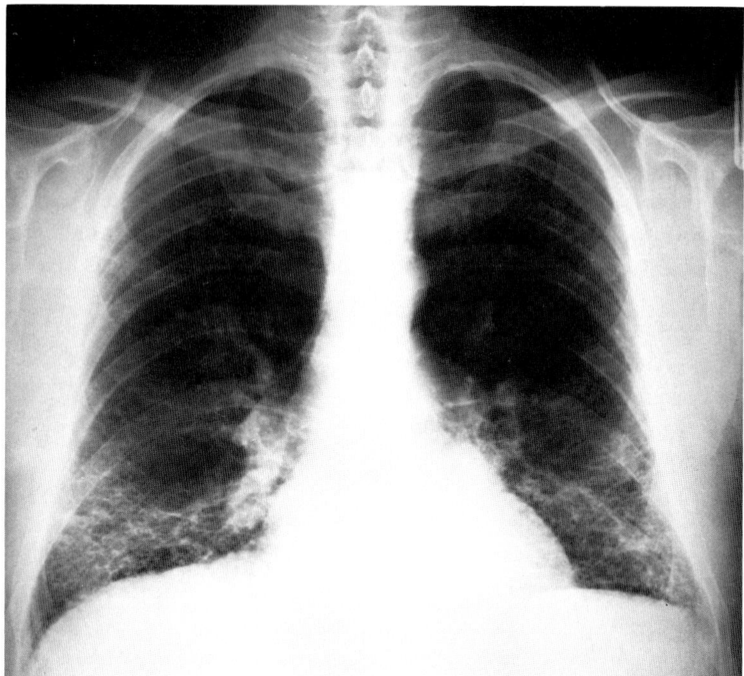

Figure 9.24. Hard metal pneumoconiosis. Irregular linear densities, predominantly basal. (Courtesy of Professor M. Lavandier, Tours, France.)

be at some risk, if associated with elevated peak air concentrations of cobalt.[29,30]

The prevalence of interstitial lung disease in tungsten carbide production is not well known. It varies from 16% reported in one study in Germany to 2% in a survey from the United States.[31] The mean duration of exposure before development of symptoms is 12 years, but the range varies from 1 month to 28 years,[32] indicating the existence of two forms of disease, one with a subacute onset and one with insidious progression.[33] The first symptoms are cough with scanty sputum followed by dyspnea on exertion. Weight loss is frequently found. Basilar rales and clubbing of the fingers occur later.

Significant reduction of vital capacity is present soon after the onset of symptoms. Other pulmonary abnormalities–ie, low carbon dioxide diffusion capacity, arterial hypoxemia–consistent with a diffuse interstitial process are less frequent.[9]

Radiologically, the characteristic findings are nodular and linear densities (bilateral and symmetric) involving major portions of both lungs, especially the lower zone (Fig. 9.24), tending to produce a shaggy appearance of the heart borders. Radiological shadowing may progress slowly or very rapidly. In advanced cases (Fig. 9.25) there may be small cystic shadows, emphysema, and pneumothorax (Fig. 9.26).

Pathologic findings have been schematically divided into two types: a subacute fibrosing alveolitis characterized by desquamation and multinucleated giant cells, and a chronic diffuse pulmonary fibrosis, with honeycomb cysts and emphysema, occurring after a few to many years of exposure.[29,30] Available evidence suggests that inhalation of finely powdered cobalt causes the pneumoconiosis, as evidenced by animal experiments. Cobalt is toxic to the lung, whereas metallic tungsten carbide is entirely inert.[34] Furthermore, cobalt is detected in bronchoalveolar lavage fluid, in urine, and in lung tissue, but only if the specimens are taken soon after the patient has stopped work (cobalt is very soluble in biological fluid).[33] More directly, intoxication by cobalt alone has been shown to produce a fibrosing alveolitis identical to that of hard metal pneumoconiosis.[35,36]

Metal and Cancer

Industrial carcinogens are responsible for only a small proportion of lung cancers (approximately 5% to 10%).[37]

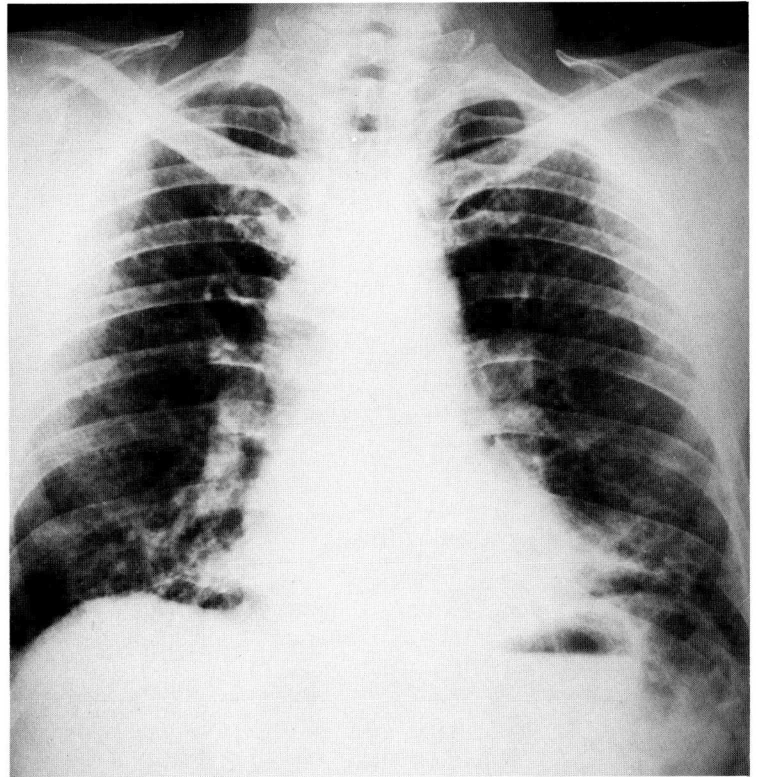

Figure 9.25. Advanced "basal fibrosis" in a case of hard metal disease.

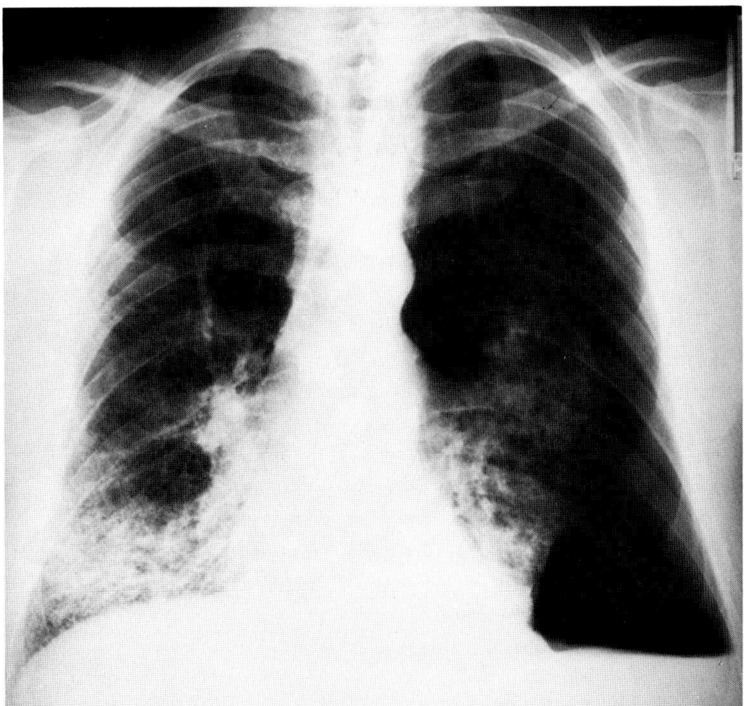

Figure 9.26. Hard metal pneumoconiosis presenting with a left pneumothorax and coarse basal infiltrates.

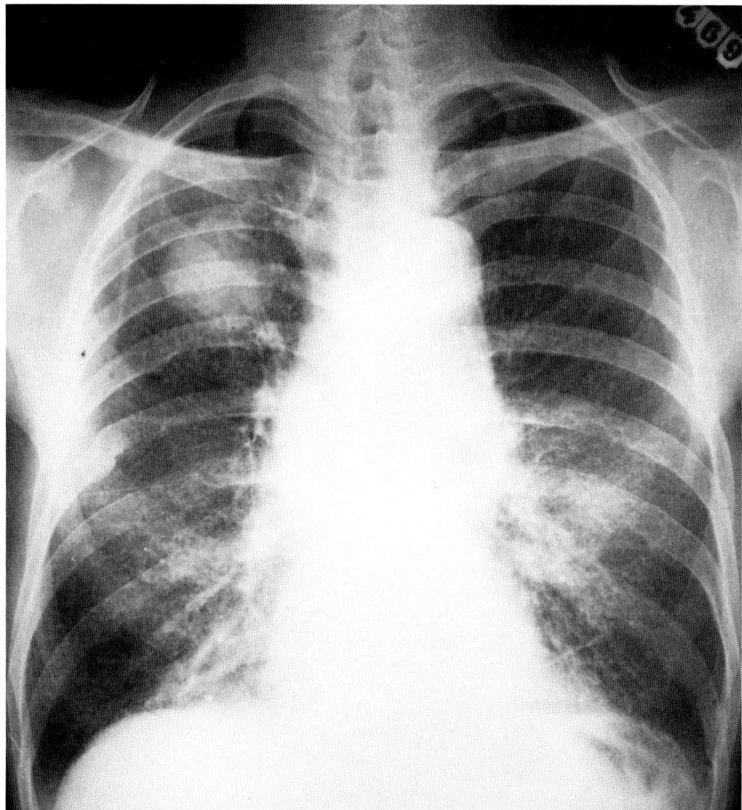

Figure 9.27. Primary lung cancer in an iron mine worker with siderosis. (Courtesy of Professor P. Lamy and Professor D. Anthoine, Nancy, France.)

Because tobacco smoke is established as the dominant respiratory carcinogen, it is difficult to evaluate the data on industrial exposure to metals if epidemiological studies, covering a sufficient period of time, demonstrate a higher prevalence of lung cancer compared with the prevalence in the general population (observed/expected ratio). However, occasionally a specific metal can be incriminated, and, more directly, experimental studies in animals may establish the carcinogenic effect of a particular metal.[38]

All histological types of lung cancer have been reported, especially of squamous (or epidermoid) type producing the appearances commonly associated with pulmonary cancers seen on chest radiographs (Fig. 9.27). Evidence for an association between metal exposure and lung cancer includes that from Cumberland[39] and from Lorraine[40] where iron miners[41] have an excess of lung cancer (observed/expected ratio 5 to 10). Heavy exposure to arsenic contributes to lung cancer in man, especially in copper-smelter workers, in workers involved in the production of insecticides containing arsenic (observed/expected ratio:7), and in agricultural workers.[42] For 50 years chromates,[43] especially chromium pigments, and biochromates have been known to be potent inducers of lung cancers in exposed workers. The observed/expected ratio varies from 30 to 50.

Nickel

In a recent study in New Caledonia, there was a threefold increase in the incidence of lung cancer among workers exposed to nickel, compared with nonworkers, when age and smoking were taken into account.[44]

Ionizing Radiation

Uranium miners have an excess of lung cancer, the gas radon seems to be the responsible agent (alpha emitters that cause dense ionization).[45]

In other types of apparently nonradioactive mines (iron, tin, silver, lead, fluospar), radioactivity may be present owing to diffusion of radon from uranium, which is present in minute amounts in all rocks.[45]

Conclusion

Organic and metallic inhalants are an uncommon cause of pulmonary disease and have widely differing radiographic appearances. The pulmonary effects are largely due to an immune response or, in the case of metal fumes, a direct toxic reaction with radiographic changes varying from minimal to gross pulmonary edema or fibrosis. The most common appearance is one of nodulation, varying from a fine ground-glass pattern to large confluent nodules with indefinite margins and a tendency to reticulonodular shadowing. Radiologists require a high index of suspicion to suggest the diagnosis of extrinsic allergic alveolitis.

It is even more difficult to diagnose the chronic fibrotic form due to the similarity to other types of late-stage pulmonary disease with emphysema and fibrosis. But early diagnosis is imperative to institute preventative measures and to treat the acute symptoms.

The possible allergens are legion and can only be confirmed or excluded by a thorough case history and detailed testing, bearing in mind the great variation from region to region and the seasonal distribution.

The conditions caused by inhalation of metallic dusts or fumes are, for the most part, more easily recognized mainly because of a definite occupational history and frequently characteristic radiographic features, particularly the asymptomatic dense nodules. "Monday fever," too, has a specific clinical picture. The devastating effects of acute metal-fume fever resembling adult respiratory distress syndrome must be borne in mind, and the late carcinogenic complications frequently produce complicated legal arguments, with the influence of cigarette smoking the contentious factor.

Chest radiographs have a most important function in reflecting the morphological changes, however nonspecific, to monitor possible progression of the disease or the effects of treatment.

The new imaging modalities have currently only a limited role in the diagnosis and management of industrial lung disease; nevertheless, the use of CT has already made a significant contribution in the study of exposure to asbestos in interstitial pulmonary fibrosis and in demonstrating secondary effects, such as bullous formation. The roles of digital radiography and magnetic resonance imaging have yet to be evaluated.

References

1. Pepys J: Hypersensitivity disease of the lungs due to fungi and organic dusts. New York, Basel, Karger, 1969.
2. Molina Cl: Broncho-pulmonary immunopathology. ed 2. Pepys J (trans). Edinburgh, Churchill Livingstone, 1984, p 260.
3. Cook PG, Wells IP, McGavin CR: The distribution of pulmonary shadowing in Farmer's lung. Clin Radiol 1988; 39:21–27.
4. Turner-Warwick M: Immunology of the lung. London, Edward Arnold, 1978.
5. Fink JN, Barboriak JJ, Sosman AJ: Immunologic studies of pigeon breeder's disease. J Allergy 1967; 1:214.
6. Bergin CJ, Muller NL: CT in the diagnosis of interstitial lung disease. Am J Radiol 1985; 145:505–510.
7. Nakata H, Kimoto T, Nakayama T, et al: Diffuse peripheral lung disease: evaluation by high resolution computed tomography. Radiology 1985; 157:181–185.
8. McLoud TC, Gaensler EA, Carrington CB: Clinics in Chest Medicine. Chest Radiology, vol 5, No 2, WB Saunders Co, 1986.
9. Parkes WR: Occupational lung disorders. ed 2. London, Butterworth, 1982.
10. Piscator M: Health hazards from inhalation of metal fumes. Environ Res 1976; 2:268–270.
10a. Baudoin J, Jobard P, Moline J, et al: Les troubles pulmonaires observés chez les ouvriers de l'industrie des métaux durs. Rev Fr Mal Respir 1975; 3(4):343–362.
11. Barnhart S, Rosenstock L: Cadmium chemical pneumonitis. Chest 1984; 86:789–791.
12. Dunphy B: Acute occupational Cadmium poisoning: a critical review of the literature. J Occup Med 1967; 9:22–26.
13. Anthony JS, Zamel N, Aberman A: Abnormalities in pulmonary function after brief exposure to toxic metal fumes. Can Med Assoc J 1978; 23:586–588.

14. Tepper LB, Hardy HL, Chamberlin RI: The Toxicity of Beryllium Compounds. Amsterdam, Elsevier, 1961.
15. Sunderman FW, Kincaid JF: Nickel poisoning—Studies on patients suffering from acute exposure to vapors of nickel carbanyl. JAMA 1954; 155:889–894.
16. Davies Tal: Manganese pneumonitis. Br J Med 1946; 3:111.
17. Armstrong CW, Moore LW, Hackler RL, et al: An outbreak of metal fume fever. Diagnostic use of urinary copper and zinc determinations. J Occup Med 1983; 25:886–888.
18. Harding HE, McLaughlin ATG, Doig AT: Clinical, radiographic and pathological studies of the lungs of electric-arc and oxyacetylene welders. Lancet 1958; ii:394–398.
19. Robertson AJ, Rivers D, Nagelschmidt G, et al: Stannosis—Benign pneumoconiosis due to tin dioxide. Lancet 1961; i:1089–1093.
20. Wilson JK, Rubin PS, McGee TM: The effects of barium sulphate on the lungs. A clinical and experimental study. Am J Roentgenol 1959; 82:84–94.
21. Doig AT: Baritosis: a benign pneumoconiosis. Thorax 1976; 31:30–39.
22. Sadoul P, Horsky P, Beigbeider R, et al: La sidérose des mineurs de fer. Arch Mal Prof 1979; 40(9-2):15–23.
23. Brun J, Cassan G, Kofman J, et al: La siderosclerose des soudeurs à l'arc à forme de fibrose interstitielle diffuse et à forme conglomerative pseudo-tumorale. Poumon Coeur 1972; 28:3–10.
24. Sanderson JT: Hazards of the arc-air gouging process. Ann Occup Hyg 1970; 11:123–133.
25. Cooper DA, Pendergrass EP, Vorwald AJ, et al: Pneumoconiosis among workers in an antimony industry. Am J Roentgenol 1968; 3:495–508.
26. Hadengue P: La stibiose: pneumopathie dûe a l'antimoine. 1980; EMC 16002, A10.
27. Vocaturo G, Colombo F, Zanoni M, et al: Human exposure to heavy metals. Rare earth pneumoconiosis in occupational workers. Chest 1983; 5:780–783.
28. Heuck F, Hoschek R: Cer-Pneumoconiosis. Am J Roentgenol 1968; 104:777–783.
29. Schepers GWH: The biological action of tungsten carbide and cobalt. Arch Ind Health 1955; 12:140–146.
30. Demedts M, Gheysens B, Nagels J, et al: Cobalt lung in diamond polishers. Am Rev Respir Dis 1984; 130:130–135.
31. Sprince ML, Chamberlin RI, Hales CA, et al: Respiratory disease in tungsten carbide production workers. Chest 1984; 86:549–557.
32. Coates EO, Watson JHL: Diffuse interstitial lung disease in tungsten carbide workers. Ann Intern Med 1971; 75:709–716.
33. Schepers GWH: The biological action of particulate cobalt metal. Arch Ind Health 1955; 12:127–133.
34. Davison AG, Haslam PL, Corrin B, et al: Interstitial lung disease and asthma in hard metal workers: bronchoalveolar lavage, ultrastructural and analytical findings and results of bronchial provocation tests. Thorax 1983; 38:119–128.
35. Metals and the lung, editorial. Lancet 1984; ii:903.
36. Cullen MR: Respiratory disease from hard metal exposure. A continuing enigma. Chest 1984; 86:513–514.
37. Harley HH: Radon and lung cancer in mines and homes. N Engl J Med 1984; 310:1525–1526.
38. Ott MG, Holder BB, Gordon HL: Respiratory cancer and occupational exposure to arsenicals. Arch Environ Health 1974; 29:250–255.
39. Paulds IS, Stewart MJ: Carcinoma of the lung in haematite miners. J Pathol Bacteriol 1956; 72:353–366.
40. Anthoíne D, Braun P, Cerveni P, et al: Le cancer bronchique des mineurs de fer de Lorraine peut-il être considéré comme une maladie profesionelle? A propos de 270 nouveaux cas observés de 1964 à 1978. Rev Fr Mal Respir 1979; 7:63–65.
41. Boyd JY, Doll R: Cancer of the lung in iron ore (haematite) miners. Br J Ind Med 1970; 27:27–105.
42. Pinto SS: Mortality experience of arsenic exposed workers. Arch Environ Health 1978; 33:325–331.
43. Langard S, Vigander T: Occurrence of lung cancer in workers producing chromium pigments. Br J Ind Med 1983; 40:71–74.
44. Lessard R, Reed D, Maheux B, et al: Lung cancer in New Caledonia, a nickel smelting island. J Occup Med 1978; 20:815–817.
45. Samet JM, Kutvirt DM, Waxweiler RJ, et al: Uranium mining and lung cancer in Navajo men. N Engl J Med 1984; 310:1481–1484.

10

Occupational Asthma

A.B. Zwi and S. Zwi

Introduction and Objectives

The aims of this chapter are firstly to describe briefly the features of "occupational asthma," including the agents involved, patterns of response, pathogenesis, and diagnosis; and then to describe the problems that may be faced by the general physician and radiologist in diagnosing a case of occupational asthma.

Definition

Bronchial asthma is characterized by increased responsiveness of the trachea and bronchi to various stimuli, manifesting as widespread narrowing of the airways with variable severity either spontaneously or as a result of therapy.[1] Bronchial asthma must be differentiated from other obstructive pulmonary diseases such as emphysema and chronic bronchitis.

Occupational asthma is a respiratory disorder characterized by reversible obstruction of airways and caused by inhalation of manufactured substances and materials or of those directly used by a worker or those incidentally present at the worksite.[2] Clinically it is manifested by chest tightness, cough, wheezing, and shortness of breath and physiologically by temporal alterations in pulmonary mechanics. Airway obstruction is initially intermittent and reversible, but continued exposure to the inciting agent may occasionally lead to irreversible obstructive airway disease and chronic respiratory symptoms.[2] Some authors include hypersensitivity pneumonitis under the broad term "occupational asthma"[3]; however, it is excluded in this discussion despite the fact that it may result from exposure to some of the same agents.

Three major factors influence the development of allergic respiratory disease: the immunologic status of the subject, the nature of the causal agent, and the circumstances under which exposure takes place.[4]

Agents Involved

A broad range of agents can cause occupational asthma. An extensive list is provided by Chan-Yeung and Lam[5] in their comprehensive review of occupational asthma.

Vegetable Origin

Substances of vegetable origin are probably the most commonly reported causes of reversible obstructive airway disease in industry.[2] Sensitization occurs to materials such as wood or wood products, cotton, flax, hemp, grain, flour, molds, coffee beans, spices, and tobacco.

Animal Origin

A broad range of animal products may lead to asthma at work, including animal hair, feathers, mites, small insects, dander, bacteria, and protein dust. Workers such as shepherds, farmers, jockeys, laboratory and research workers, animal handlers, and veterinarians are at increased risk. Proteolytic enzymes produced by *Bacillus subtilis* may cause asthma in workers manufacturing detergent.

Chemical Origin

A variety of chemicals, both simple and complex, are associated with occupational asthma, including those of low molecular weight such as formalin and sulfathiazole, or those of more complex structure such as pesticides, aliphatic polyamines, penicillin, phthalic anhydride, epoxy resins, and isocyanates.

Occupational Asthma on a Nonallergic Basis

A number of substances may lead to occupational asthma on a nonallergic basis; eg, extracts of cotton, hemp, sisal, and flax contain an active bronchoconstrictor or histamine-releasing substance, and wheat and proteolytic enzymes are also capable of producing effects due to the liberation of histamine.[2]

Acute bronchospasm may result from occupational exposure to sulfur dioxide, ammonia, hydrochloric acid, ozone, nitrogen dioxide, urea formaldehyde, organophosphate insecticides, piperazine, and thermal degradation products of polyvinyl chloride film for meat-wrapping. After a severe inflammatory reaction to an irritating gas like chlorine, attacks of bronchospasm may occur on subsequent exposure to very low concentrations of the same gas.

A variant of occupational asthma, the reactive airways dysfunctional syndrome (RADS), has been described[6]: a single exposure to a very high concentration of an irritant may precipitate a syndrome that clinically simulates acute or chronic asthma. The subjects have hyperreactive airways with no evidence for an immunologic process.[6]

Predisposing Factors

Atopy is defined as an ability to produce IgE antibodies readily on contact with common environmental allergens encountered in everyday life.[7] Atopic individuals tend to develop allergy more readily than nonatopics after short periods of exposure and with low concentrations of the responsible agent.

In some industries, there is a clear increase in the risk of sensitization in atopic individuals, for example, those exposed to biological detergents and platinum salts.[8] In cotton-exposed workers, those who are atopic seem to have increased responsiveness once sensitization has occurred.

Duration of Exposure

The development of asthma is influenced by whether exposure to the offending agent is continuous or intermittent. An allergic response cannot occur on first exposure, thus distinguishing RADS from asthma.[6] The latent interval before the development of symptoms may vary from a few weeks to many years; in industries using platinum salts sensitization usually occurs within the first 3 years of employment. Sensitization to grain dust and isocyanates may occur at any time after exposure, and sensitivity after only 10 years or more at work is not uncommon.

Smoking

Smokers appear to be more susceptible to asthma caused by agents inhaled at work and are more likely to produce specific IgE antibodies in response to certain allergens. Cigarette smoke may increase airway permeability, thus increasing antigen access to immune competent cells.[9]

Patterns of Response

Immediate, late, and dual responses may occur.[8] Immediate responses usually occur within minutes of exposure to the offending agent, are maximal at 20 minutes, and usually last for one to two hours after which recovery occurs spontaneously. Wheeze and chest tightness are almost invariably present.

Late or nonimmediate responses commonly begin several hours after exposure, are maximal at four to eight hours, and disappear after 24 hours. Late responses occur in the early hours of the morning, with a tendency, in some cases, to recur on a number of successive nights following a single challenge. Wheeze is often slight or absent, and in some cases cough may be the only symptom. The dual or combined response is the occurrence of both immediate and late responses following a single exposure.

There may be considerable variations in these patterns of response. The development of an immediate reaction in response to exposure at a workplace is strong evidence of an occupational origin. However, the commencement of symptoms at night, or even continuation into the weekend or holiday, may obscure the link between work and asthma. Furthermore, asthmatic responses may also be provoked by a range of factors such as dust, cold air, and exercise in people with occupational asthma.[5]

Four different patterns of asthmatic reactions have been described.[8] Progressive deterioration throughout the working week is apparent when symptoms and reduction in ventilation are more severe at the end of the week than at the beginning, and recovery takes less than three days. This pattern shows a "Monday best" picture.

Similar deterioration on each working day is characterized by development of symptoms during each day at work, but rapid improvement on leaving work, so that recovery is virtually complete by the time work starts again the following day.

Progressive deterioration week by week develops if recovery takes more than three days and the individual returns to work at the beginning of each week while lung function is still reduced. A gradual decline in lung function occurs until a state of "fixed" airflow obstruction is reached. On withdrawal from exposure, improvement may occur after only 10 or more days. Maximal deterioration on the first day of the working week is rare in occupational asthmas. It is, however, encountered in byssinosis, polymer-fume fever, and "humidifier fever."

Pathogenesis

A number of possible mechanisms of pathogenesis have been described.[5] Type I hypersensitivity is mediated by IgE antibodies and is commonly associated with immediate asthmatic responses. The extent of response may be reduced by sodium cromoglycate prior to exposure, although exposure is best avoided in such cases.

Type III hypersensitivity may occur in cases of occupational asthma, although this is uncertain: the asthmatic response follows some hours after exposure.

Activation of complement via an alternative pathway is another possible mechanism for the production of asthma.

The linkage of small molecular weight particles with a protein to form complete allergens may occur with metallic salts, isocyanates, and aminoethanolamine. Irritation by nonspecific irritants such as high concentrations of chlorine, formaldehyde, or phthalic anhydride may lead to the development of sensitivity to much lower doses on subsequent exposure.

The nonimmunological release of histamine is postulated to be the mechanism in at least some of the causes of occupational asthma and is regarded as important in byssinosis.

Diagnosis

Diagnosis depends largely on taking a careful history. Episodic lower respiratory tract symptoms with breathlessness, wheeze, chest tightness, and cough may occur in association with exposures at work. These symptoms may occur within minutes, hours, or even after work and may persist for several days after exposure. A history of improvement over weekends and holidays may be obtained but is not necessarily present.

The awareness of the physician of the range of substances capable of provoking asthma or access to services that provide such information will help in detecting occupational asthma.

Investigations

Skin-prick tests are useful in the detection of allergy. The correlation between skin tests and many of the agents is, however, poor.

Serology, particularly the measurement of specific IgE with radioallergosorbent test (RAST), may help confirm the presence of sensitivity to agents such as *B subtilis*, diphenylmethane diisocyanate (MDI), toluene diisocyanate (TDI), and phthalic anhydride. Sputum and blood eosinophilia are more easily available investigations but are not necessarily positive in cases of occupational asthma.

Provocation Tests

A variety of methods have been used to assess airway response to inhaled substances in workers suspected of having occupational asthma. Pre- and postexposure lung function testing with a simple spirometer may provide valuable information on airways responses to such exposure. Self-monitoring with a peak flow meter over long periods may help establish the relationship between airway narrowing and exposure to certain agents.

Provocation testing of various sorts has also been used.[7] The work environment may be simulated by a worker painting a piece of wood with a substance to which he is exposed, for example a varnish, while over a period of time, airway patency is assessed. Direct inhalation challenges may be used but should not be performed except in exceptional circumstances:[9] such as when the pattern of respiratory disease in response to a specific agent has not previously been described; when the individual reacts to an agent not previously associated with this condition; when the individual is exposed to a range of substances all capable of producing sensitization and it is necessary to establish the particular agent responsible; when there is general doubt as to the diagnosis after all other investigations have been performed; and when the symptoms that develop after exposures at work are so severe as to preclude any exposure to levels of substances such as are experienced at work.

Although provocation tests are extremely helpful in evaluating occupational asthma,[10] considerable gaps remain in our knowledge, especially in the area of diagnosis, that require further investigation.

Radiology of Occupational Asthma

In any type of asthma (including that related to occupation) the chest radiograph usually appears entirely normal. Therefore, if a patient complains of breathlessness, wheeze, cough, chest tightness, and has a normal radiograph, asthma must enter the differential diagnosis. Occupational asthma should be considered if any of the following clues are elicited on the history:

1. Exposure at work to a known cause;
2. Others at work have similar symptoms;
3. There is a temporal relationship between work and symptoms;
4. Symptoms diminish or disappear when away from work (eg, weekends, holidays);
5. Abrupt onset of asthma in an adult with no previous history of allergic disease.

When present, the radiographic signs of asthma are those of hyperinflation and air trapping. The criteria of hyperinflation[11,12] include:

1. Low diaphragm (below the sixth intercostal space anteriorly);
2. Deep retrosternal air space (> 3.5 cm);
3. Lung length the same or greater than lung width;
4. Change in ratio of lung height to width between radiographs taken during an attack of asthma and during remission;
5. Narrow heart (ie, width on or below the third percentile, or transverse diameter < 11.5 cm).

The vascular pattern throughout the lung is usually of normal caliber with normal hilar shadows, but sometimes the hilar pulmonary arteries are relatively large, indicating the presence of pulmonary hypertension. The change in vascular pattern appears to be due to reduction in size of the mid-lung and peripheral vessels.[12] These abnormalities are potentially reversible if the severity of the asthma diminishes either spontaneously or with treatment.

In asthma, the incidence of abnormalities on the radiograph is influenced by age at onset, its severity, and its constancy.[13] Hodson et al[11] studied 117 asthmatic patients over the age of 15 years and identified radiographic abnormalities in 31% of those whose asthma commenced before 15 years of age, but in none of those in whom it commenced after the age of 30 years.

In severe asthma, evidence of pulmonary hyperinflation may be detected in almost 75% of cases and it can disappear in as little as 24 hours.[14] Constant, unremitting asthma was found to be associated with radiographic abnormalities in children, whereas those with intermittent symptoms usually had normal roentgenograms even during attacks.[15]

Asthma patients who suffer repeated episodes of infection may develop bronchial wall thickening detectable on the radiograph.[16] This may be detected as two fine gently tapering linear shadows ("tramlines"), as a single thin line running alongside a pulmonary artery shadow, or as a thick-walled circle when the bronchus is seen end on.[12]

Complications of asthma that may be noted on the radiograph include pneumonia, atelectasis, mucoid impaction, mucous plugging, and pneumomediastinum and are much more common in children than in adults, possibly because of the smaller size of the airways in children. In a study of 479 roentgenograms of children with acute asthma, complications (excluding hyperinflation) were detected in 112, an incidence of 23%.[17]

Pulmonary eosinophilia may complicate asthma and be accompanied by transient or variable radiographic shadows owing to eosinophilic pneumonia. Allergic bronchopulmonary aspergillosis causes these infiltrations in most cases in Britain,[18] and the radiographs may show transient areas of consolidation, nodular shadows, parallel line or ring shadows, band shadows, and proximal bronchiectasis.[12]

Differential Diagnosis

For Fraser and Pare[13] the primary importance of chest radiography in patients with asthma is to exclude other conditions associated with diffuse wheezing. These include emphysema, chronic obstructive airway disease, bronchiectasis, and obstructions of the trachea or major bronchi. Related conditions resulting in hyperinflation and airway obstruction also require consideration, namely alpha-1-antitrypsin deficiency, cystic fibrosis, dyskinetic (immotile) cilia syndrome, and allergic bronchopulmonary aspergillosis. Occasionally left-sided heart failure, particularly due to mitral stenosis, is confused with asthma.

References

1. American Thoracic Society. Chronic bronchitis, asthma and pulmonary emphysema: A statement by the Committee on Diagnostic Standards for Nontuberculosis Respiratory Diseases. Am Rev Respir Dis 1962; 86: 762.
2. Brooks SM: Bronchial asthma of occupational origin: a review. Scand J Work Environ Health 1977; 3:53–72.
3. Fish JE: Occupational asthma: a spectrum of acute respiratory disorders. J Occup Med 1978; 24:379–386.
4. Pepys J: Occupational asthma: an overview. J Occup Med 1982; 24:534–538.
5. Chan-Yeung M, Lam S: Occupational asthma. Am Rev Respir Dis 1986; 133:686–703.
6. Brooks SM, Weiss MA, Bernstein IL: Reactive airways dysfunction syndrome (RADS). Chest 1985; 88:376–384.
7. Pepys J: Immunopathology of allergic lung diseases. Clin Allergy 1973; 3:1–22.
8. Parkes WR: Occupational Lung Disorders, ed 2. London, Butterworths, 1982, pp. 415–453.
9. Newman Taylor AJ, Davies RJ: Inhalation challenge testing. In: Weill H, Turner-Warwick M (eds) Occupational Diseases. Basel, Marcel Dekker, 1981.
10. Chan-Yeung M: Occupational asthma update. Chest 1988; 93:407–411.
11. Hodson ME, Simon G, Batten JC: Radiology of uncomplicated asthma. Thorax 1974; 29:296–303.
12. Kerr IH: Radiology. In: Clark TJH, Godfrey S (eds) Asthma, ed 2. London, Chapman and Hall, 1983, pp 111–131.
13. Fraser RG, Pare JAP: Diagnosis of Diseases of the Chest, ed 2. Toronto, WB Saunders Co, 1979, pp 1328–1351.
14. Rebuck, AS: Radiological aspects of severe asthma. Australas Radiol 1970; 14:264–268.
15. Simon G, Connolly N, Littlejohns DW, et al: Radiological abnormalities in children with asthma and their relation to the clinical findings and some respiratory function tests. Thorax 1973; 28:115–123.
16. Hodson CJ, Trickey SE: Bronchial wall thickening in asthma. Clin Radiol 1960; 11:183–191.
17. Eggleston PA, Ward BH, Pierson WE, et al: Radiographic abnormalities in acute asthma in children. Pediatrics 1974; 54:442–449.
18. McCarthy DS, Pepys J: Allergic broncho-pulmonary aspergillosis. Clin Allergy 1971; 1:261–286.

Index